Study Guide

to Accompany

Nursing Care

of Infants and Children

Third Edition

Lucille F. Whaley, R.N., M.S
Donna L. Wong, R.N., M.N.,P.N.P.

Carlene Casten, R.N., M.S.
Francine Brem, R.N., M.A.
Mary Burke, R.N., M.S.
Angela Murphy, R.N., M.S.N.
Department of Nursing, Rhode Island College
Providence, Rhode Island

The C. V. Mosby Company

ST. LOUIS · WASHINGTON, D.C. · TORONTO   1987

MOSBY

A TRADITION OF PUBLISHING EXCELLENCE

Editor: Linda Duncan
Editing and production: Editing, Design & Production, Inc.

Library of Congress Cataloging-in-Publication Data

Study guide to accompany the third edition of Nursing care of infants and children.

    To be used with: Nursing care of infants and children /
Lucille F. Whaley, Donna L. Wong. 3rd ed. 1986.
    Bibliography: p.
    Includes index.
    1. Pediatric nursing—Programmed instruction.
I. Casten, Carlene. II. Whaley, Lucille F., 1923–
Nursing care of infants and children. [DNLM: 1. Pediatric
Nursing—programmed instruction. WY 159 W552n Suppl.]
RJ245.W47 1986 Suppl. 618.92′00024613 87-1708
ISBN 0-8016-0673-X

JE/P/P 9 8 7 6 5 4 3 2   02/B/279

Acknowledgments

We wish to extend our appreciation to the following individuals for their assistance in the preparation of this manual:

To Lucille Whaley and Donna Wong for their confidence, suggestions, and support.
To our husbands and children for their patient support of this endeavor.

Preface

Purpose

Nursing Care of Infants and Children by Lucille F. Whaley and Donna L. Wong is a comprehensive textbook of pediatric nursing. This student resource manual is designed to facilitate the effective use of the textbook by students. While the purpose of most study guides is to review chapter content, this manual has been developed to enhance student learning. A new format has been created that provides the student with an opportunity to apply the concepts of pediatric nursing to both traditional and non-traditional clinical settings while utilizing the nursing process.

Organization of the Manual

Each chapter in this manual is organized to incorporate all of the learning activities that will assist students in meeting the objectives of the corresponding textbook chapter. The content of the chapters adheres to the following organizational pattern:

- "Chapter Overview," which provides a brief synopsis of the major concepts and focus of each textbook chapter.

- "Learning Objectives," which define the expected learner outcomes for each corresponding chapter.

- "Review of Essential Concepts," which provides students with an opportunity to assess their level of basic knowledge and comprehension.

- "Application, Analysis, and Synthesis of Essential Concepts," which allows students the opportunity to apply a knowledge of chapter content to specific situations and clinical settings.

- "Suggested Readings," which enables students to pursue appropriate resources for additional information.

The section entitled "Chapter Overview" highlights the major points addressed in each textbook chapter. It also identifies the relevance of the content for students and describes the anticipated student learning outcome for each chapter.

The "Learning Objectives" section defines the expected knowledge that the student should have at the completion of the corresponding chapter.

The section entitled "Review of Essential Concepts" provides students with an opportunity to assess their knowledge and comprehension of the basic sciences and humanities, as well as chapter content, through the use of test questions. Fill in the blank, true/false, matching, and short answer questions have been included for this purpose. It is important that students complete this portion of the manual prior to continuing to the section entitled, "Application, Analysis, and Synthesis of Essential Concepts." Content which will be evaluated in this section includes anatomy and physiology, developmental theories, and basic pathophysiology. Should the student be unable to correctly answer these questions, it is recommended that appropriate resources such as a pathophysiology text, humanities text, and *Nursing Care of Infants and Children* or *Clinical Handbook of Pediatric Nursing* be reviewed to establish an appropriate knowledge base.

The section of the manual entitled "Application, Analysis, and Synthesis of Essential Concepts" has been developed to bridge the gap between theory and clinical application. It offers students an opportunity to apply the concepts obtained within the chapters to specific settings. Throughout this section, the nursing process serves as the organizational framework. In some instances, students will be provided with various experiential exercises to be completed. The questions which follow these exercises evaluate information which the student should have obtained in the process of performing this assignment. However, the authors realize that some of these settings are not universally available. If this difficulty arises, students should still be able to complete the questions by utilizing *Nursing Care of Infants and Children* and applying appropriate content. When the questions are answered following the actual performance of these exercises, the student may find that additional information has been elicited. In these instances, the student should cite examples of this additional content. Another approach utilized in this section is to provide students with a specific clinical situation. The student will then be expected to answer questions related to the care of the child and/or family in this situation. The majority of questions included have a defined nursing focus. Students will be expected to assess the patient's health status, develop appropriate nursing diagnoses, outline pertinent nursing goals and interventions, and evaluate the effectiveness of the client's plan of care. The basic information necessary for the completion of this portion of the chapter will be found in *Nursing Care of Infants and Children* and also in the *Clinical Handbook of Pediatric Nursing* by Donna L. Wong and Lucille F. Whaley.

The "Suggested Readings" section is composed of a list of annotated readings that will allow the student to pursue an area of interest or serve as a resource to enhance comprehension. An attempt has been made to include the most recent nursing and research oriented articles. This section may also serve as a basis for class-room discussion related to the sections in the textbook entitled, "Questions and Controversy."

Conclusion

It is our hope that this manual, in conjunction with the third edition of *Nursing Care of Infants and Children*, will foster a new and innovative approach for student learning. Since this is a new conceptual format for student manuals in nursing, we welcome and encourage critiques and suggestions that will enable us to determine the manual's effectiveness.

Contents

Chapter 1

Perspectives of Pediatric Nursing

I. Chapter Overview

The content of this chapter provides an overview of the nursing of children from a child-centered rather than a disease-oriented approach. This viewpoint of pediatric nursing is important, because it focuses on the child as a unique individual with needs that are similar to, yet different from, those of other children. At the completion of this chapter, the student should have a knowledge of the emerging trends in the health care of children and their families. This knowledge will provide a perspective from which students may approach contemporary health care issues of pediatric nursing.

II. Learning Objectives

Upon completion of this chapter, it is expected that the student will be able to:

1. Define the terms *mortality* and *morbidity*.

2. Identify two ways that a knowledge of mortality and morbidity can improve child health.

3. List three major causes of death during infancy, childhood, later childhood, and adolescence.

4. List two major causes of illness during childhood.

5. Identify four events that were significant in the evolution of child health care in the United States.

6. Describe five broad functions of the pediatric nurse in promoting the health of children.

7. Identify the five operational phases of the problem-solving process.

8. Describe the interrelationship between accountability and primary nursing.

III. Review of Essential Concepts

1. The term *morbidity* is defined as _____.
   a. the number of individuals who have died over a specific period of time
   b. the prevalence of a specific illness in the population at a particular time
   c. disease occurring with greater frequency than the number of expected cases in a community
   d. disease occurring regularly within a geographic location

2. The major cause of death for children over the age of 1 year is _____.

3. The _____ of the child partially determines the types of injuries that are most likely to occur at a specific age.

4. The most common childhood illness is _____.
   a. cancer
   b. the common cold
   c. tonsillitis
   d. pneumonia

5. The most significant event in the reduction of mortality in children in the United States was _____.
   a. the discovery and use of immunizations and antibiotics
   b. the development of the Maternal and Child Health Program.
   c. the establishment of child labor laws
   d. the discoveries of Spitz and Robertson

6. Identify the major roles of the pediatric nurse:
   a. _____
   b. _____
   c. _____
   d. _____
   e. _____
   f. _____
   g. _____
   h. _____

7. List the five operational phases of the problem-solving process.
   a. _____
   b. _____
   c. _____

d. _____

e. _____

8. Nursing that involves 24-hour responsibility and accountability by one nurse for the care of a small group
of patients is known as _____.

IV. Application, Analysis, and Synthesis of Essential Concepts

A. **Experiential Exercise:** Spend a morning at the
Department of Health to survey the vital statistics affecting children in a given community.

1. Define the following terms:
   a. Mortality—

   b. Morbidity—

2. How might the nurse utilize the mortality and morbidity statistics in a given community to improve child
health?

3. What is the most effective approach to reducing morbidity and mortality?

B. **Experiential Exercise:** Spend a day following a
nurse in a pediatric unit or well-child clinic.

1. Briefly describe seven broad functions of the pediatric
nurse in promoting children's health.
   a. Family advocacy—

   b. Illness prevention and health promotion—

   c. Health teaching—

d. Support and counseling—

e. Therapeutic role—

f. Coordination and collaboration—

g. Health care planning—

2. State two reasons why a problem-solving process is
employed by the nurse in these settings.
   a.

   b.

3. Describe the five phases of the problem-solving process utilized by the nurse to provide optimal care for
the pediatric client.
   a. Assessment—

   b. Nursing diagnosis—

   c. Plan formulation—

   d. Implementation—

   e. Evaluation—

4. Describe the way in which primary nursing encourages
professional accountability.

V. Suggested Readings

1. Righi, F.C., and Krozy, R.E.: The child in the car: what every nurse should know about safety, Am. J. Nurs. **83**(10): 1421–1424, 1983.

This article describes the importance of child safety seat restraints. It discusses the incidence of auto accidents and evaluates the various types of child restraints available. The role of the nurse in health promotion and prevention of accidents is addressed.

2. Brodie, B.: Children: a glance at the past, Am. J. Maternal Child Nurs. **7**(4):219–225, 1982.

This entry provides an historical overview of the incidence and methods of eliminating injustices against children. It also encourages health professionals to continue the task of helping parents and society provide children with optimal quality of life.

3. Meister, S.B.: Building bridges between practice and health policy, Am. J. Maternal Child Nurs. **10**(3):155–157, 1985.

This article focuses on the need of clinicians to become involved in policy development. The relationship between DRG's and the nurse's role in defining health care practices is explored. Shaping children's health services and ensuring that new systems of reimbursement do not disrupt progress in protecting the health of children and families is stressed as a vital role of the pediatric nurse.

4. Roberts, R.B.: A model for parent education, Image **13**(3): 86–88, 1981.

This entry explores reasons for the failure of parent education programs. Various misconceptions of parents' needs by the health professional and strategies to enhance adult participation are addressed. Concrete suggestions are provided for assisting the nurse in the development of a model for parent education.

Chapter 2

Social, Cultural, and Religious Influences on Child Health Promotion

I. Chapter Overview

Chapter 2 provides an overview of the cultural, sociologic, and religious factors influencing growth and development. Since the ultimate goal of infant and child care is the promotion of optimal health and development, it is important for students to gain an understanding of children and how they grow and relate with significant persons in their environment. At the completion of this chapter, the student will have a knowledge of the social, cultural, and religious influences on health promotion of children. This knowledge will enable the student to develop nursing goals and interventions that will provide for the unique characteristics of each child.

II. Learning Objectives

Upon completion of this chapter, it is expected that the student will be able to:

1. Discuss cultural and subcultural influences on child growth and development.

2. Explain the influence that contemporary American culture exerts on the developing child.

3. Identify factors that increase the child's susceptibility to health problems.

4. Discuss the importance of the attitude of the nurse when providing multicultural health care.

III. Review of Essential Concepts

1. The _____ into which children are born outlines the roles of their parents, structures their relationships with other people, and determines much of the behavior they acquire.

2. Match each of the following concepts with the appropriate definition.

a. _____ culture

b. _____ race

c. _____ ethnicity

d. _____ socialization

a. the process by which children acquire the beliefs, values, and behaviors considered desirable or appropriate by the culture

b. the acquired knowledge people use to interpret experience and generate behavior

c. the affiliation of a set of persons who share a unique cultural, social, and linguistic heritage

d. a division of mankind possessing traits that are transmissible by descent and sufficient to characterize it as a distinct human type

3. _____ The variations in behavioral responses that children display to similar events are believed to be determined by cultures. (true or false)

4. Identify the three subcultural influences that seen to exert the greatest influence on child rearing.
   a.

   b.

   c.

5. Identify four functions of the peer subculture.
   a.

   b.

   c.

   d.

6. Identify two direct effects of discrimination.
   a.

   b.

7. Some groups of people are more _____ and others more _____ to certain illnesses than are persons from other groups.
8. List three significant factors associated with health problems.
   a.

   b.

   c.

9. When administering health care to families of various cultures, the nurse should consider:
   a.

   b.

   c.

10. _____ It is beneficial to attempt to change long-standing beliefs in order to meet the health needs of the family. (true or false)

IV. Application, Analysis, and Synthesis of Essential Concepts

A. **Experiential Exercise:** Interview parents from a variety of cultural, ethnic, economic, and religious backgrounds to determine the differences in child-rearing practices. Answer the following questions and include specific parental responses that illustrate the concepts.

1. Briefly describe the impact that cultural and subcultural factors have on growth and development.

2. What are some of the subcultural influences that may affect this family's child-rearing practices?
   a.
   b.
   c.
   d.
   e.
   f.
   g.
3. Briefly describe the influence that the following aspects of contemporary American culture have on child development.

a. The social ethic—

b. An optimistic view of the world and belief that things can be better—

c. Increasing geographic and economic mobility—

d. A basically nuclear-family orientation—

e. Influence of "experts"—

f. Schools—

g. Minority group membership—

B. **Experiential Exercise:** Spend a day in a health care center that serves a multicultural community. Answer the following questions and include specific observations as appropriate.

1. What factors increase a child's susceptibility to health problems?
   a.

   b.

2. How do the following factors contribute to the development of health problems in children from lower socioeconomic classes?
   a. Inadequate funds for food—

b. Unstructured eating patterns—

c. Inadequate preventive care—

d. Poor sanitation and crowded living conditions—

3. What two areas of religious belief should be evaluated when assessing health care practices?
a.

b.

4. Why should nurses working in a multicultural community be aware of their own attitudes and values?

5. Describe three ways in which the nurse can incorporate ethnic practices into effective health care delivery.
a.

b.

c.

V. Suggested Readings

1. O'Brien, M.E.: Transcultural nursing research: alien in an alien land, Image **13**(2): 37–39, 1981.

This entry addresses the necessity of immersing the researcher in the culture to be studied and it presents some of the potential problems with this approach to transcultural nursing research. It discusses the researcher's difficulties in gaining entrance to the study population and eliciting relevant data. The context of cultural heritage and information on health-illness socialization is presented as providing the necessary background for holistic health care.

2. Mason, D.J.: Perspectives on poverty, Image **13**(3):82–85, 1981.

This article addresses the lack of content on poverty in nursing curricula. Three perspectives from which to view poverty—cultural, situational, and adaptational—are examined. The necessity for value clarification prior to working with poor clients is cited as a major implication for nursing.

3. O'Brien, M. E.: Reaching the migrant worker, Am. J. Nurs. **83**(6): 895-897, 1983

Many of the health care problems of migrant workers and their families relate to their poverty, alienation, and seasonal mobility. Folk beliefs guide their health practices. This article explores the problems encountered by health professionals who provide care for the migrant worker population and suggests concrete methods for dealing with these problems.

4. Bonaparte, B.H.: Ego defensiveness, open-closed mindedness, and nurses' attitudes, Nurs. Res. **28**(3):166–171, 1979.

Registered nurses participated in a study to investigate nurses attitudes toward culturally different patients. Ego defensiveness and open-closed mindedness were measured. Lower ego defensiveness and open mindedness were found to result in more positive attitudes on the part of the nurses. The implications of this study for nursing practice are presented.

5. Ruiz, M.C.J.: Open-closed mindedness, intolerance of ambiguity and nursing faculty attitudes toward culturally different patients, Nurs. Res. **30**(3):177–181, 1981.

Nursing faculty were studied to determine their responses to culturally different patients. Faculty who were closed minded and intolerant of ambiguous situations were more likely to have a negative attitude toward patients on the basis of ethnicity. Implications for nursing based on the findings are presented.

Family Influences on Child Health Promotion

I. Chapter Overview

Chapter 3 provides an overview of family and parenting influences on health promotion of children. Since families assume the primary responsibility for child rearing and socialization, students need to be aware of the impact of various family structures and functions on the developing child. At the completion of this chapter, the student will have a knowledge of a variety of parenting situations that will serve as a foundation for the development of appropriate nursing strategies.

II. Learning Objectives

Upon completion of this chapter, it is expected that the student will be able to:

1. Describe the three principal family theories.

2. Demonstrate an understanding of factors in the family that influence growth and development of the child.

3. Describe the way in which children develop appropriate role behavior.

4. Identify the developmental stages of parenthood.

5. Discuss the impact of special parenting situations on the parent and child.

III. Review of Essential Concepts

1. Identify the three major family theories which are currently being utilized.
   a.

   b.

   c.

2. Match the following family theories with the appropriate defining characteristics.

a. _____ developmental

b. _____ structural-functional

c. _____ interactional

d. _____ exchange

e. _____ systems

f. _____ conflict

a. based on the assumption that individuals interact through give and take of a broad range of commodities, resources, or skills

b. defines family as a group of individuals of at least two generations with ties of affection and responsibility who live in proximity and who share mutual goals

c. employs a family life cycle approach to compare the changing structure, function, and roles of the family at various stages, with time as the central dimension

d. grounded in the Marxist philosophy of class

e. views the family as a unit of interrelating personalities

f. focuses on the interrelatedness, interdependence, and integration between the family and all aspects of society and its subcultures

3. List the three major objectives of the family in relation to children.
   a.

   b.

   c.

4. The predominant family structure in America is _____.
   a. the extended family

   b. the communal family

   c. the nuclear family

   d. the reconstituted family

5. Match the following family structures with the appropriate definition.

   a. _____ binuclear

   b. _____ extended

   c. _____ single-parent

   d. _____ communal

   e. _____ nuclear

   f. _____ reconstituted

   a. consists of a man, his wife, and their children who live in a common household

   b. a man or woman alone as head of household as a result of divorce, desertion, illegitimacy or adoption

   c. situation that allows parents to cooperate in the parenting role while terminating the spousal unit

   d. one or both of the married adults have children from a previous marriage residing in the household

   e. consists of the nuclear family, plus lineal or collateral relatives

   f. family structure in which non-related members share ownership of property and goods and share home-making and child-rearing functions

6. _____ Kin ties are stronger among middle class families than among the lower and working class families. (true or false)

7. Roles are learned through the _____ process.

8. Roles that are strictly defined by culture, in which very little deviation is allowed, are _____.
   a. achieved

   b. assumed

   c. adopted

   d. ascribed

9. Identify four elements of family configuration that influence child development.
   a.

   b.

   c.

   d.

10. _____ There is little or no evidence to support the existence of a ''parental instinct'' or ''maternal instinct''. (true or false)

11. Briefly describe the three basic goals that parents have for their children.
    a. a survival goal—

    b. an economic goal—

    c. a self-actualization goal—

12. List the four developmental stages of parenthood.
    a.

    b.

    c.

    d.

13. Identify seven factors affecting the transition to parenthood.
    a.

    b.

    c.

    d.

    e.

    f.

    g.

14. Differentiate among the following three styles of parental control.

a. Authoritarian—

b. Permissive—

c. Authoritative—

15. _____ The most successful type of child-rearing seems to be the authoritative method. (true or false)
16. Match the following types of behavioral control techniques with the appropriate defining characteristics.

a. _____ restriction

b. _____ coaxing

c. _____ postponing

d. _____ evaluation

e. _____ masking

a. the attempt to alter behavior by delay in dealing with conflict in the hope that resolution will occur without further action

b. the setting of rather narrow limits on the child's range of activities

c. the attempt by parents to elicit desired behavior by enticing the child with the promise of rewards in exchange for compliance

d. Parents attempt to manipulate a situation by withholding information or substituting incorrect information to resolve a conflict

e. Parents approve, disapprove, praise, blame, compare, or otherwise place a value judgment on the child's behavior

17. Role modification techniques are based on a

_____.

18. _____ The objectives of communication with children is to help them to behave more appropriately and to avoid conflicts. (true or false)
19. _____ Almost half the adoptable children in the United States are adopted by relatives. (true or false)
20. _____ The risks related to adoption are usually greater than those encountered in traditional families. (true or false)
21. The time of _____ may be an especially trying one for parents of adopted children.
22. Identify the factors that will influence the impact of divorce on children.

a.

b.

c.

d.

e.

23. List three complications that may be associated with divorce.

a.

b.

c.

24. List the six developmental tasks of children in response to divorce.

a.

b.

c.

d.

e.

f.

25. Briefly describe the three roles that a step-parent may assume in the process of rearing a step-child.

a.

b.

c.

26. Dual-earner families now comprise _____ of married couples in the United States.
27. _____ There is consensus that harmful effects of mothers' working outside the home are related to the quantity of time spent with the children. (true or false)

IV. Application, Analysis, and Synthesis of Essential Concepts

A. **Experiential Exercise:** After talking with children from a variety of families, answer the following questions that deal with the effects of different family structures on child development. Include specific examples to illustrate these concepts.

1. What functions should these families fulfill in relation to their children?

   a.

   b.

   c.

2. Define family structure.

3. What events might alter family structure?

4. What implication does an alteration in composition have for the family and child?

5. What are the advantages and/or disadvantages of the following types of family structure.

   a. Nuclear—

   b. Single-parent family—

   c. Extended family—

6. What impact does social class have on family structure?

7. Identify the way in which each of the following familial factors may influence the growth and development of the child.

   a. Family size—

   b. Ordinal position—

   c. Spacing of children—

   B. **Experiential Exercise:** Observe a family to determine the ways in which children develop appropriate role behavior. Answer the following questions and include specific examples which illustrate these concepts.

1. How do parents shape the roles of children?

2. Parents utilize positive and negative sanctions to ensure compliance to their norms. a. How are role behaviors positively reinforced? b. How are they negatively reinforced?

   a.

   b.

3. Describe each of the following types of roles that are learned within the family structure.

   a. Ascribed—

   b. Achieved—

   c. Adopted—

d. Assumed—

d. disengagement—

4. How does the way in which children are prepared for adult roles differ from culture to culture?

4. What factors may affect the transition to parenthood?
   a.

   b.

   c.

   d.

C. **Experiential Exercise:** Interview an expectant couple and parents with adolescent children to contrast their views of parenthood. Answer the following questions and include the parents' responses to illustrate these concepts.

   e.

   f.

1. What types of motivation may enter into a decision to initiate a pregnancy?
   a.

5. What factors influence the way in which parents rear their children?

6. When are disciplinary measures most effective?

   b.

   c.

   d.

D. **Experiential Exercise:** Talk to a single parent and dual-career parents to assess problem areas. Answer the following questions and include specific parental responses.

2. Identify the three basic goals that parents have for their children.
   a.

1. What changes or feelings accompany single parenthood?

   b.

   c.

2. Describe the impact of single parenting on the child.

3. Briefly describe the developmental stages of parenthood.
   a. anticipation—

3. Identify some of the major problems associated with dual-career families.

4. What factors influence the effect of a mother's absence from the home?
   a.

   b. honeymoon—

   b.

   c. plateau—

   c.

   d.

V. Suggested Readings

1. Sciarillo, W.G.: Using Hymovich's framework in the family-oriented approach to nursing care, Am. J. Maternal Child Nurs. **5**(4):242–248, 1980.

This article illustrates the use of a nursing model based on a developmental family framework to apply the nursing process to family-oriented care. It describes the three basic components of the model: developmental tasks, impact variables, and intervention. An actual family situation is then analyzed, utilizing the Hymovich model as the basis for family-centered care.

2. Sater, J.: Appraising and promoting a sense of self in twins, Am. J. Maternal Child Nurs. **4**(4):218–221, 1979.

A special problem in growth and development results because a twin must accomplish the dual task of perceiving himself as separate and distinct, not only from his mother but also from his twin. This article presents guidelines for assessing the mother's behavior toward twins that will promote individuation, as well as guidelines for assessing the twins' level of separation-individuation. Directions for precise nursing observations are provided.

3. Cameron, J.: Year-long classes for couples becoming parents, Am. J. Maternal Child Nurs. **4**(6):358–362, 1979.

This article describes the Childbearing Year Program, which was designed to help prospective parents deal with pregnancy and delivery. The Early Parenting component continues for 3 months after delivery to focus on the infant. The development of both the child and the parents is addressed.

4. Brockhaus, J.P.D., and Brockhaus, R.H.: Adopting an older child—the emotional process; Adopting an older child—the legal process, Am. J. Nurs. **82**(2):288–291; 292–294, 1982.

Written by experts on adoption who are also the adoptive parents of a 9-year-old child, these articles address the major crises resulting from the adoption of an older child. In the first selection, four major phases in the emotional process of adopting and being adopted are discussed in detail. The second portion gives a comprehensive view of the legal aspects of the assessment, placement, and finalization phases of the adoption process. The relevance to nursing practice is emphasized.

5. Walker, L.O.: Identifying parents in need: an approach to adoptive parenting, Am. J. Maternal Child Nurs. **6**(2):118–123, 1981.

This study was conducted to determine what parental factors are associated with the amount of need that adoptive parents experience in informational, feeling, and judgment-development areas as they adopt a child. Parental sex, parental age, number of other children, amount of previous child-care experience, and preparedness for parenthood were identified as related to parents' degree of need. The implications of these findings are presented.

6. McRae, M.: An approach to the single parent dilemma, Am. J. Maternal Child Nurs. **2**(3):164–167, 1977.

This entry addresses the issue of providing the child in the single-parent family with the essentials for normal development. Piaget's theory of intellectual development is utilized as an approach to dealing with the problems of single parenting. Short case studies are presented to illustrate the use of this method in the care of single-parent families.

7. Jackson, P.L., and Runyon, N.: Caring for children from divorced families, Am. J. Maternal Child Nurs. **8**(2):126–130, 1983.

The anxieties and problems of adjustment experienced by children during the divorce process are presented in this article. The nurse's role in reassuring and encouraging the children and in counseling the parents is addressed. An annotated bibliography of children's books on divorce is included.

8. Hanson, S.: Single custodial fathers and the parent-child relationship, Nurs. Res. **30**(4):202–204, 1981.

This study investigated the relationship between selected characteristics of single fathers and the quality of parent-child relationships to see if background characteristics could be used to predict father-child nurturance. Findings were not significant, but areas for further study were found.

Chapter 4

Growth and Development of Children

I. Chapter Overview

Chapter 4 provides an overview of the physiologic, psychologic, environmental, and social factors influencing the growth and development process. In order to be able to promote optimal health and development of both child and family, students need to understand how children grow and interact with their environment. Upon completion of this chapter, students should be aware of the theoretical foundations of all areas of development. This knowledge will serve as a basis for nursing interventions to meet the complex needs of the developing child.

II. Learning Objectives

Upon completion of this chapter, it is expected that the student will be able to:

1. Describe the major trends in growth and development.

2. Describe the overall changes in physical development that occur as the child grows.

3. Describe the alterations that occur in the major body systems during the child's growth and development.

4. Define *temperament* and recognize its influence upon parenting children of different temperament patterns.

5. Discuss the development of and the relationships among cognitive, personality, and moral development.

6. Discuss the influence of heredity and environment on the child's growth and development.

7. Demonstrate an understanding of the role of endogenous and exogenous factors in the physical and emotional development of the child.

8. Describe the role of play in the growth and development of the child.

9. List three universal needs of children.

III. Review of Essential Concepts

1. Match the following terms with their correct definitions:

a. _____ growth and development

b. _____ growth

c. _____ maturation

d. _____ developmental task

e. _____ development

f. _____ differentiation

a. an aging or an increase in competence and adaptability

b. a gradual growth and expansion involving a change from a lower to a more advanced stage of complexity

c. implies a change in quantity and results when cells divide and synthesize new proteins, reflected in an increased size and weight of the whole or any of its parts

d. a biologic description of the processes by which early cells and structure are modified to achieve specific, characteristic physical and chemical properties

e. a set of skills and competencies peculiar to each developmental stage that children must master in order to deal effectively with their environment

f. the sum of the numerous changes that take place during the lifetime of an individual

2. Fill in the ages denoted by each of the following periods of development.
   a. prenatal period:
   b. neonatal period:
   c. infancy:
   d. early childhood:
   e. toddler period:
   f. preschool period:
   g. middle childhood or school age:

h. prepubertal period:

i. adolescence:

3. List the three directional trends in growth and development.

   a.

   b.

   c.

4. Those times in the lifetime of an organism when it is more vulnerable to positive or negative influences are called _____.

5. For each of the following stages of development, match the body part in which growth predominates.

a. _____ prenatal   a. trunk

b. _____ infancy   b. head

c. _____ early and middle   c. shoulder and hip breadth
         childhood
                                     d. legs
d. _____ adolescence

6. The most prominent feature of childhood and adolescence is _____.

7. List the two concurrent processes that comprise skeletal growth and development in the healthy child.

   a.

   b.

8. _____ Lymphoid tissue follows a growth pattern that is similar to that of other body tissues. (true or false)

9. Name the four major stages into which development of dentition is sometimes divided.

   a.

   b.

   c.

   d.

10. _____ is the dramatic acceleration of the growth rate that follows periods of illness or malnutrition and usually continues until the child's individual growth pattern is resumed.

11. The basal caloric requirement for infants is about _____ to _____ kcal/kg of body weight and decreases to _____ to _____ kcal/kg at maturity.

12. Identify the four steps in the developmental sequence of motor behavior.

   a.

   b.

   c.

   d.

13. Identify the temperamental category that is described by each of the following:

a. _____   highly active, irritable, and irregular in habits; adapts slowly to new routines, people, or situations

b. _____   reacts negatively and with

c. _____   mild intensity to new stimuli; quite inactive and moody but shows only moderate irregularity in functions

even-tempered, regular and predictable in his habits; positive approach to new stimuli; open and adaptable to change

14. List the five stages of psychosexual development and the ages encompassed by each.

   a.

   b.

   c.

   d.

   e.

15. For each of the following age groups, identify Erikson's stage of psychosocial development.

   a. Birth to 1 year _____

   b. 1 to 3 years _____

   c. 3 to 6 years _____

   d. 6 to 12 years _____

   e. 12 to 18 years _____

   f. early adulthood _____

   g. young and middle adulthood _____

   h. old age _____

16. Match the following stages of cognitive development with the appropriate defining characteristics (answers may be used more than once; more than one answer may apply).

a. _____ sensorimotor stage

b. _____ preoperational stage

c. _____ concrete operations

d. _____ formal operations

a. predominant characteristic is egocentricity

b. stage in which thought is characterized by adaptability and flexibility

c. progression from reflex activity to imitative behavior

d. thought becomes increasingly logical and coherent; problems are solved in a concrete, systematic fashion

e. child begins to develop a sense of self as he differentiates self from environment

f. can think in abstract terms, use abstract symbols, and draw logical conclusions

g. child considers points of view other than his own; thinking becomes socialized

h. child is unable to see things from any perspective other than his own; thinking is concrete; there is a lack of conservation or reversibility

17. Identify the stage of moral development that is described by each of the following statements.
    a. _____—Children conform to rules imposed by authority figures and are culturally oriented to the labels of good/bad and right/wrong.
    b. _____—Children endeavor to define moral values and principles that are valid and applicable beyond the authority of the groups and persons holding these principles.
    c. _____—Children are concerned with conformity and loyalty, actively maintaining, supporting, and justifying the social order as well as personal expectations of those who are significant in their lives.

18. What factors must be present in order for the acquisition of language to occur?
    a.
    b.
    c.
    d.

19. _____ It is commonly accepted that the end product of development results from either heredity or environment. (true or false)

20. _____ Probably the single most important influence on growth is nutrition. (true or false)

21. Identify four factors that may result in malnutrition.
    a.

    b.

    c.

    d.

22. The most prominent feature of emotional deprivation, particularly during the first year, is _____
_____.

23. Match the following types of play with their defining characteristics.

a. _____ solitary play

b. _____ cooperative play

c. _____ onlooker play

d. _____ associative play

e. _____ parallel play

   a. Child watches what other children are doing but makes no attempt to enter into the play activity

   b. Child plays alone and independently with toys different from those by other children within the same area

   c. Child plays independently among other children with toys that are like those that the children around him are using, neither influencing nor being influenced by the other children

   d. Child plays with other children, engaging in a similar or identical activity in which there is no organization, division of labor, or mutual goal

   e. Child plays in a group with other children with discussion and planning of activities for accomplishing an end

24. List seven specific goals that play serves to develop throughout childhood.
    a.
    b.
    c.
    d.
    e.
    f.
    g.

25. Identify the six universal needs of infants and children.
    a.
    b.
    c.
    d.
    e.
    f.

IV. Application, Analysis, and Synthesis of Essential Concepts

A. **Experiential Exercise**: Observe a child from each age group: infant, toddler, preschool, school-age, and adolescent.

1. Why is it necessary to have an understanding of patterns of development before assessing a child's developmental status?

2. Match the following developmental characteristics to the age groups in which they occur. (answers may be used more than once; more than one answer may apply).

a. _____ infant

b. _____ toddler

c. _____ preschooler

d. _____ school-age child

e. _____ adolescent

    a. 50% of adult height attained

    b. yearly weight gain of 2 to 3 kg.

    c. birth length doubled

    d. rapid growth of trunk

    e. rapid growth of legs

    f. legs appear bowed

    g. shoulder and hip growth increase

3. Identify the psychosocial conflict of each age group and provide a specific intervention that will assist in the resolution of this conflict.
   a. infant—

   b. toddler—

   c. preschool—

   d. school-age—

   e. adolescent—

4. What behavior might be observed in each age group that would indicate the level of spiritual development?
   a. infant—

   b. toddler—

   c. preschool—

d. school-age—

e. adolescent—

5. Identify the two major factors to be considered in selecting toys for children.
   a.

   b.

B. **Experiential Exercise**: Interview the parents of a newborn regarding the infant's temperament.

1. What is the significance of assessing a child's temperament?

2. Identify behavioral characteristics that would indicate the temperament pattern of each child:
   a. the easy child—

   b. the difficult child—

   c. the slow-to-warm-up child—

C. **Experiential Exercise:** Spend a day in a children's hospital or an acute-care pediatric unit.

1. Identify nursing interventions designed to meet each of the following universal needs of children:
   a. physical and biologic needs—

b. love and affection—

c. security—

d. discipline and authority—

e. dependence and independence—

f. self-esteem—

2. Why is it particularly important to meet the universal needs of children during illness?

V. Suggested Readings

1. Betz, C.L.: Faith development in children, Pediatr. Nurs. 7(2):22–25, 1981.
   This article discusses the characteristics of Fowler's five stages of faith development in children: the undifferentiated, intuitive-projective, mythical-literal, synthetic-convention, and individuating-reflexive stages. Questions to be incorporated in the social and health history regarding the child's and family's religious beliefs are presented. Nursing interventions designed to support the child in each stage are outlined.
2. Snyder, C., Eyres, S.J., and Barnard, K.: New findings about mothers' antenatal expectations and their relationship to infant development, Am. J. Maternal Child Nurs. 4(6):354–357, 1979.
   Parents who are ignorant of the capabilities of their infants and of parenting skills miss opportunities for promoting development. This study describes how a mother's expectations are related to the quality of the early environment that she provides and to the way in which her child develops. Specific implications for prenatal teaching are discussed.
3. Johnston, M.: Toward a culture of caring: children, their environment, and changing, Am. J. Maternal Child Nurs. 4:210–214, 1979.
   A children's health care environment that supports the child and contributes to recovery is described in detail in this selection. Concepts considered in its planning include choice, privacy versus isolation, comfort, appropriateness, stimulation, developmental support, and individual importance versus group efficiency. The importance and functions of a play area are discussed.
4. Webster-Stratton, C., and Kogan, K.: Helping parents parent, Am. J. Nurs. 80:240–244, 1980.
   Video tapes of parents and children in a parenting clinic were used to select examples of behavior to be reviewed with parents. Parent-child interactions were then utilized as the medium for training parents to cope with disturbing behaviors and prevent interpersonal disturbance. A written list of suggestions was then provided. Three cases that illustrate the use of this system and the five specific areas of parent training are described in detail.
5. Slevin K.F.: Motherhood, culture, and change, Pediatr. Nurs. 8(6):405–408, 1982.
   This entry explores the ways in which cultural expectations affect motherhood. The changing definition of motherhood in the United States and its consequences, both positive and negative, are discussed. The article concludes with implications for the pediatric nurse in helping families to choose mothering options that fit their individual situations.
6. Hollen, P.: Parents' perceptions of parenting support systems, Pediatr. Nurs. 8:309–313, 1982.
   This study of parenting support systems determined that physicians were perceived as being utilized for support or information 8.5 times more often than were nurses. It found behavioral and growth-and-development concerns to be of greater interest to parents than illness. The implications of the study for increased nursing awareness of and participation in parental support activities is discussed.

Chapter 5

Hereditary and Prenatal Influences on Health Promotion of the Child and the Family

I. Chapter Overview

This chapter addresses the relationship of genetics and the environment as they influence the development of the child before birth. Genetic disease is present in a significant portion of the population. Thus, it is important that students understand abnormal prenatal development as a basis for caring for children with frequently encountered congenital problems. At the completion of this chapter, students should have knowledge of the genetic and prenatal influences on the developing child, methods of prevention, and treatment modalities. This will enable students to deal with hereditary or other congenital disorders as they impact upon both the child and the family.

II. Learning Objectives

Upon completion of this chapter, it is expected that the student will be able to:

1. Differentiate among the classes of genetic disorders.

2. Demonstrate an understanding of the processes responsible for chromosomal aberrations.

3. Describe the basic patterns of inheritance.

4. Determine the risk of recurrence of a disorder caused by a single gene.

5. Differentiate between fraternal and identical twins.

6. Explain the relationship between genetic and environmental factors in the causation of defects or disease.

7. List the major protocols utilized in the therapeutic management of genetic disease.

8. Differentiate between the terms *eugenics* and *euthenics*.

9. Define the terms related to prenatal development.

10. Describe the way in which the environment influences development and differentiation.

11. Identify the purposes of screening for the detection of genetic disease.

12. Discuss the role of the nurse in genetic counseling.

III. Review of Essential Concepts

1. Match the following terms related to genetic disorders with their correct definitions.

a. _____ phenotype

b. _____ congenital

c. _____ genetic

d. _____ genotype

e. _____ familial

f. _____ heterozygous

g. _____ multifactorial

h. _____ cytogenetic disorders

i. _____ homozygous

a. disorder caused by a single harmful gene, several genes, or by a deviation in chromosome number or structure

b. having the same genes at a given position on a pair of chromosomes

c. physical and/or chemical characteristics of the individual produced by the interaction of the environment and the genotype

d. disorders that result from a complex interaction of both genetic and environmental factors

e. condition present at birth that may be brought about by nongenetic causes, genetic causes, or a combination of these.

f. genetic constitution that determines the physical and chemical characteristics of an individual

g. having dissimilar genes at a given position on a pair of chromosomes

h. a disorder that runs in families or is present in more members of a family than would be expected by chance

i. deviations in either the structure or number of chromosomes

2. _____ Maldistribution of chromosomes owing to the failure of the process of separation and migration during cell division is known as translocation. (true or false)

3. _____ An individual whose cells display mixed chromosomal counts is known as a mosaic. (true or false)

4. _____ Both non-disjunction and translocation are related to increasing parental age. (true or false)

5. The first and the most common disorder in which an associated chromosomal abnormality was demonstrated is _____.
   a. Klinefelter syndrome
   b. Down syndrome
   c. Turner syndrome
   d. fragile X-syndrome

6. Conditions that can be directly attributed to a single gene are distributed in families in characteristic patterns according to the _____.

7. _____ The phenomenon of gene mutation is most apparent in autosomal dominant disorders. (true or false)

8. Using the following key, match the identifying initials of the type of inheritance pattern or patterns with each of the listed characteristics that its posessor may exhibit.
   autosomal-dominant inheritance: A-D
   autosomal-recessive inheritance: A-R
   X-linked dominant inheritance: X-D
   X-linked recessive inheritance: X-R

a. _____ All of the daughters but none of the sons of an affected male are affected.

b. _____ Affected individuals have an affected parent.

c. _____ Males and females are affected with equal frequency.

d. _____ Affected individuals are principally males.

e. _____ All children of two affected parents are affected.

f. _____ Unaffected children of an affected parent have unaffected children.

g. _____ There is usually no evidence of the trait in previous generations.

h. _____ Daughters of an affected male are carriers.

i. _____ Affected individuals have unaffected parents.

j. _____ Each child of a heterozygous affected parent has a 50% chance of possessing the defective gene.

9. _____ twins are always alike in both gene complement and physical characteristics.

10. One of the characteristics of dizygotic twinning is that it _____.
    a. occurs increasingly with advancing maternal age
    b. is unaffected by heredity
    c. accounts for approximately one-third of twin births
    d. occurs with relatively uniform frequency in all races

11. _____ The most reliable physical means to distinguish types of twins are blood group comparisons. (true or false)

12. Match the following terms related to congenital anomalies with their definitions.

a. _____ dysplasia

b. _____ disruption

c. _____ atrophy

d. _____ sequence

e. _____ syndrome

f. _____ polytropic field defect

g. _____ deformation

h. _____ malformation

a. decreased development of a mass of tissue or an organ as a result of a decrease in cell size and/or number

b. pattern of multiple anomalies thought to be pathogenetically related and not known to represent a single sequence or polytropic field defect

c. an abnormal form, shape, or position of part of the body caused by mechanical forces

d. an abnormal organization of cells into tissues and its morphologic result

e. morphologic defect resulting from the extrinsic breakdown of an originally normal developmental process

f. a morphogenic defect resulting from an intrinsically abnormal developmental process

g. pattern of anomalies derived from the disturbance of one developmental field

h. pattern of anomalies derived from a single known or presumed prior anomaly or mechanical factor

13. _____is the improvement of the race through altering the genetic makeup of the individual; _____ is the improvement of the human race by modifying the environment.

14. An example of positive eugenics would be _____.
    a. special schools for the deaf
    b. sterilization
    c. hormone replacement
    d. cloning

15. Fill in the correct term for each of the following definitions related to prenatal development:
    a. an increase in cell numbers: _____
    b. an increase in cell size: _____
    c. process by which early cells are systematically modified and specialized to form the tissues of an individual: _____
    d. period of prenatal development during which the beginnings of all major organ systems are formed: _____

16. _____ The sensitive periods for all organs and parts of the developing organism occur simultaneously. (true or false)

17. _____ refers to a disturbance of prenatal growth processes that produces a structural or functional defect.

18. The teratogenic effect of drugs is not believed to have an effect on the developing fetus until day 15 of gestation when _____ begins to take place.

19. List the three purposes of genetic screening.
    a.

    b.

    c.

20. _____ is a communication process that deals with the human problems associated with the occurrence or risk of occurrence of a genetic disorder in a family.

21. _____ In estimating the degree of risk of recurrence of genetic disorders, it is known that, in general, the more definite and clear-cut the genetics, the more hopeful the outlook. (true or false)

22. An example of a random-risk disorder would be _____.
    a. congenital heart disease
    b. Duchenne-type muscular dystrophy

c. abnormality resulting from maternal rubella
d. cleft lip and palate

IV. Application, Analysis, and Synthesis of Essential Concepts

A. **Experiential Exercise**: Care for a child with a congenital or genetic disorder. Answer the following questions and include specific examples related to the client that illustrate these concepts.

1. Distinguish between *congenital* and *genetic* disorders by defining each term.
   a. Congenital—

   b. Genetic—

2. Provide the correct classification for each of the following genetic disorders by filling in the letter of the appropriate category of its cause from the key below.
   Chromosomal aberration: C
   Mutation of a gene or genes: G
   Multifactorial: M
   a. _____ hemophilia
   b. _____ Down syndrome
   c. _____ muscular dystrophy
   d. _____ cleft lip or palate
   e. _____ diabetes mellitus
   f. _____ cystic fibrosis
   g. _____ phenylketonuria
   h. _____ congenital hip dysplasia
   i. _____ Turner syndrome
   j. _____ congenital heart disease

3. What two factors are required for the appearance of clinical manifestations in multifactorial disorders?

4. The following are modalities that are currently utilized in the treatment of genetic disorders. For each treatment modality, supply at least two genetic disorders in which it may be used.
   a. surgical repair—

b. diet modification—

c. product replacement—

d. removal of toxic substances—

e. transplantation—

f. gene transfer—

B. **Clinical Situation**: Billy, a 3-year-old boy with hemophilia, is admitted to the hematology unit of Children's Hospital for treatment of hemarthrosis. Billy, who has an older brother and sister, is the only family member in whom the diagnosis of hemophilia has been made.

1. What is the cause of Billy's disorder?

2. Identify the possible status of each of Billy's family members in regard to hemophilia.
   a. father:
   b. mother:
   c. brother:
   d. sister:
3. If Billy were to have children as an adult, what would their status be in regard to hemophilia?
   a. sons:
   b. daughters:
4. What significance does genetic screening have for the following family members?
   a. sister—

b. parents—

C. **Experential Exercise**: Spend a day in a genetic counseling clinic.

1. List five goals that nurses and other trained genetic counseling professionals help clients to achieve.
   a.

   b.

   c.

   d.

   e.

2. What are the three overall objectives of genetic counseling?
   a.
   b.
   c.
3. From what sources does the genetic counseling professional obtain information to determine risks of recurrence?
   a.
   b.
   c.
4. Identify four potential roles of nurses in relation to genetic counseling.
   a.
   b.
   c.
   d.
5. What are some important considerations for the nurse and other genetic counseling professionals in meeting the emotional needs of families with a genetic disorder?

6. List four barriers to effective counseling.
   a.

b.

c.

d.

V. Suggested Readings

1. Gaffney, S.E.: Intrauterine fetal surgery: The ramifications for nurses, Am. J. Maternal Child Nurs. **10**(4):250–254, 1985.

This article describes the attempts made to date at intrauterine fetal surgery to correct or treat hydrocephalus, diaphragmatic hernia, and hydronephrosis. The nurse's role as a support person, patient advocate, and care giver prior to, during, and following the surgery, is examined. Ethical and legal issues related to the surgery are raised.

2. Weeks, H.F.: Perinatal pharmacology, Am. J. Maternal Child Nurs. **5**(2):143, 1980.

This edition of the feature "MCN Pharmacopeia" lists the three mechanisms of prenatal drug interactions and describes the five FDA categories to indicate a drug's potential for causing birth defects. The potential effects of drugs used during and after labor and delivery are described. Medications of particular concern are noted.

3. Wicklund, S.: Special report: Drugs for two in pregnancy, Am. J. Nurs. **82**:980–981, 1982.

This selection presents a list of medications in several drug families that provide the required therapeutic action and are relatively safe during pregnancy. Categories included are antibiotics, antituberculous drugs, analgesics, antihypertensives, anticoagulants, anticonvulsants, antiemetics, psychotropics, antidiabetics, antithyroid drugs, antiasthmatic drugs, cardiac glycosides, and diuretics.

4. Luke, B.: Maternal alcoholism and fetal alcohol syndrome, Am. J. Nurs. **77**:1924–1926, 1977.

This article describes the pattern of craniofacial, limb, cardiovascular, growth, and developmental defects associated with maternal alcoholism. Alcohol-associated illnesses, which should alert health professionals to maternal alcoholism are listed. The correction of resulting complications such as malnutrition, anemia, and seizures is discussed, and supportive services are outlined.

5. Stagno, S.: Toxoplasmosis, Am.J. Nurs. **80**:720–722, 1980.

Congenital toxoplasmosis as a cause of severe anomalies in the fetus is described in terms of its epidemiology and clinical spectrum. The use of diagnostic procedures and treatment of toxoplasmosis acquired during pregnancy are discussed. Preventive measures to protect seronegative pregnant women are suggested.

6. McKay, S.R.: Smoking during the childbearing year, Am. J. Maternal Child Nurs. **5**(1):46–50, 1980.

This selection describes the effects of maternal smoking on both mother and fetus. Nursing interventions to educate the smoker to its dangers and help alter smoking habits are discussed. Throughout the article, the nurse's responsibility to influence smoking mothers is emphasized.

7. Davies, B.L., and Doran, T.A.: Factors in a woman's decision to undergo genetic amniocentesis for advanced maternal age, Nurs. Res. **31**(1):56–59, 1982.

This is a study of a small sample of women that was conducted to identify factors in their decisions to undergo genetic amniocentesis because of advanced child-bearing age. Formal religious affiliation seemed to be less important than the need for reassurance that the child was free from Down syndrome, personal hardship in dealing with an affected child, and the opportunity to choose abortion. Implications for practice are discussed.

8. Hammer, R.M., and Tufts, M.A.: Chorionic villi sampling for detecting fetal disorders, Am. J. Maternal Child Nurs. **11**(1):29–31, 1986.

The procedure utilized in chorionic villi sampling is described in detail in this article. The possible complications of the procedure as well as its disadvantages are presented. The advantages of chorionic villi sampling over amniocentesis and implications for its future use are explored.

9. Tishler, C.L.: The psychological aspects of genetic counseling, Am. J. Nurs. **81**:733–734, 1981.

This selection utilizes a review of literature to illustrate some of the adverse reactions to attempted genetic counseling. It then explores the basic reasons for having babies and relates these to the stages of acceptance of genetic counseling. Intensive group therapy is explored as an approach to genetic counseling. The importance of avoiding bias and maintaining confidentiality is stressed.

10. Williams, J.K.: Pediatric nurse practitioners' knowledge of genetic disease, Pediatr. Nurs. **9**(2):119–121, 1983.

This study determined that while there was a strong support for genetic counseling nationally, there was inconsistent knowledge about the genetic clinical disorders and risk factors. At the same time, it found that pediatric nurse practitioners saw themselves as ideal providers of the supportive care for children with birth defects and their families. It was concluded that pediatric nurse practitioners should have more opportunities to learn genetic counseling.

Chapter 6

Communication and Health Assessment of the Child and the Family

I. Chapter Overview

Chapter 6 introduces an essential component of the nursing of children and their families, communication. It is important, because it is an essential skill in the assessment process and may be crucial to the establishment of a trusting relationship with children and their families. Guidelines for health and nutritional assessment are also presented. At the completion of this chapter, the student should have knowledge of the communication process with children and their families, and a foundation for the performance of a health and nutritional assessment in the clinical area.

II. Learning Objectives

Upon completion of this chapter, it is expected that the student will be able to:

1. Outline guidelines for communication and interviewing.

2. Identify communication strategies for interviewing parents.

3. Outline guidelines for using an interpreter.

4. Identify communication strategies for communicating with children of different age groups.

5. Describe four communication techniques that are useful with children.

6. State the components of a complete health history.

7. Identify the methods utilized to assess the nutritional status of the child.

III. Review of Essential Concepts

1. The four prerequisites to establish a setting conducive to the interviewing process are

a.

b.

c.

d.

2. Various communication strategies are useful when interviewing parents. Identify the purpose of each strategy listed below.
a. Encouraging the parent to talk.—

b. Directing the focus.—

c. Listening—

d. Silence—

e. Being empathetic—

f. Providing reassurance—

g. Defining the problem—

h. Solving the problem—

i. Providing anticipatory guidance—

j. Avoiding blocks to communication—

3. _____ Talking more than the interviewee does is a method to prevent blocks in the communication process. (true or false)
4. Guidelines to be followed when interviewing through an interpreter include: _____
   a. directing questions during the interview to the interpreter
   b. asking questions about sex, which may embarrass the interpreter
   c. using a different interpreter on subsequent interviews
   d. explaining the purpose of the interview to the interpreter
5. Match the communication strategy to the age group that it is best used with:

_____ infants
_____ young child
_____ school-age child
_____ adolescence

a. told what they will do and how they will feel
b. cuddling
c. told what is going on and why it is being done
d. being attentive and not prying

6. _____ Neurolinguistic programing is a communication strategy in which:
   a. The nurse listens carefully and reflects back the feelings and content of the statements to the client.
b. Books are used in a therapeutic and supportive manner.
   c. The nurse presents statements and has the client fill in the blanks.
   d. The nurse uses the same sensory mode as the client.
7. Three non-verbal methods of communication that are utilized with young children are _____.
8. _____ An important component of the personal-social portion of the health history is the assessment of the home and community environment. (true or false)
9. The nine major components of a health history for the child and family include:
   1.
   2.
   3.
   4.
   5.
   6.
   7.
   8.
   9.
10. _____ The purpose of a nutritional assessment is to evaluate how much weight a child needs to gain. (true or false)
11. A thorough nutritional assessment includes

_____.

12. _____ A method utilized in the clinical examination portion of the nutritional assessment is:
    a. fundoscopy
    b. arthroscopy
    c. anthropometry
    d. biopsy

IV. Application, Analysis, and Synthesis of Essential Concepts

A. **Experiential Exercise**: Interview a preschool child and his family.

1. It is important to establish a setting for the interview. What is the first thing that should be said to establish this setting?

2. What blocks to communication may occur during the interview?

3. What communication techniques are effective in encouraging communication with the parents and child?

4. Why is it important to include the parents in the problem-solving process?

B. **Clinical Situation:** Mrs. Fernandez brings her daughter Susan, age 18 months, to the pediatric child clinic for an annual check-up. It is the first time that they have visited the clinic. Mrs. Fernandez' English is poor. The Fernandezes have been living in the United States for 6 months. An interpreter will be available for the interview.

1. In addition to the general guidelines for interviewing, what six principles should be employed when utilizing an interpreter?
   a.
   b.
   c.
   d.
   e.
   f.

2. During the interview Mrs. Fernandez focuses her comments on the other four children. How might the nurse redirect the focus of the interview?

3. What portion of the past-history section of the health history is of particular importance because Susan has been in this country only 6 months?

4. What information in the family history section of the health history should the nurse obtain from Mrs. Fernandez?

C. **Clinical Situation:** Gwen, age 8, was referred to the nutrition clinic by the nurse practitioner. The nurse was concerned because Gwen's weight was above the 90th percentile for her age. A complete nutritional assessment was performed.

1. What factors should be included in a dietary history of Gwen?

2. Identify three methods that Gwen's mother can use to record Gwen's dietary intake.

3. Anthropometry was performed on Gwen. Why?

4. What should Gwen be told about the nutritional assessment process.

5. The results of the nutritional **assessment** revealed that Gwen's mother knows little about nutrition and that Gwen's obesity is the result of her excessive intake of nutrients. Develop two nursing diagnoses based on the assessment results.
   a.
   b.

V. Suggested Readings

1. Farr, K.: Communication pitfalls in routine counseling, Pediatric Nursing. **5**:55–57, 1979.
   This article is an excellent supplement to the material in the text on interviewing techniques. It explores factors that may influence the interviewing process, aids and blocks to communication, and errors that are commonly made.
2. Brockopp, D.Y.: What is NLP? American Journal of Nursing. **83** (7): 1012–1014.
   Neurolinguistic programming is explained. The article defines this method, explains the basis for the technique, and explores why it works. The types of people and the words they might use to indicate the sensory mode they are using are presented.
3. Knowles, R.D.: Building rapport through neurolinguistic programming. American Journal of Nursing. **83** (7):101–1014.
   This is a companion article to the one written by Brockopp. Predictors of the types of communication strategies utilized by people in the three sensory modalities are presented. The article also provides some techniques that facilitate the use of NLP in practice.
4. McLeavey, K. A.: Children's art as an assessment tool. Pediatric Nursing. **5** (2): 9–14,1979.
   The use of drawing as a tool to assess development and emotional state is explained. Criteria used to evaluate the drawings and examples that illustrate them are presented.

5. Baer, E.D., McGowan, M.N., and McGivern, D.O.: Taking a health history. American Journal of Nursing. **77**(7):1190–1193, 1977.
This article combines communication techniques with the obtaining of a health history. It explores communication strategies such as open ended questions, the importance of the introduction and blocks to the communication process. The various components of the health history are presented.

Physical and Developmental Assessment of the Child

I. Chapter Overview

Chapter 7 provides the theoretical basis for the performance of a complete pediatric physical assessment and a developmental assessment. Since assessment is the first step in the nursing process, procedures and skills that aid in obtaining accurate and complete data are crucial to students. This chapter provides the base for the performance of a complete physical and developmental assessment in the practicum setting.

II. Learning Objectives

Upon completion of this chapter, it is expected that the student will be able to:

1. Identify three circumstances that may indicate the need for an alteration in the schedule of preventive child health services.

2. Prepare children for a physical examination according to their developmental needs.

3. Define the four traditional categories of assessment skills.

4. Perform a physical examination in a sequence appropriate to the child's age.

5. Recognize expected normal findings for children at various ages.

6. Record the physical examination according to the traditional format.

7. Perform a developmental assessment using a standard screening test such as the Denver Developmental Screening Test.

II. Review of Essential Concepts

1. Three circumstances that indicate the need for additional visits for preventive health care services include:
   a.
   b.
   c.

2. Five goals that serve as a basis for modifying the normal examination sequence in children are:
   a.
   b.
   c.
   d.
   e.

3. List the methods the nurse might use to facilitate the examination process.
   a.
   b.
   c.
   d.
   e.
   f.

4. _____ Percussion is an assessment skill that involves the use of sight to make judgements. (true or false)

5. _____ The sounds that are obtained by auscultation are usually described in terms of intensity, pitch, duration, and quality. (true or false)

6. List the sequence of events in the physical assessment of a child.
   a.
   b.
   c.
   d.
   e.
   f.
   g.
   h.
   i.
   j.
   k.
   l.
   m.
   n.
   o.
   p.

q.

r.

s.

7. The best order for taking the vital signs in the infant is _____.

8. _____ In general, children whose growth pattern should be followed closely include:
   a. those whose height and weight fall between the 50th and 90th percentile for their age
   b. those whose pattern of growth resembles their parents'
   c. those who fail to show rapid weight gain in the toddler and school-age years
   d. those who show a sudden decrease in a previously steady pattern

9. Respirations in the infant are counted _____, because they are irregular.

10. _____ Areas that are assessed in the general appearance section of the physical exam include:
    a. weight
    b. posture
    c. apical pulse
    d. color

11. Match the abnormal color change with its correct definition

_____ cyanosis	a. small pinpoint hemorrhages
_____ erythema	b. blue tinge to skin
_____ jaundice	c. redness of the skin
_____ petechie	d. yellow staining of the skin

12. _____ Criteria that are utilized when referring a 3-year-old for further evaluation of visual acuity include:
    a. 20/10 vision on the Snellen Chart
    b. 20/40 vision on the Snellen Chart
    c. 20/30 vision on the Snellen Chart
    d. 20/50 vision on the Snellen Chart

13. _____ Respirations in the older child are primarily abdominal. (true or false)

14. _____ Pubic hair begins to appear in girls between the ages of 13 and 16 years. (true or false)

15. What should be recorded when assessing the head of an 8-month-old infant?

16. It is important to record the presence of _____ reflexes if the child is beyond infancy.

17. _____ The Denver Developmental Screening Test is composed of four major categories: fine motor-adaptive, cognitive, reflexive and language. (true or false)

18. The Denver Developmental Screening Test can be used to assess the development of children of ages _____.

19. _____ Delays on the Denver Developmental Screening Test are defined as the failure to perform any item passed by 90% of children of the same age. (true or false)

20. _____ A screening test that can be utilized to assess the development of a child 4 years of age is
    a. McCarthy Scale
    b. Caudwell Home Scale
    c. Bayley Scale
    d. Brazelton Scale

IV. Application, Analysis, and Synthesis of Essential Concepts

A. **Clinical Situation**: Tia Vang, age 3, is brought to the pediatric clinic for a routine physical exam. Tia has been in this country for 1 year, and Tia's father has been unable to immigrate to this country from Cambodia. Tia's immunizations are up to date. This is Tia's first visit to the clinic.

1. Why will it be necessary to suggest to Mrs. Vang that Tia be brought to the clinic more frequently?

2. What preventive health care measures would you accomplish at this visit?

3. Tia refuses to look at you during the health history interview. What behaviors might indicate her readiness to cooperate during the physical exam and how might you facilitate this process?

4. How might you help Tia relax to aid in the process of palpation?

5. Tia's height and weight are below the 5th percentile for children her age. What additional information should you assess before diagnosing that Tia's growth is not normal?

6. What method would you use to assess Tia's height?

7. Why would you not want to take Tia's temperature orally?

8. How should Tia's vision be assessed?

B. **Experiential Exercise**: Perform a physical assessment on an infant and a school age child.

1. What area do you assess after you assess each child's general appearance?

2. How do you obtain each child's height and how is it recorded?

3. By what method do you obtain the heart rate in each child?

4. Data that you obtain when you assess the school age child's behavior include:

5. You assess the external auditory structures and visualize the internal landmarks. What did you forget to as-

sess and what method could you use in each of the children?

6. You assess the heart sounds for _____.

7. The school-age child appears to have an arrythmia. How do you determine whether this is a sinus arrythmia?

8. How do you record your evaluation of the deep tendon reflexes?

C. **Experiential Exercise**: Perform a developmental assessment on a toddler and preschool child.

1. What do you tell the child's parent before the test is begun?

2. What information do you obtain from the child's parent at the conclusion of the test?

3. How do you determine that a delay is present?

4. How do you score items on the Denver Developmental Screening Test?

5. What should you do if the results of the screening

exam are abnormal **and the** child's mother states that his behavior was **typical?**

V. Suggested **Readings**

1. Bausell, R. B.: A **national** survey assessing pediatric preventive behaviors, **Pediatr. Nurs.** **11**:443–446,1985.

   This article reviews **the survey** research conducted by Louis Harris and Associates **on the** extent to which parents comply with the suggested **preventive health** care practices for their children. The sample of **the survey** method of collection, results, and limitation of **the study** are presented. The author also discusses the application of the results to clinical practice.

2. Performing **palpation**, Nursing 83. **13** (1):68–69.

   The article **defines** palpation, identifies the types of palpation, explores the **methods** used to perform this technique and provides the reader **with** guidelines on what to look for when **performing** this assessment skill.

3. Performing percussion, Nursing 83. **13** (1):63–64

   The types of **percussion**, definition of this skill, method utilized to perform **the technique**, what the various sounds mean, and characteristics of **the sounds** obtained are explored in this excellent supplement **to the** text.

4. Yoos, L.: A **developmental** approach to physical assessment, MCN. **6**:168–70, 1982.

   This excellent article examines how developmental differ-

ences affect the physical assessment process. **The author** integrates developmental theory with the exam **process** to explain the different methods appropriate for children **of various** ages.

5. Moss, J.R.: Helping young children cope **with the** physical examination, Pediatr. Nurs. **7** (2):17–20, **1981.**

   The effect of development on the examination **process** is examined in this article. Developmental theory is **presented as a** basis for problems encountered in the assessment **process. The** author addresses the need for modifying the examination sequence and proposes sequences based on the **responses of the** child.

6. Brown, M.S., and Collar, M.: Effects of prior **preparation** on the preschoolers' vision and hearing screening, MCN. **7**(5):323–328,1982.

   The author identifies the importance of screening in children and adressess why early detection is important. A **method** to improve the screening process is explored as a basis for this research study. Application of the findings of **the research** is presented.

7. Holland, S.H.: 20/20 vision screening, **Pediatr. Nurs.** **8**(2):81–87, 1982.

   The various methods that can be used to assess visual acuity in the child are presented. Common errors in the visual screening process are examined. An excellent supplement to the text.

8. Castigila, P.T., and Petrina, M.A.: Selecting a developmental screening tool, Pediatr. Nurs. **11**(1):8–16, 1985.

   This excellent article explores all aspects of the screening process. The author identifies methods to select tools, and adresses the rationale of developmental screening. A review of all developmental tools is provided as well as the sources for obtaining the tools.

Chapter 8

Health Promotion of the Newborn and the Family

I. Chapter Overview

Chapter 8 introduces the nursing considerations of caring for the infant and family, during delivery and in the neonatal period. Profound physiologic and psychologic changes occur as the neonate adjusts to extrauterine life. Students need to be aware of these changes so they can assess the neonate's successful adaptation and help the parents adjust to family life. At the completion of this chapter the student will know the necessary nursing care for the neonate and his family. This knowledge will enable the student to assess the neonate and his family and to formulate nursing goals and interventions that will promote the normal physiologic and psychologic adjustment and development.

II. Learning Objectives

Upon completion of this chapter, it is expected that the student will be able to:

1. Identify the principal cardiorespiratory changes that occur during transition to extrauterine life.

2. Identify the immature physiologic functioning of each body system and its significance to nursing care of the neonate.

3. Perform an initial and transitional assessment of the newborn based on the Apgar score and periods of reactivity.

4. Perform a newborn physical assessment based on recognition of expected normal findings.

5. Administer safe care to the neonate during delivery and in the nursery.

6. Assess and promote parent-infant attachment behavior.

7. Identify the components that should be included in the discharge planning for the newborn and family.

III. Review of Essential Concepts

1. The respiratory changes that occur during the transition to extrauterine life include:_____.

2. _____ A change in the cardiovascular system that occurs after birth involves an increase in pressure on the right side of the heart. (true or false)

3. _____ The most important factor controlling the closure of the ductus arterious is:
   a. increased oxygen concentration of the blood
   b. deposition of fibrin and cells
   c. fall of endogenous prostaglandin
   d. presence of metabolic acidosis

4. Factors that predispose the neonate to heat loss include:
   a.
   b.
   c.
   d.

5. _____ A limitation of the newborn's gastrointestinal system includes:
   a. the inability to digest disaccharides
   b. decreased transit time of food passing through the stomach and colon
   c. increased storage of glycogen
   d. deficiency of the enzyme lipase

6. _____ The kidney of the neonate is unable to concentrate urine. (true or false)

7. The five items that are included in the Apgar score are:_____.

8. The maximum score that an infant can receive on the Apgar is _____.

9. For the first _____ hours the infant is in the first period of reactivity.

10. Behaviors seen during the second period of reactivity include:

11. List the six external physical signs of the Dubowitz Scale:

12. _____ The normal head circumference of the neonate is 20 to 21 inches. (true or false)
13. _____ The normal pulse rate of the neonate is 120 to 140 beats/min. (true or false).
14. _____ A reflex that should be present in the normal neonate is:
    a. Landau
    b. Moro
    c. parachute
    d. neck-righting
15. Areas to be assessed in the general appearance section of the newborn assessment include:

16. The purpose of assessing the umbilical cord is to determine the presence of _____.
17. _____ The state of regular sleep is characterized by closed eyes, irregular breathing, muscle twitching and reactions to external stimuli. (true or false).
18. Four nursing goals that are the basis for safe and effective care of the neonate are:

19. The use of soap is discouraged in the newborn period because it interferes with _____.
20. _____ Vitamin K is administered to the newborn to prevent the occurrence of disseminating intravascular coagulation. (true or false)
21. _____ Cow's milk is not suitable for the infant's nutrition because it _____.
    a. has too few calories per ounce
    b. has too much protein
    c. is too dilute
    d. has too much calcium
22. _____ The process of the father's attachment to the newborn is called engrossment. (true or false)
23. Variables that may influence the attachment process include:

24. The reasons that discharge planning and care at home are of increasing importance are that

25. Common concerns or problems during the period immediately after discharge include:

IV. Application, Analysis, and Synthesis of Essential Concepts

A. **Experiential Exercise**: Perform an initial and transitional assessment on a newborn based on Apgar score and periods of reactivity.

1. The five areas you assess to determine the Apgar score include:

2. The infant received a score of 1 on the heart rate category of the Apgar. This indicates that the neonate's heart rate was _____.
3. The infant had little difficulty adjusting to extrauterine life. The Apgar score for this infant would be between _____.
4. What behaviors do you observe to indicate that the infant is in the first period of reactivity.

5. _____ An appropriate nursing intervention in the first stage of reactivity would include:
   a. performance of inital bath
   b. instillation of eye drops before child has contact with the parents
   c. allowing mother to breast feed
   d. minimizing contact with parents until temperature has stabilized

B. **Experiential Exercise:** Determine a neonate's gestational age.

1. Assessment of gestational age is important because

2. The optimal time for the assessment of gestational age is between _____.
3. The six neuromuscular signs that you assess include:

4. _____ The infant receives a score of 3 on the square-window item. This indicates that the angle between the hypothenar eminence and the ventral aspect of the forearm is 30 degrees. (true or false)
5. _____ An infant who receives a total score of 30 on the Dubowitz Scale would have a gestational age of:
   a. 28 weeks   c. 36 weeks
   b. 34 weeks   d. 40 weeks.
6. You plot the infant's height, weight, and head circumference on standardized graphs. You determine that the infant is normal for gestational age because

_____.

C. **Experiential Exercise:** Perform a physical assessment on a newborn.

1. The head circumference of the infant you assess should be between _____. If the head circumference is significantly smaller than the chest circumference _____.

2. You note that the infant's legs appear to be extended; the legs are abducted and the thighs are rotated. What information would you need before you determined whether this is an abnormal finding?

3. An assessment of the heart yields the presence of a functional murmur. This type of murmur is common in the the newborn period because of the _____ _____ through the openings in the fetal heart.

4. What areas do you assess when you examine the eyes of the neonate?

5. How do you determine that the infant is in the ''alert inactivity'' behavioral state?

D. **Clinical Situation:** Baby Boy Florenz is a 1-day-old infant who is rooming in with his mother. Baby Florenz is a term infant who received a normal newborn examination. He is the first child.

1. Formulate at least three nursing diagnoses for Baby Florenz during the newborn period.
   a.

   b.

   c.

2. Three nursing goals to protect the neonate from injury are:
   a.
   b.
   c.

3. _____ An appropiate nursing intervention to prevent the infant from losing heat by the means of radiation is:
   a. rapidly drying the skin after delivery
   b. placing the infant away from walls
   c. placing the infant on a covered surface
   d. transporting the neonate in a crib with solid sides

4. List the nursing interventions that should be utilized to maintain a patent airway in Baby Florenz.
   a.
   b.
   c.
   d.

5. What is the rationale for keeping clothes and blankets loose?

6. Why should the administration of silver nitrate or antibiotics to the eyes be delayed 1 hour.

7. What criteria could be utilized to evaluate nursing interventions aimed at maintaining a patent airway in the transition period?

8. What areas should be included in the discharge planning of Baby Florenz and his parents?

E. **Clinical Situation:** The Cohens have just had their first baby, Sarah. The infant received a normal newborn exam. The Cohens have been attending parenting classes in the hospital and feel comfortable about the routine care of their infant.

1. What behaviors might be assessed to determine if the Cohens have attached to Sarah?

2. Why is it important to know the Cohens' relationship to their own parents?

3. Formulate one nursing diagnosis related to the attachment process.

4. Develop six nursing interventions to facilitate the attachment process.

   a.

   b.

   c.

   d.

   e.

   f.

V. Suggested Readings

1. Arnold, H.W., Putnam, N.J., Barnard, and others: The newborn. Transition to extra-uterine life. Am. J. Nurs. **65**(10):77–80, 1965.

   The article provides a discussion of the need for a transitional nursery. The many changes that the infant must accomplish are reviewed. The care that the infant should receive as well as the findings or observations that occur in transition are discussed to help the nurse anticipate problems.

2. Davis, V.: The structure and function of brown adipose tissue in the neonate, JOGN **9** (6): 368–372, 1980.

   This excellent article reviews the principles and conditions of newborns that predispose them to problems of thermoregulation. It also explores the mechanisms that help the newborn to maintain a stable temperature.

3. Judd, J.M.: Assessing the newborn. Nursing 85 **12**:34–41, 1985.

   This article provides a comprehensive discussion of the assessment of the newborn. It reviews the basic principles of examination and provides the reader with a list of equipment. A complete discussion of the normal findings provides a basis for practicing in the clinical area.

4. Kuller, J.M., Lund, C. and Tobin, C.: Improved skin care for premature infants. MCN **8**, (3): 200–203, 1983.

   Although the focus of this article is the premature infant, the principles that are addressed are applicable to the normal newborn. There are excellent guidelines and interventions that can be put directly into practice.

5. Sasso, S.C.: Erythromycin for eye prophylaxis. MCN **9**: 417, 1984.

   The uses, administration and contraindications of erythromycin are discussed. Nursing interventions are discussed. A good overview of ophthalmia neonatorum.

6. Gibbons, M.B.: Circumcision: the controversy continues. Pediatr. Nurs. **10**:103–110, 1984.

   This is an excellent detailed article on the controversy surrounding routine circumcision. It is the result of a task force study. It discusses the procedure and reviews the hygiene of the circumcised and uncircumcised infant. The complications of circumcision are also discussed.

7. Cronenwett, L.R., and Kunst-Wilson, W.: Stress, social support and the transition to fatherhood. Nurs. Res. **30** (4):196–201, 1981.

   The authors develop a framework for viewing the transition to fatherhood. The stress associated with this role change and the importance of a support network are addressed.

8. Nugent, J.K.: The Brazelton neonatal Behavioral Assessment Scale: implication for intervention. Pediatr. Nurs. **7**:18–21, 1981.

   A detailed description of the scale is provided as well as what can be assessed using the scale. The method of scoring the scale and the importance of teaching parents about their infants are addressed. While it is not the focus of the article, the use of the scale as a teaching and intervention tool is described.

Chapter 9

Health Problems of the Newborn

I. Chapter Overview

Chapter 9 introduces nursing considerations essential to the care of the newborn who has health problems. While many of these problems may be effectively resolved in the neonatal period, students need to be aware that some of the long-term sequelae may persist throughout life. At the completion of this chapter, the student will have a knowledge of health problems commonly encountered in the neonatal period. The student will be able to develop nursing goals and interventions to provide support for the normal development of the newborn and to assist parents in coping with the added stresses of a neonatal health problem.

II. Learning Objectives

Upon completion of this chapter, it is expected that the student will be able to:

1. Recognize birth injuries that are commonly observed in the newborn.

2. Recognize common health problems that occur in the newborn.

3. Identify neonatal problems that are related to physiologic factors.

4. Describe nursing responsibilities in the care of the child with an inborn error of metabolism.

II. Review of Essential Concepts

. Soft-tissue injury usually occurs when there is some degree of disproportion between the _____ and the _____ .

. The most commonly observed scalp lesion is _____, a vaguely outlined area of edematous tissue situated over the portion of the scalp that presents during a vertex delivery.
   a. caput succedaneum
   b. hydrocephalus
   c. cephalhematoma
   d. subdural hematoma

3. Fracture of the _____ is the most common birth injury.

4. Loss of movement on the affected side of the face and an absence of wrinkling of the forehead would be indicative of _____ .

5. Nursing care of the neonate with brachial palsy is primarily concerned with _____ of the affected arm.

6. Candidiasis and impetigo are two infections that commonly afflict neonates. Match the following statements with the appropriate infectious process. Mark C if the answer is candidiasis and I if the answer is impetigo.
   a. _____ Candida albicans is the causative organism.
   b. _____ Group A beta-hemolytic streptococci and *staphylococcus aureus* are the causative organisms.
   c. _____ The infection is characterized by vesicular lesions.
   d. _____ The infection is characterized by white, curdy patches that cannot be scraped from mucous membranes.
   e. _____ This infection frequently follows prolonged antibiotic therapy.
   f. _____ This infection is usually treated with systemic and local antibiotics.
   g. _____ The isolation technique of choice is wound and skin precautions.

7. _____ refers to an increased bilirubin level in the blood.

8. A serum bilirubin level of more than _____ in a full-term infant may cause brain damage.

9. The major clinical manifestation of hyperbilirubinemia is _____ .

10. Why do most newborns experience elevated bilirubin levels?

11. A common treatment for hyperbilirubinemia that involves the use of intense fluorescent light is called

    _____ .

12. The treatment of hypocalcemia in the neonate involves the intravenous administration of

    _____ .

13. List the two precautions that should be instituted when administering intravenous calcium gluconate.
    a.

    b.

14. _____ The two principal causes of hypoglycemia in the neonate are decreased amounts of stored glycogen and an increased use of blood glucose. (true or false)

15. Prevention of hypoglycemia involves reducing nonessential _____ by maintaining the newborn's body temperature and ensuring _____ through initiation of early feeding.

16. _____ Phenylketonuria (PKU) is inherited as an autosomal-recessive trait. (true or false)

17. The hepatic enzyme, _____, is absent in PKU.

18. The most effective method of identifying neonates with PKU is through _____.

19. _____ Infants with galactosemia usually display notable abnormalities at birth. (true or false)

IV. Application, Analysis, and Synthesis of Essential Concepts

A. **Clinical Situation:** Baby Boy Jacobs is admitted to the newborn nursery following an uncomplicated vertex delivery. During the initial assessment it is noted that he has a caput succedaneum over the right frontal area.

1. Differentiate between the following types of head trauma that can occur during the birth process.
   a. Caput succedaneum—

   b. Cephalhematoma—

2. Identify the two major nursing goals associated with the care of the neonate with birth-related head trauma.
   a.
   b.

B. **Experiential Exercise:** Care for a hospitalized child with a candida infection.

1. Which children are particularly at risk for the development of candidiasis?
   a.
   b.
   c.
   d.

2. Formulate at least four nursing diagnoses appropriate for an infant with candidiasis.
   a.

   b.

   c.

   d.

   e.

C. **Clinical Situation:** Mrs. Jackson brings her 6-week-old daughter to the dermatology clinic because of a crusty, weeping rash on the infant's neck. A diagnosis of impetigo is made.

1. Briefly state the two major elements of the therapeutic management of impetigo.
   a.
   b.

2. Develop a set of at least four home care instructions that should be given to Mrs. Jackson.
   a.

   b.

   c.

d.

D. **Experiential Exercise:** Care for a neonate who is receiving phototherapy.

1. What two factors are primarily responsible for the development of physiologic jaundice in the newborn?
   a.
   b.
2. When would the nurse expect the following phases of physiologic jaundice to occur in the full-term infant?
   a. Onset—
   b. Peak—
   c. Resolution—
3. When would the nurse expect the following phases of physiologic jaundice to occur in the premature infant?
   a. Onset—
   b. Peak—
   c. Resolution—
4. Identify the nursing interventions associated with the care of the child receiving phototherapy.
   a.
   b.
   c.
   d.
   e.
5. Identify the rationale for each of the interventions listed in the previous question.
   a.

   b.

   c.

   d.

   e.

E. **Experiential Exercise**: Spend a day in a PKU clinic.

1. Describe the principal screening method used in the newborn nursery to detect phenylketonuria.

2. Which infants should be retested within 2 weeks?
   a.
   b.
   c.
3. Why is urine testing not considered a reliable method of screening in the newborn?
   a.

   b.

4. What two criteria must the nurse consider in assessing the dietary management of PKU?
   a.
   b.
5. Why must the child with PKU be monitored frequently for urinary phenylpyruvic, blood phenylalanine, and height and weight measurements?

6. Listed below are a series of problems associated with the management of PKU. Provide a possible nursing intervention that might help alleviate each.
   a. Lofenalac, the formula used in infancy, is expensive.

   b. Lofenalac tends to have a lumpy texture.

   c. The formula has a distinctive odor and taste.

   d. Compliance with the diet is difficult after infancy.

   e. The affected child may bear an affected offspring.

V. Suggested Readings

1. Tufts, F., and Johnson, F.: Neonatal jaundice and phototherapy, Can. Nurse **75**:45–47, 1979.

This entry reviews bilirubin metabolism, the factors that predispose to the development of jaundice, and the potential consequences of jaundice in the newborn. It then discusses phototherapy as the treatment of choice, with particular emphasis on its nursing implications.

2. Taur, K.M.: physiologic mechanisms in childhood hypoglycemia, Pediatr. Nurs. **9**(5):341–344, 1983.

This article describes the mechanisms of glucose homeostasis. It provides an etiologic classification of hypoglycemia in infants and children and alerts the nurse to specific contributing factors and manifestations.

3. Wyatt, D.S.: Phenylketonuria: the problems vary during different developmental stages, Am. J. Maternal Child Nurs. **3**(5):296–302, 1978.

Phenylketonuria is concisely explained and its basic treatment outlined. Each developmental age is then presented as having its unique problems arising from the management of PKU. Concrete suggestions are provided for helping the child and family to cope with these situations.

4. Smith, E.J.: Galactosemia: an inborn error of metabolism, Nurse Pract. **5**:8–9, Mar./Apr. 1980.

This article utilizes a case-study approach to present the symptoms, diagnosis, and treatment of galactosemia. It describes the nurse's role in the continuing education, counseling, and support of the family.

The High-Risk Newborn and Family

I. Chapter Overview

Chapter 10 is concerned with the neonate at high risk for morbidity and mortality because of conditions that are superimposed on the normal course of events associated with birth. The improvement and advances of medical technology now afford many of these infants effective treatment and increase their chances of survival. Students need to be familiar with the conditions and care of the high risk infant and family, because the required nursing care is complex. Many of these infants will have long-term sequelae that require continuous care. This chapter will expose the student to the conditions and circumstances that place these infants at risk and to the interventions associated with their care. At the completion of the chapter the student will have a foundation for high-risk infant care that can be built upon in the practicum setting.

Learning Objectives

Upon completion of this chapter, it is expected that the student will be able to:

1. Describe three ways in which high-risk infants may be classified.

2. Outline a general plan of care for the high-risk infant.

3. Contrast the characteristics of premature, full-term, and postmature infants.

4. Develop a care plan to meet the needs of an infant at high risk.

5. Develop a plan of care to meet the needs of an infant with a high-risk condition of maternal origin.

II. Review of Essential Concepts

1. List at least three preconceptional factors that can predispose the infant to high-risk status.

2. _____ The presence of two umbilical arteries may be associated with fetal anomalies. (true or false)

3. The high-risk infant may be classified according to _____.

4. _____ A Level I facility has the capacity to care for complex neonatal complications. (true or false)

5. The limits on the cardiac monitor are usually set at _____.

6. List the observations that are crucial in the care of ill newborns.

7. Items to be included in the gastrointestinal assessment of the infant include

8. _____ One of the reasons that thermoregulation is a problem in the low-birth-weight infant is:
   a decreased metabolic rate
   b. greater muscle mass
   c. large amounts of brown fat
   d. poor reflex control of capillaries

9. Extracelluar water content is _____ in a preterm than in a full-term infant.

10. Soap or detergent should not be used to clean the skin of the preterm infant, because they interfere with the _____ .

11. _____ An indication that the preterm infant can breast feed is:
   a. presence of a rooting reflex
   b. weigh at least 1250 g
   c. presence of a suck reflex
   d. an intolerance to formula

12. Six factors that effect the growth and development of the preterm infant include:

13. _____ The presence of avoidance behavior during a stimulation session suggests that the interventions should be continued. (true or false)
14. Match the characteristics on the left with type of maturity on the right.

_____ abundant lanugo   a. premature

_____ presence of subcuta-   b. postmature
      neous fat
                             c. term
_____ cracked skin

15. _____ Infants who are receiving theophylline for the treatment of apnea should be monitored closely for:
    a. bradycardia
    b. congestive heart failure
    c. tachycardia
    d. cyanosis
16. _____ A factor in the pathophysiology of respiratory distress syndrome is
    a. decreased pulmonary vascular resistance
    b. failure to establish a functional reisidual capacity
    c. presence of surfactant.
    d. nonreactivity of the baroreceptors.
17. _____ The diagnosis of sepsis is always made on the basis of blood cultures. (true or false)
18. Complications of sepsis that the nurse should look for include:_____.
19. Clinical manifestations of necrotizing enterocolitis include:

20. Feedings are withheld in infants who have suffered asphyxia, because

21. _____ Apnea may be a clinical manifestation of a patent ductus arteriosus. (true or false)
22. _____ A medication used in the therapeutic management of a PDA includes:
    a. theophylline
    b. indomethacin
    c. inderal
    d. prostaglandin E
23. The most common cause of anemia in the preterm infant is: _____.
24. The clinical manifestations of an intraventricular hemorrhage include _____.
25. The most important factor influencing the well-being of the fetus of a diabetic mother is _____.
26. _____ A characteristic clinical manifestation of the infant of a diabetic mother not under complete control is:
    a. hyperglycemia
    b. loss of subcutaneous fat
    c. absence of vernix caseosa

    d. macrosomy for gestational age
27. Paregoric is administered to decrease _____ of the infant of a heroin-addicted mother.
28. _____ A complication of maternal smoking is a small-for-gestational-age infant. (true or false)

IV. Application, Analysis, and Synthesis of Essential Concepts

A. **Clinical Situation**: Care for a high-risk infant.

1. What is the best method to utilize in classifying the high-risk infant?

2. Why is the prevention of infection such an important goal for the high-risk infant?

3. What interventions do you utilize to maintain the thermal stability of the infant?
   a.
   b.
   c.
   d.
4. What is the rationale for determining the point of maximum intensity in the assessment of the infant's cardiovascular status?

5. The nursing diagnosis for the nursing goal of providing nutrition is:

6. What assessment parameter could you utilize to determine if the infant was getting adequate nutrition?

7. How do you evaluate whether the interventions are successful in preventing skin breakdown?

8. Interventions used to provide visual stimulation include:
   a.
   b.

9. Three nursing goals developed to prevent an alteration in family process include:
   a.
   b.
   c.
10. What is the rationale for encouraging the parents to visit the infant?

B. **Clinical Situation:** Tommy is an infant who is 43 weeks gestation. He was admitted to the ICU with a diagnosis of meconium aspiration syndrome. Tommy is experiencing severe respiratory distress and has been placed on a ventilator.

1. What physical characteristics are assessed in Tommy that lead the nurse to determine that he is postmature?

2. The etiology of the hyperinflation and air trapping that occur with this syndrome is:

3. The items that should be included in the *respiratory* assessment of this infant include:
   a.
   b.
   c.
   d.
   e.
   f.
   g.
4. Why is mouth care an important intervention for Tommy?

5. Identify at least four nursing interventions to support respiratory effort.
   a.
   b.
   c.
   d.
   e.
   f.
6. How would the nurse know that Tommy can have his oxygen concentration lowered?

7. Why is conservation of energy an important nursing goal for Tommy?

C. **Clinical Situation:** Cindy is a premature infant in the ICU. She has recovered from her respiratory distress and has been diagnosed as having an intraventricular hemorrhage. She is suspected of having sepsis.

1. Postnatally, Cindy may have obtained her infection as a result of:

2. What findings were observed that suggest sepsis?

3. The most important nursing goal in caring for Cindy is: _____.
4. Identify the nursing goals associated with Cindy's care.
   a.
   b.
   c.
   d.
5. What nursing interventions may have contributed to Cindy's developing an intraventricular hemorrhage?

D. **Clinical Situation:** Michael is a premature infant who experienced severe asphyxia at birth. Oral feedings were started within the first 24 hours. He is now having problems with feedings. Necrotizing enterocolitis (NEC) is suspected. He is also anemic.

1. What factor in Michael's history predisposes him to the development of NEC?

2. The most important nursing responsibility when caring for infants who are at risk for developing NEC is _____.

3. Nursing interventions that would alert the nurse to the presence of NEC include:

4. List the nursing interventions that are used when NEC is suspected.
   a.
   b.
   c.
   d.
   e.
   f.
   g.
5. How would you evaluate whether the infant is receiving adequate hydration?

6. Why is anemia a common problem for the preterm infant?

7. The most important nursing consideration in the prevention of anemia is _____.

8. List the nursing interventions the nurse might use to detect anemia?
   a.
   b.
   c.
   d.
   e.

E. **Clinical Situation:** Terry is a 3 day-old infant born to a mother who developed diabetes during pregnancy. Terry was admitted to the ICU for observation.

1. Why is hypoglycemia a common occurrence in infants of diabetic mothers?

2. Why is feeding begun so early with these infants?

3. *Nursing responsibilities* for the infant of a diabetic mother include monitoring the infant for signs of: _____.

4. List the nursing interventions that should be included in preparing the parents for discharge of the infant:
   a.
   b.
   c.
   d.
   e.

5. How would you evaluate whether the interventions were successful in preparing the parents for discharge?

V. Suggested Readings

1. Sandelowski, M.: Perinatal nursing: whose specialty is it anyway? MCN. **8**:317–322, 1983

   The author reviews the "new" specialty, perinatal nursing. A review of its development is provided, and the author asks some relevent questions about the development of the specialty.

2. Scharping, E.M.: Physiologic measurements of the neonate. MCN. **8**:70–73, 1983

   This is an excellent supplement to the text. The article stresses the importance of early recognition and discusses in detail the assessment of temperature, pulse respiration and blood pressure in the neonate. Differences between the neonate and adult are provided.

3. Bragdon, D.B.: A basis for the nursing management of feeding the premature infant. JOGN **12**:51s–57s.

   Feeding the premature infant may require modification of routine practices. This article reviews the nutritional needs of these infants, explores the methods used, and discusses common feeding problems that can occur.

4. Blackburn, S.: Fostering behavioral development of high-risk infants JOGN Nursing **12**: 76s–86s, 1983.

   This article is an extension of text material. It stresses the need for assessment and individualization of any stimulation program. The article provides nursing interventions that can be used in an infant-stimulation program.

5. Nugent, J.: Acute respiratory care of the newborn. JOGN Nursing **12**:31s–44s, 1983.

   Respiratory diseases are extremely common in neonates. The author briefly reviews many common ones and provides the reader with a detailed discussion of the methods, indications, and uses of respiratory assistance. Nursing interventions are provided in detail as well.

6. Cohen, M.A.: The use of prostaglandins and prostaglandin inhibitors in critically ill neonates. MCN. **8**:194–199, 1983.

   There is increasing use of these medications in the ICU. The article explores the uses, indications, dosages and nursing considerations of caring for an infant who is recieving these medications.

7. Braune, K., and Lacey, l.: Common hemotologic problems of the immediate newborn period. JOGN Nursing **12**:19s–26s, 1983.

   The article reviews the most common problems that may occur. A discussion of the causes and prevention is provided along with nursing interventions that can be used to care for infants with hematologic problems.

8. Carey, B.: Intraventricular hemorrhage in the preterm infant. JOGN Nursing **12**:60s–68s, 1983.

   A complete discussion of this disorder is provided in this article. It reviews the incidence, causes, pathophysiology, diagnosis and treatment of this disease. An excellent supplement to the text.

9. Burn, E.M.: Diabetes mellitus and pregnancy, Nurs. Clin. N.A. **18**:673–685, 1983.

   A comprehensive review of the classifications of diabetes during pregnancy, as well as the effects of pregnancy on diabetes, the effects of diabetes on pregnancy, and the effects of diabetes on the fetus. The management of the diabetic mother in the antenatal and postpartum period is discussed.

Conditions Caused By Problems in Physical Development

I. Chapter Overview

Chapter 11 introduces nursing considerations essential to the care of the child who has a congenital malformation. Since these defects account for a substantial number of the health problems of infants, it is important for students to be aware of the need for immediate, temporary, and permanent intervention. At the completion of this chapter, the student will understand the structural and physiologic changes associated with the various congenital malformations and will be able to develop appropriate nursing interventions for a child with a congenital health problem.

II. Learning Objectives

Upon completion of this chapter, it is expected that the student will be able to:

1. Describe the role of the nurse in dealing with parents upon the birth of a child with a defect.

2. Formulate a nursing care plan for the preoperative and postoperative care of a child with a myelomeningocele.

3. Describe the preoperative and postoperative care of a child with hydrocephalus.

4. Differentiate between the various congenital skeletal defects.

5. Design a teaching plan for the parents of a child with a congenital skeletal deformity.

6. Outline a plan for teaching the parents pre- and postoperative care of a child with a cleft lip or palate.

7. Compare the pre- and postoperative care of an infant with a structural defect of the gastrointestinal tract.

8. Describe the various types of hernias.

9. Discuss the preoperative preparation of the parents of and the child with a structural defect of the genitourinary tract.

10. Discuss the role of the nurse in helping the parents to cope with the problems of a newborn with ambiguous genitalia.

11. Identify factors in the prenatal environment that may have an adverse effect on the developing fetus.

III. Review of Essential Concepts

1. The birth of an infant with a defect evokes the same psychologic reaction as the _____.

2. _____ refers to a hernial protrusion of a sac-like cyst containing meninges, spinal fluid, and a portion of the spinal cord with its nerves through a defect in the vertebral column.
   a. Rachischisis
   b. Meningocele
   c. Encephalocele
   d. Myelomeningocele

3. An important nursing intervention when caring for a child with a myelomeningocele in the preoperative stage would be _____.
   a. applying a heat lamp to facilitate drying and toughening of the sac.
   b. assessing sensory and motor function frequently to monitor for signs of impairment.
   c. applying a diaper to prevent contamination of the sac.
   d. placing the child on his side to decrease pressure on the spinal cord.

4. _____ is a condition caused by an imbalance in the production and absorption of cerebrospinal fluid in the ventricular system, usually under increased pressure.

5. Although the causes of hydrocephalus are varied, the result is either:
   a.
   b.
6. The most frequently observed clinical manifestations of hydrocephalus in the infant include:
   a.
   b.
   c.
   d.
   e.
   f.
7. _____ The signs and symptoms of hydrocephalus in early to late childhood are caused by increased intracranial pressure. (true or false)
8. _____ In infancy, the diagnosis of hydrocephalus is based on head circumference that crosses one or more grid lines on the measurement chart within a period of 2 to 4 weeks. (true or false)
9. List the three degrees of congenital hip dysplasia.
   a.
   b.
   c.
10. In the child between birth and 2 months of age, subluxation and the tendency to dislocate are most reliably demonstrated by the _____ and _____ tests.
11. Match the following types of club foot positions with their defining characteristics.

a. _____ talipes varus
b. _____ talipes equinus
c. _____ talipes valgus
d. _____ talipes calcaneus

   a. plantar flexion in which the toes are lower than the heel
   b. an eversion or bending outward
   c. dorsiflexion, in which the toes are higher than the heel
   d. an inversion or bending inward

12. Therapeutic management of congenital club foot involves:
    a.
    b.
    c.
13. The major potential handicap for a child with a cleft palate is _____.
14. The immediate nursing problems in the care of an infant with cleft lip and palate deformities are related to _____ the infant.
15. Two clinical manifestations that may indicate the presence of esophageal atresia in an infant are:
    a.
    b.
16. List the three ''C's'' of a tracheoesophageal fistula.

a.
b.
c.
17. _____ is the obstruction or absence of a portion of the bile ducts.
18. Match the following types of hernias with the appropriate defining characteristics.

a. _____ umbilical hernia
b. _____ diaphragmatic hernia
c. _____ gastroschisis
d. _____ hiatal hernia
e. _____ inguinal hernia
f. _____ omphalocele

   a. protrusion of the abdominal organs through an abnormal opening in the diaphragm into the thoracic cavity
   b. involves the sliding of the cardiac end of the stomach through the esophageal hiatus
   c. results from incomplete closure of the fascial ring causing protrusions of the omentum and intestine through the opening
   d. serious congenital malformation in which a variable amount of abdominal contents protrudes into the base of the umbilical cord
   e. herniation through a defect in the abdominal wall that permits extrusion of abdominal contents without involving the umbilical cord.
   f. occurs when abdominal fluid or a portion of the intestine is forced into the proximal portion of the processus vaginalis

19. _____ refers to a condition in which the urethral opening is located behind the glans penis or anywhere along the ventral surface of the penile shaft.
20. List the diagnostic tools that may be used to determine sex and assist in making a gender assignment in a child with ambiguous genitalia.
    a.
    b.
    c.
    d.
    e.
    f.
    g.
21. Identify the microbial agents that comprise the TORCH complex.

a.

b.

c.

d.

e.

22. _____ The effects of fetal alcohol syndrome are reversible. (true or false)

23. The major emphasis in the management of fetal alcohol syndrome is placed on _____.

IV. Application, Analysis, and Synthesis of Essential Concepts

A. **Clinical Situation:** Adam Barnes, a newborn, is transferred to the pediatric unit for surgical evaluation of a myelomeningocele. Following an initial assessment, it is noted that Adam has an associated hydrocephalus. The Barneses have accompanied their child and are visibly upset.

1. Identify three nursing goals for Adam's initial care.
   a.
   b.
   c.

2. The early prognosis for the child with myelomeningocele depends on:
   a.
   b.

3. Myelomeningocele is one of the most common causes of _____ in childhood, and the prognosis for children who survive the early complications depends on the severity of their _____.

4. Appropriate nursing interventions for Adam's preoperative care include:
   a.
   b.
   c.
   d.
   e.
   f.

5. If Adam's hydrocephalus were allowed to progress, what clinical manifestations would he exhibit?
   a.
   b.
   c.
   d.
   e.
   f.

6. Postoperative nursing interventions for the child with hydrocephalus include _____.
   a. observing for signs of increased intracranial pressure
   b. positioning child with the head of the bed elevated 45 degrees
   c. positioning the child on the affected side to facilitate drainage

d. administering sedatives to decrease discomfort

7. Identify a nursing diagnosis appropriate for Adam's parents at this time.

8. For each of the following nursing goals, identify at least two appropriate nursing interventions to be utilized when caring for Adam's family.
   a. Deal with the family's anxiety about recurrence in future children—

   b. Prepare family for child's discharge—

   c. Provide anticipatory guidance—

   d. Facilitate developmental progress—

   e. Support parents—

   f. Coordinate services—

B. **Experiential Exercise:** Care for a child with congenital hip dysplasia.

1. During the infant assessment process, what clinical signs could indicate congenital dislocation of the hip in the newborn?
   a.
   b.
   c.

2. The two objectives of therapeutic management for congenital hip dysplasia are:
   a.
   b.

3. A major nursing goal when preparing the child for discharge is:

4. What instructions should be incorporated into a teaching plan for the parents of a child who is being discharged with a reduction appliance such as a Pavlik harness?

a.

b.

c.

d.

e.

C. **Experiential Exercise:** Care for a child with a cleft lip or palate.

1. Identify two immediate nursing problems in the care of an infant with a cleft lip and palate deformity.
   a.
   b.
2. Why does feeding pose a special challenge to the nurse?

3. How is feeding best accomplished in the preoperative period?

4. The major nursing goal in the postoperative period is directed toward _____.
5. Identify the rationales for each of the following nursing interventions utilized in the postoperative care of the child with cleft lip or palate.
   a. Place in partial side-lying position—

   b. Apply jacket or arm restraints—

   c. Rinse mouth before and after feedings—

   d. Keep suture site clean of formula and drainage—

   e. Modify feeding techniques—

f. Remove restraints periodically and provide adequate stimulation—

D. **Clinical Situation:** Angela Smith is 24 hours old. Following her initial feeding of dextrose and water in the newborn nursery, Angela began to cough and choke and became cyanotic. She has been transferred to the pediatric Intensive Care Unit for surgical evaluation of a tracheoesophageal fistula.

1. How is a diagnosis of esophageal atresia established?

2. The therapeutic management of esophageal atresia is directed toward
   a.
   b.
3. Identify at least two interventions for each of the following nursing goals related to the preoperative care of the child with tracheoesophageal fistula.
   a. Facilitate ventilation—

   b. Prevent aspiration pneumonia—

4. Following Angela's surgery, the nurse is developing a plan for her care. Match each intervention to the appropriate rationale. (Answers may be used more than once.)

RATIONALE	INTERVENTIONS
a. _____ maintenance of fluid and electrolyte balance	a. Administer gastrostomy feeds.
	b. Provide tactile stimulation.
b. _____ prevention of wound infection	c. Weigh daily.
c. _____ maintenance of nutrition	d. Suction secretions frequently.
d. _____ promotion of adequate ventilation	e. Monitor operative site for drainage.
e. _____ maintenance of comfort	f. Position for optimal lung expansion.
	g. Administer mouth care.
	h. Obtain specific gravity.

E. **Experiential Exercise:** Care for a child who is undergoing surgery for the repair of hypospadias.

1. List the principal objectives of surgical correction.
   a.

   b.

   c.

2. Why is circumcision contraindicated in an infant with hypospadias?

3. What is the preferred time for surgical repair?

4. What two types of information should be included when preparing the parents and child for the surgical correction of hypospadias?
   a.
   b.
5. Formulate at least three nursing diagnoses related to the postoperative care of the child with hypospadias.
   a.

   b.

   c.

   d.

V. Suggested Readings

1. Jackson, P.: When the baby isn't perfect, Am. J. Nurs. **85**:396–399, 1985.

This article describes the various reactions that a set of parents experienced following the birth of a child with a defect. It is written by a pediatric nurse and provides insight into the stressors that parents must cope with following the birth of such an infant.

2. Swagman, A.: Caring for limb-deficient children and their families, Am. J. Maternal Child Nurs. **11**(1):46–52, 1986.

This article addresses the various causes and classifications of limb malformations. Care of the family is discussed in terms of explaining the child's problem, displaying respect for the child and family, providing emotional support, and offering corrective assistance. Surgical intervention and follow-up care for specific defects is described. The role of the nurse is discussed throughout the article.

3. Moynihan, P., and Gerraughty, A.: Diaphragmatic hernia: low stress equals higher survival, Am. J. Nurs. **85**:662–665, 1985.

This selection reviews the factors that contribute to the poor survival rate of infants with diaphragmatic hernia. Techniques to identify risks and minimize stress are described. The nurse's role in maintaining contact with and supporting parents during the separation phase is emphasized. The need for further advances is identified.

4. Hazle, N.: An infant who survived gastroschisis, Am J. Maternal Child Nurs. **6**(1):35–40, 1981.

This article provides a description of gastroschisis, its immediate nursing management, and long-term problems. It utilizes a case study approach to present a nursing care plan for an infant following surgical correction of this defect. Discharge planning, follow-up care, and the potential for long-term problems are also described.

5. Stevens, M.S., and Reinitz, M.: Nursing a child through exstrophic bladder reconstruction surgery, Am. J. Maternal Child Nurs. **5**(4):265–270, 1980.

Exstrophy of the bladder and associated anomalies are described in this article. The responsibility of the nurse in teaching the parents about their baby's special needs and preparing both the child and parents for corrective surgery is discussed. Nursing care during the stages of surgery and preparation for discharge is described.

6. Devore, N.E., Jackson, V.M., and Piening, S.L.: TORCH infections, Am. J. Nurs. **83**:1660–1665, 1983.

This article summarizes information specific to the five types of organisms that comprise the TORCH complex. A detailed chart displays pertinent information regarding both the maternal and perinatal aspects of the disorders. The importance of follow-up care for resulting chronic sequelae is stressed.

7. Stephens, C.J.: The fetal alcohol syndrome: cause for concern, Am. J. Maternal Child Nurs. **6**(4):251–256, 1981.

This entry presents a detailed description of the fetal alcohol syndrome and explores factors related to the consumption of alcohol by pregnant women. It also describes the nurse's responsibility in assessment, counseling, and referral. The importance of prevention is addressed.

Chapter 12

Health Promotion of the Infant and Family

I. Chapter Overview

Chapter 12 explores infancy, the period from birth to 12 months. The focus of this chapter is the normal progression of growth and development and the fostering of optimal health in the infant through anticipatory guidance of the parents. Infancy is the period of the fastest gain in physical size and of the most dramatic developmental achievements of the entire life span. It is characterized by an orderly progression of physical, cognitive, and social maturation which may be susceptible to positive and negative influences. Upon completion of this chapter the student should have the necessary information base to counsel parents on optimal development and to integrate it in the clinical setting.

II. Learning Objectives

Upon completion of this chapter, it is expected that the student will be able to:

1. Identify the major biologic, psychosocial, cognitive, and social developments of the first year.

2. Relate parent-child attachment, separation anxiety, and stranger fear to developmental achievements during infancy.

3. Identify how the infant's temperament can influence child-rearing practices.

4. Provide anticipatory guidance for parents on common concerns during infancy.

5. Provide parents with feeding recommendations for infants in the first and second halves of infancy.

6. Develop guidelines for parents regarding sleep disturbances in infants.

7. List recommendations for parents on dental health during infancy.

8. Outline immunization requirements during infancy.

9. Administer immunizations safely.

10. List the general contraindications to immunizations.

11. Provide anticipatory guidance to parents regarding accident prevention, based on the infant's developmental achievements.

12. Provide anticipatory guidance to parents to foster optimal health and development in their infant

III. Review of Essential Concepts

1. An infant who is 6 months of age should have _____ his birth weight.

2. Binocularity should be well established by the age of _____.

3. _____ A physiologic characteristic of a 4-month-old is:
   a. the presence of iron deficiency anemia
   b. presence of drooling
   c. eruption of the first tooth
   d. adult level of fat absorption

4. List two reasons why infants are susceptible to dehydration.
   a.
   b.

5. _____ The fine motor development of a 3-month-old can best be described by
   a. the ability to transfer objects
   b. the desire to grasp an object
   c. the ability to voluntarily grasp an object
   d. the presence of a pincer grasp

6. _____ The gross motor development of a 6-month-old can best be described by
   a. the ability to roll from back to abdomen
   b. the ability to sit unsupported
   c. the ability to crawl
   d. the ability to pull self to standing position

7. _____ The infant is in Erikson's stage of oral development. (true or false)

8. _____ Piaget's stage of secondary circular reactions is characterized by:
   a. totally autistic behavior
   b. recognizing familiar behavior
   c. showing stranger anxiety
   d. becoming bored when left alone

9. The two components of cognitive development that are necessary for attachment are
   a.
   b.

10. _____ At 3 months, the infant displays a definite preference for the mother. (true or false)

11. Separation anxiety is defined as:

12. _____ An 8-month-old infant's language ability can best be described as:
    a. the ability to say dada
    b. the ability to understand no
    c. the ability to say mama
    d. the ability to respond to own name

13. List the social developmental milestones of a 6-month-old infant.
    a.
    b.
    c.

14. Appropriate toys for a 4-month-old child are:

15. How should the parents of a temperamentally active child modify their child-rearing practices.

16. _____ Problems with dental development are associated with the use of a pacifier. (true or false)

17. A quick guide to assessment of deciduous teeth during the first year is _____.

18. The main reason for shoes when the child has started walking is for_____.

19. Human milk is deficient in the mineral _____ and supplements of _____ per day should be given

20. _____ The amount of formula that a 6-month-old should be taking at each of five feedings is 8 oz. (true or false)

21. List the reasons why it is not advisable to introduce solid foods to a 3-month-old infant.
    a.
    b.
    c.
    d.

22. The first solid that is introduced is _____ because of its high _____ content.

23. _____ Each new solid food is introduced alone for 4 to 7 days, to detect food allergies. (true or false)

24. _____ The management of night crying includes:
    a. putting child in own bed when asleep
    b. arranging a separate sleeping area
    c. placing child in parents' bed for comfort
    d. rocking child until asleep

25. _____ During infancy teeth are cleaned with a soft toothbrush. (true or false)

26. _____ A 7-month-old's immunization record should read:
    a. DTP at 2, 4 months; TOPV at 2,4 months
    b. DTP at 2, 4 months; TOPV at 2, 4, 6 months
    c. DTP at 2, 4, 6 months; TOPV at 2, 4 months
    d. DTP at 2 months; TOPV at 2,4,6 months

27. Common reactions to a DTP immunization include

28. _____ A contraindication for all immunizations is
    a an upper respiratory infection
    b. antibiotic therapy
    c. steroid therapy
    d. gastritis

29. The leading cause of fatal injury in children under 1 year of age is _____.

30. _____ Guidelines to prevent accidental injuries in a 2-month-old child include:
    a. teaching child to swim to prevent drowning
    b. using a pillow to prevent aspiration
    c. using warm mist vaporizer to prevent chilling
    d. shaking baby powder on own hands first to prevent choking

31. _____ Guidance in discipline should begin in the second half of the first year. (true or false)

IV. Application, Analysis, and Synthesis of Essential Concepts

A. **Clinical Situation:** Mrs. Backer brings 7-month-old Jerry to the well-child clinic for his check-up. During the course of the examination Mrs. Backer says that Jerry is teething, has shown little interest in breast feeding, and cries when she leaves the room. She has been reading *Parents* magazine and is concerned that Jerry is not "doing" what the magazine states he should be "doing."

1. Jerry was 7 pounds at birth. At this visit he weighs 16 pounds. Is his weight normal for his age?

2. What fine motor, gross motor, language, and social developmental milestones does the nurse assess in Jerry that lead to a determination that Jerry is developing normally?

3. What nursing intervention might you suggest to Mrs. Backer regarding Jerry's crying when she leaves the room?

4. List the interventions that Mrs. Backer could implement to relieve teething pain.

   a.

   b.

5. What might Jerry's lack of interest in breast feeding indicate, and what interventions should you suggest to Jerry's mother?

6. List the interventions that Mrs. Backer can use to promote good dental health in Jerry.

   a.

   b.

   c.

   d.

   e.

7. What are the major nursing goals in the anticipatory guidance of Jerry?

B. **Clinical Situation:** Rachel is a 4-month-old infant who is at the clinic for her check-up. Rachel's mother states that she is having difficulty managing Rachel, because nothing she tries works twice, and she is concerned about Rachel's sleeping pattern

1. What behaviors are assessed to determine whether Rachel is in Piaget's stage of secondary circular reactions?

2. List the nursing interventions used to assist Rachel's mother in caring for Rachel.

   a.

   b.

   c.

3. What should the nurse assess regarding Rachel's sleeping pattern?

   a.

   b.

   c.

   d.

   e.

4. Rachel's mother will start Rachel on solid foods before the next check-up. What guidance should be given to her?

   a.

   b.

   c.

   d.

   e.

   f.

5. Anticipatory guidance for Rachel's mother should focus on:

   a.

   b.

   c.

   d.

C. **Experiential Exercise:** Administer immunizations to an infant.

1. What factors do you need to assess in the infant that might prevent you from administering immunizations?

2. What are the two nursing interventions that should be utilized to properly administer immunizations?

3. What is the safest site for administration of immunizations in the infant?

4. What are the nursing interventions that are associated with a DTP vaccine administration?

   a.

   b.

   c.

   d.

D. **Experiential Exercises**: Teach the parents of an

infant who is 8 to 12 months old how to prevent accidental injury to their child.

1. What developmental landmarks do you assess in the infant that predispose him to injury?

2. What interventions might you suggest to prevent burns in the child?
   a.
   b.
   c.
   d.
3. What is the rationale for keeping the bathroom door closed?

4. List the interventions that you would teach to prevent bodily damage:
   a.
   b.
   c.
   d.
5. Why is choking still such a problem in this age group?

6. What is the rationale for not administering medications as candy?

7. How might you evaluate whether your teaching plan was successful?

8. The parents inform you that their infant frequently spends time at the grandparents' home. What nursing intervention should you suggest to them?

V. Suggested Readings

1. Zigler, E., and Lang, M.E.: The emergence of "superbaby": a good thing? Ped. Nurs. **11** (5): 337–342, 1985.
   This excellent article reviews the research on early stimulation programs. It describes such programs, reviews the research and critiques the methods. It can be a source when questions regarding such programs arise.
2. Nelms, B.C.: Attachment *vs* spoiling. Ped. Nurs. **9** (1): 49–51,1983

Parents are often concerned about spoiling the infant. Nelms reviews what attachment is and how it can be fostered and provides anticipatory guidance to teach parents about this process and the child's emotional development. She differentiates attachment from "spoiling."
3. Chess, S., and Thomas,A.: Temperamental differences: a critical concept in child health care. Ped. Nurs. **11**(3):167–172, 1985.
   A definition of the concept and the three groups are provided. The role of temperament in well-child care is explored, as well as specific interventions for parents. Case studies are provided to illustrate the importance of the concept to practice.
4. Anderson, G.C.: Pacifiers: the positive side. MCN **11**(2):122–24, 1986.
   The author reviews the research on sucking needs in the infant and the use of pacifiers as a means of self-regulatory sucking. The article can provide students with a source for parents' questions about their use.
5. Smith, D.P.: Myths about day care: fact or reality. Ped. Nurs. **10**(4):278–280, 1984.
   This article provides the basis for effective counseling on day care. It identifies the myths and reviews the research as well as providing research on children's adjustment to day care. It provides the reader with guidelines and questions to use in evaluating day care facilities.
6. Reifsnider, E., and Meyers, S.T.: Employed mothers can breast feed too! MCN. **10**(4),256–260, 1985.
   The article explores the problems associated with working and breast feeding with women who were successful. The items that were most helpful and hindering are presented. Nursing interventions are addressed to assist the woman who wishes to continue breast feeding when she returns to work.
7. Bishop, W.S.; Weaning the breast-fed toddler or preschooler. Ped. Nurs. **11**(3), 211–214, 1983.
   A definition is provided as well as the period in which weaning commonly occurs. The factors to consider as to the timing of weaning are addressed. Approaches to the topic and anticipatory guidance for parents are provided. Although the topic is an older child, the concepts are applicable to infants.
8. Edgil, A.E., Wood, K.R., and Patterson, D.P.: Sleep problems of older infants and preschool children. Ped. Nurs. **11**(2): 87–91, 1985.
   This excellent study explores the problem of night waking in children of two age groups. It was designed to describe the problem from the mothers' perspective, to identify children who were described as having problems, and to identify interpersonal, intrapersonal and extrapersonal systems for preventing sleep problems and to identify domestic settings that may relate to the sleep problem.
9. Kronmiller, J.E., and Nirschl, R.F.: Preventive dentistry for children. Ped. Nurs. **11** (6);446–453, 1985.
   This article explores preventive dentistry for children of all ages. It identifies dental problems during childhood and prophylaxis for all children.
10. Mansell, K.A.: New immunization against H. *influenzae* Type B. Ped. Nurs. **11**(6):433–438, 1985.
    The article reviews the problem of bacterial meningitis and the types and incidence of HiB disease. A description of the vaccine, its effectiveness, recommendations and limitations is provided.

11. Nachem, B., and Bass, R.A.: Children aren't being buckled up. MCN **9**(5):320–324, 1984.

An excellent article that can be the basis of teaching plans. A review of the problem and methods for teaching are discussed in detail. The article provides nursing goals and interventions to assist in the teaching process.

12. Keim, K.A.: Preventing and treating plant poisonings in young children. MCN **8**(4)287–290, 1983.

This article discusses an often overlooked area of child safety. It explores the problem, provides principles of plant toxicity, addresses resources and describes emergency treatment.

Health Problems During Infancy

I. Chapter Overview

Chapter 13 introduces common health problems of the first year. They are usually influenced by environmental factors affecting the physical or psychologic development of the child due to the infant's immature physiologic system. Some have no "etiology." Students need to be aware of these health problems because most of them are amenable to prevention, and prompt identification and treatment will avert problems later in life. At the completion of this chapter the student should have the foundation to prevent and provide nursing care to children with common health problems and their families.

II. Learning Objectives

Upon completion of this chapter, it is expected that the student will be able to:

1. Recognize children at risk for developing nutritional disturbances.

2. Outline a nutritional counseling plan for the parents of a child with a nutritional disturbance.

3. Outline a dietary plan for parents when the infant is sensitive to milk.

4. Distinguish among the common feeding problems of infancy.

5. Identify measures that can be used to alleviate colic.

6. Outline a feeding plan for the child with rumination.

7. Identify characteristics of failure-to-thrive children and their families.

8. Develop a nursing care plan to meet the physical and emotional needs of the failure-to-thrive child and parents.

9. Compare the manifestations of age-related skin disorders in children.

10. Outline a plan of care for a child with eczema.

11. Develop a nursing care plan to meet the immediate and long-term needs of the family who has lost a child to sudden infant death syndrome.

12. Develop nursing care for the child who has infantile apnea and his family.

13. Describe the characteristics of autistic children.

III. Review of Essential Concepts

1 List the factors that predispose infants to the development of nutritional disturbances.
   a.
   b.
   c.
   d.
   e.

2. _____ Vitamin D is necessary for the absorption of calcium and phosphorus in the body. (true or false)

3. Vitamin excess if often a result of _____.

4. _____ The deficiency of Vitamin C is referred to as:
   a. rickets
   b. scurvy
   c. pellegra
   d. beriberi

5. _____ Excess sodium in the diet may lead to the development of hypotension. (true or false)

6. The clinical manifestations of a zinc deficiency include:

7. Sources of iron in the diet include:

8. _____ Kwashiorkor is defined as
   a. deficiency of calories

b. deficiency of calories and protein

c. deficiency of fats and carbohydrates

d. deficiency of protein with adequate calories

9. The diagnosis of cow's milk intolerance is initially made _____

10. _____ A formula that is a suitable cow's milk substitute is:

   a. Ensure

   b. Advance

   c. Isomil

   d. SMA

11. Match the feeding problem on the left with its definition on the right column.

_____ regurgitation   a. paroxysmal abdominal pain

_____ spitting up   b. voluntary return of food into the mouth

_____ colic

_____ rumination   c. return of undigested food from the stomach

     d. dribbling of unswallowed formula

12. List the measures used in the management of colic.

   a.

   b.

   c.

   d.

   e.

   f.

13. _____ Rumination is usually considered to be the result of disturbed parent-child relationship. (true or false)

14. The primary objective in the nursing care of the child who is ruminating is

15. _____ A clinical criteria that can be utilized in the diagnostic evaluation of nonorganic failure to thrive is:

a. evidence of systemic disease

b. developmental retardation persisting with adequate stimulation

c. weight above the 10th percentile

d. presence of significant psychosocial interruption

16. _____ A characteristic of children who fail to thrive is their intense interest in social interaction. (true or false)

17. Parents of the failure-to-thrive infant are usually

18. The most important nursing goal for the failure-to-thrive infant is _____.

19. List the guidelines that should be utilized for the feeding interaction of the failure-to-thrive infant.

   a.

   b.

   c.

   d.

   e.

   f.

   g.

20. Match the skin disorders on the right with their clinical manifestations on the left.

_____ appears on scalp, face, arms, and legs. Lesions are red, have papules and vesicles, and are itchy   a. seborrheic dermatitis

     b. atopic dermatitis

     c. diaper dermatitis

_____ appears on the scalp, eyelids, and external ear canal. Lesions are thick, yellowish, scaly

_____ appears on convex surfaces or in skin folds

21. The first goal in the treatment of eczema is _____.

22. List the measures used in the therapeutic management of eczema.

   a.

   b.

   c.

   d.

   e.

   f.

23. The three groups of children who are considered at risk for SIDS are

24. One approach to the nursing care for families of SIDS infants is based on

25. One of the most important aspects of the care of the parents following a SIDS death is

26. _____ Parents of a SIDS infant who are in the impact phase of the crisis are characterized by:
    a.
    b.
    c.
    d.

27. _____ Infantile apnea is defined as the cessation of breathing for at least 10 seconds. (true or false)

28. The most widely used test in the diagnostic evaluation of infantile apnea is the _____.

29. The therapeutic management of the infant with apnea involves the use of _____.

30. Three safety measures that should be discussed with parents of the infant being monitored at home are:

31. List the five criteria for the diagnosis of infantile autism.
    a.
    b.
    c.
    d.
    e.

32. _____ A predominant characteristic of infantile autism is:
    a. abnormal concern for varied stimulation
    b. presence of stranger anxiety at an early age
    c. extreme interpersonal isolation
    d. social advancement that stops at 7-month level

IV. Application, Analysis, and Synthesis of Essential Concepts

A. **Clinical Situation:** Mr. Bacon brings his 10-month-old into the pediatric clinic for the well-child visit. Upon examination it is noted that the child's weight gain has leveled off and he exhibits signs of a thiamine deficiency. The Bacons belong to the Seventh Day Adventist faith.

1. What risk factors should the nurse have assessed in previous well-child visits that might have prevented the nutritional problems?

2. It is important that during the nutritional assessment of the Bacon's infant that the nurse assess

    _____.

3. List the items that would be included as interventions to help alleviate the nutritional problems of the Bacon's infant:

a.
b.
c.
d.
e.
f.

4. How would you evaluate whether your interventions were successful in treating the nutritional problem?

B. **Clinical Situation:** A home visit has been scheduled to assist Mrs. Stone in caring for her 5-month-old infant, Andrew, who has atopic dermatitis. The infant is also suspected of having cow's milk sensitivity.

1. The principal nursing objective in caring for the child with a cow's milk sensitivity is _____.

2. Four nursing interventions that should be utilized when counseling parents about milk sensitivity are:
    a.
    b.
    c.
    d.

3. Formulate at least three nursing diagnoses that pertain to the child who has eczema:
    a.
    b.
    c.
    d.
    e.
    f.

4. The nursing goal for the nursing diagnosis of skin integrity impairment of . . . would be; _____.

5. How would you evaluate whether the interventions that were developed to encourage play activities were successful?

6. List the interventions that you could teach Mrs. Stone to provide hygienic care to Andrew.
    a.
    b.
    c.
    d.

C. **Experiential Exercise:** Care for a child who has nonorganic failure to thrive and his family.

1. Identify three nursing goals for the nursing diagnosis of potential for trauma, neglect.
    a.
    b.
    c.

2. What characteristics did you assess in the infant that are indicative of failure-to-thrive infants?

3. To evaluate whether the interventions have been successful in alleviating the nutritional problem you would evaluate whether

4. List the interventions that should be utilized to provide a nurturing environment.
   a.
   b.
   c.
   d.
   e.
   f.
5. Develop one nursing diagnosis that could be used when working with the parents

6. Rumination is often seen in the failure to thrive infant. List the three nursing interventions that are specific to restoring a normal eating pattern:
   a.
   b.
   c.

D. **Clinical Situation:** Mrs. Ryan brings 2-month-old Sean to the clinic for his well-child visit. Upon examination you discover that Sean has severe diaper dermatitis. Mrs. Ryan reports that Sean has been having severe crying episodes in the evening and wonders whether he has colic.

1. How was the diagnosis of diaper dermatitis made?

2. Nursing interventions for diaper dermatitis are aimed at altering _____.
3. What interventions might you suggest to Mrs. Ryan to treat and prevent the diaper rash?
   a.
   b.
   c.
   d.
   e.
4. The initial step in managing colic is _____
_____.

5. Mrs. Ryan is breast-feeding Sean. What interventions might you suggest to her regarding her diet in order to treat Sean's colic?

E. **Clinical Situation:** Mr. and Mrs. Cohen arrive in the Emergency Room with their infant. The Cohen's discovered that their infant stopped breathing and called the rescue team, but the child could not be resuscitated.

1. List the interventions that should be used to support the parents on the discovery of the infant.
   a.
   b.
   c.
2. In addition to supporting the parents another nursing goal to meet the immediate needs of the family who have lost a child from SIDS is_____
3. What interventions could be used to help the parents adjust to the loss?
   a.
   b.
   c.
4. What problems might occur with the Cohen's other children as a result of this crisis?

F. **Experiential Exercise:** Care for a child with infantile autism.
1. What behaviors in the infant do you assess that are characteristic of infantile autism?

2. The child's intellectual functioning is assessed. The majority of autistic children _____
3. The goals used in the management of autism include

G. **Clinical Situation:** Tommy, a 1-month-old infant, is admitted to the hospital for a diagnostic work-up for infantile apnea. Tommy's parents called the pediatrician when they noticed that Tommy had periods where he stopped breathing and turned "blue."

1. Nursing interventions aimed at supporting the parents of the infant with infantile apnea are

2. Why is safety a major area of nursing intervention if the infant is to be home monitored?

3. What is the rationale for informing the local utility and rescue squad of the home monitoring?

4. To lessen the continuous responsibility of monitoring for the parents nursing interventions should be aimed at

5. Tommy's mother informs the nurse that he vomits small amounts of formula after he feeds. How can the nurse distinguish between vomiting and spitting up?

V. Suggested Readings

1. Rudy, C.A.: Vegetarian diets for children, Pediatr. Nurs. **10**(5): 329–337, 1984

    This comprehensive article reviews the various types of diets, explores the reasons for selecting vegetarian diets, and presents the advantages and disadvantages of these diets. The article provides an extensive discussion of the means of preventing nutritional disturbances when a child is consuming this type of diet.

2. White, J.E. and Owsley, V.B.: Helping families cope with milk, wheat, and soy allergies, MCN **8** (6):423–428, 1983.

    The authors provide an excellent discussion of the etiology of food allergies, methods used to evaluate their presence, signs and symptoms of allergies and ways that parents can adapt to allergies. An excellent source of nursing interventions.

3. DellaPorta, M. and Guida, D.A.: Slow weight gain in the breast-fed infant: management options, Pediatr. Nurs. **10**(2):117–120, 1984.

    The slow weight gain of some breast-fed babies is discussed. The need to readjust our beliefs about weight gain patterns is also presented. The nursing management of the infant is explored in detail. Management options are presented to assist the student with counseling of mothers.

4. Rowell, P.A.: Infantile colic: reviewing the situation, Pediatr. Nurs. **4** (3):20–21, 1978.

    Colic is a common problem and an article that reviews the problem so completely should be useful. A description of colic, its occurrence, management and treatment is provided.

5. Yoos, L.: Taking another look at failure to thrive, MCN **9**(1): 32–37, 1984.

    This excellent article is a supplement to text material. It provides a definition, reviews potential etiologies, discusses the methods used to diagnose this problem and provides the reader with a comprehensive assessment tool. The article also explores interventions that are utilized with these children and families.

6. Cordell, A.S., and Aploita, R.: Family support in infant death. JOGN Nursing **10**(4):281–285, 1981.

    The needs of grieving families are explored. The article describes a program to assist these parents and, in the process, explores the needs and reactions of the grieving parents.

7. Rehm, R.S.: Teaching cardiopulmonary resuscitation to parents. MCN **8**(6):411–416, 1983

    A step-by-step guide for students is provided. The program where the guide is used is discussed.

8. Graber, H.P.: and Balas-Stevens, S.: A discharge tool for teaching parents to monitor infant apnea at home. MCN **9**(3):178–180, 1984.

    The need for home monitoring is discussed. This article reviews the steps in the discharge planning and provides a comprehensive tool that can be used in the clinical setting.

9. Zoltak, B.B.: Autism: recognition and management. Pediatr. Nurs., **12**(2):90–96, 1986.

    The characteristics of autistic children are presented as well as the possible causes of the disorder. The behaviors exhibited by autistic children in all age groups are presented in detail. This article provides a discussion of the diagnosis and management of autism and of the nursing interventions.

Chapter 14

Health Promotion of the Toddler and Family

I. Chapter Overview

Chapter 14 presents the issues relevant to the toddler period of development. Since this is a time of accelerated psychosocial, cognitive, and adaptive changes, students need to be aware of behavior problems that may occur. At the completion of this chapter, the student will understand the toddler's needs and be aware of areas of special concern to parents. This knowledge enables the student to develop nursing goals and interventions that provide support for the normal development of the toddler and help parents to cope with the associated developmental difficulties.

II. Learning Objectives

Upon completion of this chapter, it is expected that the student will be able to:

1. Identify the major biologic, psychosocial, cognitive, and adaptive developments during the toddler years.

2. Relate separation anxiety and negativism to developmental tasks.

3. Recognize signs of readiness for toilet training and offer parents guidance for training.

4. Prepare toddlers for the birth of a sibling.

5. Provide parents with guidelines for limit setting and discipline, including management of temper tantrums.

6. Provide parents with feeding recommendations.

7. Outline a preventive dental hygiene plan for toddlers.

8. Provide anticipatory guidance to parents regarding accident prevention based on the toddler's developmental achievements.

III. Review of Essential Concepts

1. The toddler period is that time between _____ and _____.

2. The growth rate slows considerably during the toddler years, and the birth weight is quadrupled by _____ years of age.

3. _____ When plotted on height and weight graphs, the toddler's growth curve is usually a steady, upward curve which is step-like in nature. (true or false)

4. Why does the toddler exhibit a squat, pot-bellied appearance?

5. Visual acuity of _____ is achieved during the toddler years, although _____ is considered acceptable.

6. One of the most prominent changes of the gastrointestinal system is the voluntary control of

_____.

7. The major gross motor skill acquired during the toddler years is _____.

8. Identify the seven major developmental tasks that must be dealt with during the toddler years.
   a.
   b.
   c.
   d.
   e.
   f.
   g.

9. According to Erikson, the developmental task of toddlerhood is acquiring a sense of _____ while overcoming a sense of _____ and _____.

10. Identify two characteristics that are typical of toddlers in their quest for autonomy.
 a.
 b.
11. According to Freud, the child of 2 years is in the _____ stage.
 a. oral
 b. anal
 c. oedipal
 d. latency
12. A child of 21 months would be expected to be in Piaget's stage of _____.
 a. tertiary circular reactions
 b. preoperations
 c. coordination of secondary schemata and their application to new situations
 d. secondary circular reactions
 e. invention of new means through mental combinations
13. At approximately 2 years of age the child enters the _____ of cognitive development.
14. Briefly describe the following types of speech used by the toddler:
 a. Egocentric—

 b. Socialized—

15. A toddler's reasoning can best be described as being _____.
 a. transductive
 b. inductive
 c. deductive
16. Match the following terms related to toddler behavior with their definitions.

a. _____ transductive reasoning
b. _____ centration
c. _____ ritualism
d. _____ animism
e. _____ negativism
f. _____ egocentrism

 a. the undeviating and repetitive sequence of events that the toddler utilizes to structure his life and maintain reliability
 b. thinking that progresses from the particular to the particular
 c. the inability to envision situations from perspectives other than one's own
 d. the tendency to focus on one aspect rather than considering all possible alternatives
 e. strongly expressed opposition to everything in the environment
 f. attribution of life-like qualities to inanimate objects

17. At the toddler stage of moral development, whether an action is good or bad depends on whether it results in _____ or _____.
18. _____ The development of body image closely parallels cognitive development. (true or false)
19. Briefly describe the two phases of the toddler's task of differentiation of self from significant others.
 a. Separation—

 b. Individuation—

20. _____ The most striking feature of language development in the toddler is the number of new vocabulary words acquired. (true or false)
21. The typical child of 2 years has a vocabulary of approximately _____ words, and approximately _____ percent of this speech is understandable.
22. In the realm of personal-social behavior, the toddler's developing skills of _____ are evident in all areas.
23. The child of 2 years can be expected to _____.
 a. use expressive jargon
 b. build a tower of 8 cubes
 c. have a vocabulary of 500 words
 d. run fairly well with wide stance
24. The solitary play of infancy progresses to _____ play in the toddler.
25. The age of _____ is a particularly integrated period of developmental achievement.
26. Physical and psychological readiness for toilet training is not completed until the _____.
27. _____ Bowel training is usually accomplished before bladder training in the toddler. (true or false)
28. Sibling rivalry seems to be most pronounced in the _____ child and in children under _____ years of age.
29. _____ It is advisable to prepare the toddler for the birth of a sibling at least 6 months in advance. (true or false)
30. Distinguish between the following terms.
 a. Limit-setting—

b. Discipline—

31. List the five functions of limit setting and discipline.
   a.

   b.

   c.

   d.

   e.

32. _____ is an element which should be included in the discipline of a toddler.
   a. Consistency in enforcing rules
   b. Delayed punishment for wrong doing
   c. Increased opportunity for negative responses
   d. Explanation of the reasons for punishment
   e. Varying approaches to limit setting
33. The decreased nutritional requirements of the toddler are manifested in a phenomenon known as

   _____.
34. A good rule of thumb in determining the appropriate serving size for a toddler is to give _____ of food for each year of age.
35. The toddler should see a dentist after the first teeth erupt and no later than the age of _____ years, when primary dentition is completed.
36. The most effective methods for placque removal are _____ and _____.
37. When adequate amounts of _____ are ingested before the eruption of teeth, the enamel is more resistant to caries.
38. _____ Fluoride rinses are recommended as a means of reducing caries in children under 4 years of age. (true or false)
39. _____ is a statement that accurately describes nursing-bottle caries.
   a. Nursing-bottle caries occurs in children between 8 and 18 months of age.
   b. The syndrome is distinguished by protruding upper front teeth resulting from sucking on a hard nipple.
   c. The syndrome does not occur when the child has been breast fed.
   d. Giving a bottle of milk at nap or bedtime predisposes the child to this syndrome.
40. _____ cause more deaths in children 1 to 4 years of age than in any other childhood period except adolescence.
41. What is the implication of the previous statement?

42. Briefly describe the Rule of Fours that applies to the use of car restraint systems.

43. _____ are the most common type of thermal injury in children.
44. The major reason for accidental poisoning in young children is _____.

IV. Application, Analysis, and Synthesis of Essential Concepts

A. **Clinical Situation:** A young mother brings her 2-year-old son, David, into a well-child clinic for a routine check-up. The child is apprehensive and clings to his mother. Height and weight are obtained; the child's height is 35 in (89 cm) and his weight is 30 lb (13.64 kg).

1. Plot David's height and weight on a growth chart. How do his measurements compare to the norms for this age?
   a. Height—
   b. Weight—
2. David's mother is concerned because he has gained only 2 pounds and grown 2 inches since his 18-month check-up. What information should be provided to this mother regarding toddler growth patterns?

3. Identify three developmental milestones that David should have accomplished in the following areas.
   a. Gross motor development—

   b. Fine motor development—

c. Language development—

c.

d.

. David's mother states that when he is with other children of his age, he plays near them but makes no attempt to interact with them. What information regarding the toddler's play habits should be provided?

. What information should be provided to David's mother regarding the selection of appropriate play activities?
a.

b.

c.

David is not yet toilet trained. His mother asks when she should begin trying to train him. The nurse's most appropriate response would be _____.
a. David will need to be able to sit on the toilet for long periods of time.
b. A factor in successful training is the child's desire to please the mother by controlling impulses to defecate and urinate.
c. Bladder training should be attempted first since the child usually has a stronger and more regular urge to urinate.
d. Attempts to begin toilet training before age 3 are usually unsuccessful because myelinization of the spinal cord is incomplete.
David's mother asks questions about dental care. List four components of a preventive dental hygiene plan for a toddler.
a.

b.

B. **Experiential Exercise:** Interview the parents of a toddler about negativism, management of temper tantrums, methods of discipline, and eating patterns. Answer the following questions and include specific responses that illustrate these concepts.

1. How is negativism most often manifested in the toddler?

2. The most effective method of dealing with negativism is to reduce the opportunity for a _____.
3. How does negativism contribute to the toddler's acquisition of a sense of autonomy?

4. Why are temper tantrums so prevalent in the toddler age group?

5. What information should be assessed before offering guidance to parents regarding the management of temper tantrums?
a.
b.
c.
6. Identify two goals that are accomplished by dealing calmly with temper tantrums.
a.
b.
7. The initial nursing goal in the area of discipline is to help parents _____.
8. When disciplining a toddler, it is important to _____.
a. be consistent when enforcing rules
b. delay punishment for wrongdoing
c. increase the opportunity for negative responses
d. explain the reasons for punishment
e. vary the approaches to limit setting
9. Identify four reasons why the practice of time-out avoids many of the problems of other disciplinary approaches.
a.
b.
c.
d.

10. Why does physiologic anorexia occur in the toddler?

11. Identify four eating behaviors that are characteristic of the toddler.
    a.
    b.
    c.
    d.

12. Why is nutritional counseling for parents with toddlers an important nursing intervention?

d. Place all toxic agents out of reach in a locked cabinet.

e. Place child-protector caps on all medicines and poisons.

f. Cover electrical outlets with protective plastic caps

g. Avoid giving sharp or pointed objects.

h. Keep tablecloth out of child's reach.

C. **Experiential Exercise:** Assess the home of a toddler for the presence of potential safety hazards. Answer the following questions and include specific examples that illustrate these concepts.

1. Identify the two key determinants in injury prevention.
   a.
   b.

2. Why is there a critical increase in injuries during the toddler years?

3. What categories of injuries are common during the toddler years?
   a.
   b.
   c.
   d.
   e.
   f.

4. Identify at least five factors in the home that could pose a safety hazard to the toddler.
   a.
   b.
   c.
   d.
   e.

5. Match the following developmental accomplishments with the appropriate safety measures. Answers may be used more than once.

a. _____ walks, runs, climbs

b. _____ exhibits curiosity

c. _____ pulls objects

d. _____ puts things in mouth

a. Closely supervise when near a source of water.

b. Choose toys without removable parts.

c. Turn pot handles toward back of stove.

V. Suggested Readings

1. Pontious, S.L.: Practical Piaget: helping children understand Am. J. Nurs. **82**:114–117, 1982.

   This article reviews the major concepts related to Piaget's stages of cognitive development. It contrasts the cognitive abilities of the preoperational and concrete-operational child. It utilizes a chart to illustrate characteristics of children's thinking in the areas of perception, thought, reasoning, and language. The theory is applied to the use of words to describe and explain hospital procedures at the child's level of reasoning.

2. Horner, M.M.E., and McClellan, M.A.: Toilet training: ready or not? Pediatr. Nurs. **7**(1):15–18, 1981.

   This article presents a nursing protocol developed by the authors and utilized in practice to determine readiness for toilet training. Developmental considerations are discussed and a flow chart is provided which defines critical decision points. This too can be used as a basis for anticipatory guidance of parents who are considering toilet training.

3. Honig, J.C.: Preparing preschool-aged children to be siblings, Am. J. Maternal Child Nurs. **11**(1):37–43, 1986.

   In this selection, the reactions of young children to the birth of a sibling are examined. This provides a framework for a program for siblings-to-be that is designed to help children cope with the birth of a sibling. A complete curriculum and annotate bibliography supplement the description of one successful sibling preparation program.

4. Lamontagne, L.L., Mason, K.R., and Hepworth, J.T.: Effects of relaxation on anxiety in children: implications for coping with stress, Nurs. Res. **34**(5):289–292, 1985.

   This study suggests that relaxation training may have implications for relieving childhood stress and improving coping. It found that children can learn stress management techniques if given the opportunity. Since behavior patterns that influence health are formed during childhood, future research in this area is recommended.

5. Swanson, J.: A toddler's eating habits, Pediatr. Nurs. **5**:(1):52–53, 1979.

   The eating behavior of the toddler is described in this article in relation to normal growth and development. Eating practices that are often a source of concern to parents are discussed, and practical suggestions are offered for their resolution.

6. Nachem, B., and Bass, R.A.: Children still aren't being buckled up, Am. J. Maternal Child Nurs. **9**(5):320–323, 1984.

This entry provides background information which establishes the importance of the use of child restraint devices. The types of devices are described, and a chart compares their advantages and disadvantages. The role of the nurse in parent education is stressed throughout. A care plan is provided which addresses common problems with restraint devices.

Chapter 15

Health Promotion of the Preschooler and the Family

I. Chapter Overview

Chapter 15 focuses on the development of the child in the preschool period, which spans the ages of 3 to 5 years. Since this period completes what is considered to be the most critical period of emotional and psychologic development, students need to be aware of some of the issues for this age group. Upon completion of the chapter, the student will have a knowledge of the preschooler's needs and be aware of the areas that are of special concern to parents. This knowledge will enable the student to develop nursing goals and interventions that provide support for the normal development of the preschooler and assist parents in coping with associated developmental difficulties.

II. Learning Objectives

Upon completion of this chapter, it is expected that the student will be able to:

1. Identify the major biologic, psychosocial, cognitive, spiritual, and adaptive developments during the preschool years.

2. List the benefits of imaginary playmates.

3. Prepare preschoolers for nursery or day care experience.

4. Provide parents with guidelines for sex education.

5. Recognize causes of stuttering during the preschool years.

6. Offer parents suggestions for preventing speech problems.

7. Provide parents with guidelines for dealing with fears and sleep problems.

8. Recognize feeding patterns of preschoolers.

9. Provide anticipatory guidance to parents regarding accident prevention based on the preschooler's developmental achievements.

III. Review of Essential Concepts

1. The preschool years, a period from _____ years of age to the completion of the _____ year, comprises the end of early childhood.

2. During the preschool years, physical growth continues to _____ and _____.

3. A great deal of learning takes place during the preschool years. Identify three types of knowledge that are attained during this period.

   a.

   b.

   c.

4. According to Erikson, the chief psychosocial task of the preschool period is acquiring a sense of

   _____ .

5. A major task for preschoolers is the development of the _____, or _____.

6. According to Freud, the preschool child is in the _____ stage.

   a. oral
   b. anal
   c. oedipal
   d. latency

7. The two stages that comprise Piaget's preoperational phase are:
   a.
   b.
8. Identify one of the major transitions that occurs during the preoperational stage of development.

9. The preschooler's ability to only think of one idea at a time is known as _____ .
10. _____ The preschool child has achieved the cognitive ability known as conservation. (true or false)
11. The preschooler's thinking is often described as _____ since they believe that thoughts are all-powerful.
12. Briefly describe the naive instrumental orientation stage of moral development.

13. _____ Preschoolers have poorly defined body boundaries and little knowledge of their internal anatomy. (true or false)
14. List two examples that demonstrate that the preschool child has relinquished much of the stranger anxiety and fear of separation of earlier years.
    a.
    b.
15. _____ During the preschool years, vocabulary increases dramatically. (true or false)
16. _____speech is a common characteristic during the early preschool years.
17. The typical child of 5 years can be expected to have a vocabulary consisting of at least _____ words.
18. How does the preschooler differ from the toddler in demonstrating a sense of autonomy?
    a.
    b.
19. The type of play that is most apparent during the preschool years is _____ play.
20. _____ A helpful rule in planning creative activities for the preschooler is one simple project per year of age. (true or false)
21. The appearance of imaginary playmates usually occurs between the ages of _____ to _____ years.
22. Identify three functions that are served by imaginary playmates.
    a.
    b.
    c.
23. The child of 4 years of age can be expected to _____.
    a. walk down stairs using alternate footing
    b. tie shoelaces

   c. use sentences of 6 to 8 words
   d. question what parents think
24. List three opportunities that nursery schools and day-care centers provide for children.
    a.
    b.
    c.
25. What factors should parents consider when choosing a preschool or day-care program?
    a.
    b.
    c.
    d.
    e.
    f.
    g.
    h.
    i.
26. In terms of overall evaluation of a program, the most important factor is _____ of the facility.
27. List the two rules that govern answering a child's questions about sex or other sensitive issues.
    a.
    b.
28. _____ in the preschool child is a normal part of sexual curiosity and exploration.
29. A gifted child is usually categorized as having an intelligence quotient of _____ or above.
30. Identify 3 factors that tend to increase aggressive behavior in children.
    a.
    b.
    c.
31. The most critical period for speech development occurs between _____ and _____ years of age.
32. Why is stuttering a common occurrence during the preschool years?

33. The best therapy for speech problems is _____ and _____ .
34. Identify two measures that often help prevent stress in the child's life.
    a.
    b.
35. Identify some of the child's most common fears during the preschool years.
    a.
    b.
    c.
    d.
    e.

f.

36. Identify the most effective way to help children overcome their fears.

37. Nutritional requirements for preschoolers are similar to those for _____. _____ years of age is a period for the resurgence of finicky eating. The child of _____ is influenced by the food habits of others and is ready for the social side of eating.

38. What fact should be stressed to parents of preschoolers in the course of nutritional counseling?

39. Identify five reasons why preschool children are subject to sleep disturbances.
    a.
    b.
    c.
    d.
    e.

40. Why is dental care essential for the preschool child?
    a.
    b.

41. _____ During the preschool years, the emphasis on injury prevention is placed on education for safety and potential hazards. (true or false)

IV. Application, Analysis, and Synthesis of Essential Concepts

A. **Clinical Situation:** Frank Squire, who will be 5 years old next month, is brought to the pediatrician's office by his mother for a well-child visit. Height and weight are obtained. The child's height is 42 in. (106.6 cm) and his weight is 39 lbs (17.69 kg).

1. Plot Frank's height and weight on a growth chart. How do his measurements compare to the norms for this age?
   a. Height—
   b. Weight—

2. What information could be given to Frank's mother regarding the physical growth of the preschooler?

3. Prior to the physical examination, the nurse questions Mrs. Squire about Frank's developmental progress.

Identify three developmental milestones that Frank should have accomplished in the following areas.
a. Gross motor development—

b. Fine motor development—

c. Language development—

4. Mrs. Squire says that Frank spends most of his time playing with his imaginary friend, Oscar. She wonders if this phase will pass. What information should be given to her?

5. Mrs. Squire states that Frank has several toys but only plays with a few. What types of playthings and activities could be recommended to foster Frank's development?
   a. Physical play—

   b. Dramatic play—

   c. Creative play—

   d. Quiet play—

6. Mrs. Squire is very concerned about child safety. What developmental achievements make Frank more prone to injury?

B. **Experiential Exercise:** Interview the parents of a child who attends a preschool program. Answer the following questions and include specific responses that illustrate these concepts.

1. What is the most important aspect of a preschool or day-care program?

2. What specific factors should be considered when selecting a preschool program?
   a.
   b.
   c.
   d.
   e.
   f.
   g.
   h.
   i.

3. What should parents do when visiting a facility they are considering for their child?
   a.
   b.
   c.
   d.

4. How should parents prepare the child for the preschool experience?
   a.

   b.

   c.

   d.

. How can the parents provide support for the child on the first day of school?
   a.

   b.

   C. **Experiential Exercise:** Interview the parents of a preschool child about the following common parental concerns: sex education, sleep disturbances, and eating patterns. Answer the following questions and include specific responses that illustrate these concepts.

1. Why is the preschool stage of development appropriate for beginning sex education?

2. What two mistakes should parents avoid when answering their children's questions about sex?
   a.
   b.

3. Identify the rationales for each of the following interventions which promote the sex education of the preschool child.
   a. Determining what the child thinks—

   b. Being honest—

4. What sleep problems occur in this age group that might concern parents?

5. What interventions could be suggested to parents to deal with this problem?
   a.
   b.
   c.
   d.
   e.

6. What is the primary concern of parents regarding the preschool child's diet?

7. Describe one intervention that might decrease this parental concern.

V. Suggested Readings

1. Betz C.L.: Faith development in children, Pediatr. Nurs. **7**(2):22–25, 1981.
   This article discusses the characteristics of Fowler's five stages of faith development in children: undifferentiated, intuitive-projective, mythical-literal, synthetic-convention, and individuating-reflexive. Questions to be incorporated in the social

and health history regarding the child's and family's religious beliefs are presented. Nursing interventions that are designed to support the child in each specific stage are outlined.

2. Mitchell, S.: Imaginary companions: friend or foe? Pediatr. Nurs. **6**(6):29–30, 1980.

The author examines the phenomenon of the imaginary playmate as it occurs in children, beginning with the preschool years. The purposes these companions serve and factors that seem to be associated with their appearance are explored. Elements to be included when counseling parents about their children's imaginary companions are presented.

3. Chabin, M.: Hospital-supported child care, Am. J. Nurs. **83**:548–552, 1983.

This selection documents the fact that child care problems are related to both initial and continued withdrawal from the nursing work force. It addresses how some hospitals have offered assistance by establishing day-care programs and explores what some of these programs have encountered. It briefly describes the various types of hospital-supported services: on-site centers, subsidies, priority placement, family day care, information and referral programs, vendor-payment programs, pooling resources, and flexible benefits.

4. Mayer, G.G.: Choosing daycare, Am. J. Nurs. **81**:346–348, 1981.

The author briefly surveys the various day-care options, listing their advantages and disadvantages. She then presents her own six objectives for a day-care setting, elaborating on each of them. Additional considerations of nurses who are seeking day care are delineated. A message from a day-care director for working mothers addresses issues related to their feelings about working and day care.

5. Aquilino, M.L., and Ely, J.: Parents and the sexuality of preschool children, Pediatr. Nurs. **11**(1):41–46, 1985.

This article reports on a survey of 81 parents of preschool children about the sexual activity and curiosity of 3- to 5-year-olds. It was determined that most of the parents were knowledgeable and responded positively to situations involving normal preschool sexual activities but that their comfort with childhood sexuality varied. The implications for presenting information to parents about childhood sexuality are presented.

6. Miller, S.R.: Children's fears: a review of the literature with implications for nursing research and practice, Nurs. Res. **28**(4):217–223, 1979.

This article reviews studies about children's fears from a developmental perspective. It concludes that children's fears change with age, becoming more complex, varied, and realistic as the child develops. It recommends that such variables as sex, social class, family relationships, and the media be included in future longitudinal studies. Several examples are cited which apply knowledge of childhood fears to nursing practice.

7. Edgil, A., Wood, K., and Smith, D.: Sleep problems of older infants and preschool children, Pediatr. Nurs. **11**(2):87–89, 1985.

This article examines current knowledge about the various early childhood sleep disturbances that are sources of major concern to parents. It then focuses upon a study designed to identify sleep behaviors described by mothers as problems, sleep goals that mothers have for their children, family consequences of children's sleep problems, various systems involved in promoting or preventing sleep problems, and environmental factors related to sleep problems. The findings, their significance to nursing practice, and implications for future research are described in detail.

8. Inglis S.: The nocturnal frustration of sleep disturbance, Am. J. Maternal Child Nurs. **1**(5):280–287, 1976.

The author reviews some of the potential causes of sleep problems in children and methods that have been utilized to manage them. She then describes a modified counseling approach that a group of nurses developed, using the principles of behavior modification and environmental modification. She introduces cases studies of three distinct types of sleep disturbances, to illustrate the use and effectiveness of this approach.

Chapter 16

Health Problems of Early Childhood

I. Chapter Overview

Chapter 16 introduces nursing considerations essential to the care of the young child experiencing health problems. While many of these problems can be effectively managed in the home environment, students need to be aware that there is a potential for long-term consequences if appropriate interventions are not instituted promptly. At the completion of this chapter, the student will have a knowledge of commonly encountered health problems of early childhood. This knowledge will enable the student to develop nursing goals and interventions directed at returning the child and family to a state of optimal health.

II. Learning Objectives

Upon completion of this chapter, it is expected that the student will be able to:

1. Recognize the major communicable diseases of childhood.

2. List three principles of nursing care of children with communicable diseases.

3. Describe the nursing care of the child with conjunctivitis.

4. Discuss the nursing care of the child who has a pinworm infestation and his family.

5. Identify four principles in the emergency treatment of poisoning.

6. Describe the nursing care of the child with lead poisoning.

7. State three factors known to be associated with child abuse.

8. State four areas of the history that should arouse suspicion of abuse.

9. Describe the nursing care of the abused child.

III. Review of Essential Concepts

1. Match the following terms related to communicable diseases with their definitions.

a. _____ communicable disease

b. _____ epidemic

c. _____ endemic

d. _____ pandemic

e. _____ incubation period

f. _____ period of communicability

g. _____ prodromal period

h. _____ mode of transmission

a. a disease occurring regularly within a geographic location

b. time interval between infection or exposure to disease and appearance of initial symptoms

c. mechanism by which an infectious agent is transported from reservoir to susceptible human host

d. interval of early manifestations of disease to time when overt clinical syndrome is evident

e. disease occurring in greater than the expected number of cases in a community

f. illness caused by a specific infectious agent or its toxic products through a direct or indirect mode of transmission of that agent from a reservoir

g. disease affecting large portions of the population throughout the world

h. time or times during which infectious agent may be transferred directly or indirectly from infected person to another person

2. List the four nursing goals in the care of the child and family with a communicable disease.
   a.
   b.
   c.
   d.
3. The principal nursing intervention in communicable diseases is

4. Identify four factors that are helpful in identifying communicable diseases in children.
   a.
   b.
   c.
   d.
5. Primary prevention of communicable disease rests almost exclusively on _____.
6. Nursing interventions to prevent the spread of communicable disease include:
   a.
   b.
7. List the three groups of children who are at risk for developing serious or fatal complications from communicable diseases.
   a.
   b.
   c.
8. Define conjunctivitis.

9. Identify the most common causes of conjunctivitis in the following groups.
   a. Recurrent conjunctivitis in infants—

   b. Acute conjunctivitis in children—

10. The distinguishing symptom of bacterial conjunctivitis is _____.
11. _____ Viral conjunctivitis usually occurs in association with an upper respiratory infection. (true or false)
12. _____ The chief sign of conjunctivitis caused by a foreign body is the presence of such symptoms as tearing, pain, and inflammation in both eyes. (true or false)
13. Bacterial conjunctivitis is usually treated with _____.
    a. corticosteroids
    b. topical antibacterial agents
    c. oral antibiotics
14. The two major nursing goals in the care of the child with conjunctivitis are:
    a.
    b.
15. An important nursing goal in bacterial conjunctivitis is

16. _____ constitute the most common infections in the world.

17. Identify two reasons why young children are at risk for parasitic infections.
    a.
    b.
18. List five factors to consider when planning the eradication of a parasitic organism or prevention of infection.
    a.
    b.
    c.
    d.
    e.
19. Most parasitic infections result from _____ of parasite eggs.
20. Nursing responsibilities related to parasitic intestinal infections are directed toward:
    a.
    b.
    c.
21. The nurse's most important function in relation to parasitic infections is

22. _____ is the most common intestinal parasitic pathogen in the United States.
23. _____ or _____ is the most common helminthic infection in the United States.
24. _____ The principal symptom of pinworms is intense perianal itching. (true or false)
25. List six symptoms that might indicate the presence of pinworms in a young child who has difficulty verbalizing.
    a.
    b.
    c.
    d.
    e.
    f.
26. The most common test for diagnosing pinworms is the _____.
27. The drug of choice in the treatment of pinworms is _____.
28. Briefly describe the Poison Prevention Packaging Act of 1970.

29. Identify the developmental characteristics of young children which predispose them to poisoning by ingestion.
    a.

b.

c.

d.

30. List the four principles of emergency treatment following the ingestion of toxic agents.
   a.
   b.
   c.
   d.
31. The preferred method of inducing vomiting at home is through the administration of _____.
32. Identify the indications for gastric lavage.
   a.
   b.
   c.
33. _____ Vomiting is indicated in the treatment of corrosives ingestion. (true or false)
34. The immediate danger from most hydrocarbons is _____.
35. _____ Ingestion of plant parts is the most common cause of childhood poisoning. (true or false)
36. List three reasons for the decline in the incidence of acute salicylate poisoning in children.
   a.
   b.
   c.
37. Which two salicylate products are of particular concern in acute ingestion?
   a.
   b.
38. The most impressive clinical manifestation of salicylate overdose is _____.
39. _____ Acute salicylate poisoning is considered a more serious intoxication than chronic ingestion. (true or false)
40. _____ is the most common drug poisoning among children and produces _____ damage.
41. Initial management for acetaminophen poisoning is _____ or _____ if the child is treated within 2 hours of the ingestion. If treatment is delayed longer than 2 hours, _____ is administered.
42. What nursing interventions should be emphasized in the care of the child with iron poisoning?
   a.
   b.

43. What three general factors are related to the ingestion of lead?
   a.
   b.
   c.
44. When the chronic ingestion of lead stops, it takes the body _____ as long to excrete the stored lead as it did to accumulate it.
45. List the two most frequently used procedures for routine lead screening.
   a.
   b.
46. For each of the following classifications, provide the child's risk status and need for further testing.
   a. Class IV—

   b. Class III—

   c. Class II—

   d. Class I—

47. _____ Lead poisoning exists when a child has an E.P. level of equal to or greater than 250 mcg/dl and a confirmed blood lead level of equal to or greater than 50 mcg/dl (true or false)
48. List three commonly used chelating drugs.
   a.
   b.
   c.
49. _____ is a broad term that includes intentional physical abuse or neglect, emotional abuse or neglect, and sexual abuse of children, usually by adults.
50. _____ Child neglect involves more children than any other form of child maltreatment. (true or false)
51. What three broad factors seem to predispose children to maltreatment?
   a.
   b.
   c.
52. The most important criterion on which to base the decision to report child maltreatment is _____.
   a. inappropriate parental concern for the degree of injury
   b. refusal of parents to sign for additional tests or agree to necessary treatment
   c. incompatibility between the history given and the injury sustained
   d. conflicting stories about the "accident" from parents or child
   e. unavailability of the parents for questioning
53. The child-abuse victim usually _____.
   a. belongs to a low socioeconomic population
   b. readily identifies the abusing parent
   c. in no way contributes to the abusing situation

d. is wary of physical contact with adults

54. Identify three broad nursing goals associated with child maltreatment.
    a.
    b.
    c.

55. List five types of sexual abuse.
    a.
    b.
    c.
    d.
    e.

56. _____ Seductiveness by the child usually initiates incest. (true or false)

IV. Application, Analysis, and Synthesis of Essential Concepts

A. **Clinical Situation:** Mrs. Braun brings her 4-year-old daughter, Jill, to the pediatric clinic. She tells the nurse practitioner that Jill has been scratching herself around the anus and has been sleeping restlessly. A tentative diagnosis of pinworm infection is made.

1. How would a diagnosis of pinworms be confirmed?

2. For each of the following nursing goals associated with a pinworm infection, provide at least 3 nursing interventions.
    a. Identify the parasite—

    b. Eradicate the organism—

    c. Prevent reinfection—

B. **Experiential Exercise:** Spend a day in the Emergency Room to observe the types of poisoning that occur and their emergency treatment. Answer the following questions and include specific examples that illustrate these concepts.

1. What is the most important principle in dealing with poisoning?

2. What life support measures may be necessary following the ingestion of poisoning?

3. Identify at least three nursing interventions for each of the following areas of emergency treatment.
    a. Assessment—

    b. Gastric decontamination—

    c. Family support—

    d. Prevention of recurrence—

4. Salicylates and acetaminophen are the two most commonly ingested drugs among children. Match the following statements regarding ingestion with the appropriate drug. Mark A if the answer is acetaminophen and S if the answer is salicylates.
    a. _____ Hyperventilation is the most impressive clinical manifestation.
    b. _____ N-acetylcysteine (Mucomyst) is the antidote
    c. _____ In chronic overdose, it can cause bleeding tendencies.
    d. _____ Excretion is facilitated by the administration of sodium bicarbonate.
    e. _____ Acute overdose results in hepatic damage.

5. In formulating nursing interventions following salicylate injection, the nurse should know that _____.
    a. vomiting should never be induced
    b. particular attention should be given to the rate and depth of respirations

c. hepatic damage is a direct result of salicylate ingestion
d. the toxic effect is lessened if the aspirin ingested is of the time-released type

6. What four questions that would assess parents' knowledge should be included in a parent education program regarding accidental poisoning preparedness?

a.

b.

c.

d.

C. **Experiential Exercise:** Assess a specific child's environment with regard to its potential for lead poisoning. Answer the following questions and include specific examples that illustrate these concepts.

1. When assessing the child's environment, what environmental factors would alert the nurse to the potential for lead poisoning?
a.
b.
c.
d.
e.
f.

2. In this assessment, what characteristics of the child and parents should be noted?
a. Child—

b. Parents—

3. What early signs of lead poisoning should the nurse be alert to when performing an assessment?
a.

b.

c.

d.

4. If, during the assessment, the presence of lead poisoning is suspected, what should the nurse's initial goal be?

5. Once it has been determined that a child has lead poisoning, how is the course of therapy determined?

6. According to the CDC's classification, what therapeutic management would be initiated in each of the following situations?
a. Class IV (urgent risk)—

b. Class III (high risk)—

c. Class II (moderate risk)—

d. Class I (low risk)—

7. The nurse is developing a care plan for a child with lead poisoning which includes the interventions listed below. Match each intervention to its appropriate rationale. (Answers may be used more than once.)

INTERVENTIONS	RATIONALE
a. _____ Measure intake and output.	a. Prevents tissue damage
b. _____ Make home visits.	b. Protects from toxic side effects of chelation therapy
c. _____ Rotate injection sites.	c. Monitors for side effects of chelation therapy
d. _____ Apply heat to injection site.	d. Provides relief of pain
e. _____ Remove sources of lead from home.	e. Prevents recurrence of poisoning
f. _____ Avoid activity that places strain on painful muscle area.	
g. _____ Collect urine specimens.	
h. _____ Institute seizure precautions.	
i. _____ Palpate muscle area before preparing injection site.	
j. _____ Have emergency equipment at bedside.	

D. **Experiential Exercise:** Care for a child who is hospitalized as a result of maltreatment. Answer the following questions and include specific examples that illustrate these concepts.

1. Identify characteristics in each of the following areas that can be used to assess the vulnerability of families to abuse.
   a. Parents—

   b. Child—

   c. Environment—

2. What two factors are used as diagnostic tools in determining child abuse?
   a.
   b.
3. Identify at least five areas that should arouse suspicion of abuse when the nurse is obtaining a history.
   a.
   b.
   c.
   d.
   e.
   f.
   g.
   h.
   i.
4. Develop four nursing diagnoses that could be used as a basis for the care of an abusing family.
   a.
   b.
   c.
   d.
5. Why are accurate nurses' notes essential to any suspected maltreatment situation?

6. For each of the following nursing goals, identify two evaluation criteria that indicate the achievement of these goals.

   a. Protect from further abuse—

   b. Prevent recurrence—

   c. Provide therapeutic environment while hospitalized—

   d. Promote a sense of parental adequacy—

   e. Educate parents—

   f. Lessen environmental crises—

7. List three services the nurse may utilize as sources of interventions to help parents achieve major self-changes.
   a.
   b.
   c.

V. Suggested Readings

1. Fleming, J.W.: Common dermatologic conditions in children, Am. J. Maternal Child Nurs. **6**(5):346–354, 1981.
   This article opens with a detailed description of the structure and function of the skin which is designed to serve as a basis for the assessment of skin lesions. The specific types of lesions are then described in terms of type, size, configuration, distribution, location, color, communicability, and cause. A series of color photographs illustrates the most common childhood diseases that produce skin eruptions. Nursing management of the various conditions is discussed.
2. Jackson, M.M., and Lynch, P.: Infection control: too much or too little? Am. J. Nurs. **84**:208–211, 1984.
   This entry discusses the concerns of nurses and other hospital personnel about contracting an infectious disease from a patient and transmitting infections from one patient to another. Guidelines are provided for making decisions about what precautions should be taken in the delivery of care, regardless of whether the patient is on specific infection control precautions. The new recommendations in the latest edition of the Center for Disease Control's *Guideline for Isolation Precautions in Hospitals* are described.
3. Henley, M., and Sears, J.R.: Pinworms: a persistent pediatric problem, Am. J. Maternal Child Nurs. **10**(2): 111–113, 1985.

This selection reviews studies that address the epidemiology, symptomatology, and therapeutic management of pinworm infections. It describes the life cycle of the pinworm and relates this to its communicability. The problems associated with diagnosis are discussed. A chart clearly presents relevant information about the medications utilized in treatment. The importance of parent education regarding hygienic practices is stressed.

4. Foster, S.D.: In case of an emergency: ipecac syrup, Am. J. Maternal Child Nurs. **7**(4):227, 1982.

This edition of the MCN pharmacopoeia succinctly reviews nursing responsibilities related to poison prevention and the importance of recommending that ipecac syrup be kept in the homes of young children. It provides detailed information about the action, dosage, precautions, and contraindications of which the nurse should be aware when teaching parents to use ipecac syrup.

5. Keim, K.A.: Preventing and treating plant poisonings in young children, Am. J. Maternal Child Nurs. **8**(4):287–289, 1983.

This article addresses the fact that ingested house plants are one of the most common sources of childhood poisoning. It presents a list of principles of plant toxicity and supplies an annotated reference list of poisonous plants. Emergency interventions and nursing responsibilities when a toxic plant is ingested are described.

6. Christensen, M.L, Schommer, B.L., and Velasquez, J.: An interdisciplinary approach to preventing child abuse, Am. J. Maternal Child Nurs. **9**(2):108–112, 1984.

This entry describes a special project designed to identify families at risk for abusing or neglecting their infants and to prevent abuse through outreach, teaching, counseling, and advocacy for the first 2 years of the child's life. Members of the public health nursing and of the human services departments of one county staffed the project. The combined efforts of these two disciplines proved to be beneficial to both the clients and the professionals who participated.

7. Velasquez, J., Christensen, M.L., and Schommer, B.L.: In-

tensive services help prevent child abuse, Am. J. Maternal Child Nurs. **9**(2):113–117.

This article reports the evaluation of the project described in the entry above. The evaluation determined that intensive, early intervention with high-risk mothers resulted in a reduced incidence of abuse, neglect, and out-of-home placements. It also found that normal growth and development of the infants was promoted. To a lesser extent, the project was also successful in improving the mothers' parenting skills and their use of support networks.

8. Holter, J.C.: Child abuse, Nurs. Clin. North Am. **14**(3):417–427, 1979.

This article provides a comprehensive overview of the subject of child abuse, addressing its definition, incidence, pattern, and characteristics. Child abuse legislation is summarized. A case study is used as a basis for discussion of intervention strategies and problems encountered by health professionals in dealing with abusive families.

9. Nalepka, C., O'Toole, R., and Turbett, J.P.: Nurses' and physicians' recognition and reporting of child abuse, Iss. Compre. Pediatr. Nurs. **5**:33–44, 1981.

This study compares how nurses and physicians in practice reach the judgment of possible child abuse. It compares the relationship between theories of family violence and professional understanding of child abuse, examines how professional knowledge is used in diagnostic behavior, and analyzes how diagnostic behavior affects diagnosis of child abuse. The differences found and their implications for practice are discussed.

10. Miller, E.L.: Interviewing the sexually abused child, Am. J. Maternal Child Nurs. **10**(2):103–105, 1985.

This selection begins with a brief review of the aspects of child sexual abuse that make the interview process particularly painful. Techniques, such as playing with anatomically correct dolls and drawing, are suggested for uncovering the facts. The importance of accurately recording the child's words and describing the child's actions during the interview is stressed. The nurse's role is emphasized throughout the article.

Chapter 17

Health Promotion of the School-Age Child and Family

I. Chapter Overview

Chapter 17 discusses the school-age period, the ages from 6 to 12. Because this developmental stage is characterized by greater social awareness and social skills, it is important for nursing students to understand the roles of peer and family relationships, school, and play, in the socialization process. At the completion of this chapter, the student will have a knowledge of the child's growth and development and be aware of areas of special concern to parents. This knowledge will enable the student to develop nursing goals and interventions that foster health maintenance behavior in school-age children and their families.

II. Learning Objectives

Upon completion of this chapter, it is expected that the student will be able to:

1. Describe the physical, cognitive, and moral changes that take place during the middle childhood years.

2. Describe ways to assist a child in developing a sense of accomplishment.

3. Demonstrate an understanding of the changing interpersonal relationships of the school-age child.

4. Discuss the role of the peer group in the socialization of the school-age child.

5. Outline an appropriate health teaching plan for the school-age child.

6. Plan a sex education session for a group of school-age children.

7. Describe the attitude of the child toward personal care and responsibility during the school-age years.

8. Discuss the major responsibilities of the parents in fostering development in the school-age years.

III. Review of Essential Concepts

1. According to Freud, the school-age child is in the _____ stage.
   a. oral
   b. anal
   c. oedipal
   d. latency

2. The middle years begin with the shedding of the _____ and end at puberty with the acquisition of the final _____.

3. _____ During the school-age years, a child will grow approximately 2 inches per year and will almost triple in weight. (true or false)

4. Identify the three most pronounced physiologic changes that indicate increasing maturity in the school-age child.
   a.
   b.
   c.

5. The preadolescent years, ages _____ to _____, are years of transition.

6. The average age of puberty in girls is _____, and in boys it is _____.

7. According to Erikson, the developmental task of middle childhood is acquiring a sense of _____.
   a. trust
   b. autonomy
   c. initiative
   d. industry

8. Failure to develop a sense of accomplishment results in a sense of _____.

9. _____ In the process of self-evaluation, children actively strive to come up to internalized goals or levels of attainment that they hope to achieve. (true or false)

10. According to Piaget, the school-age child is in the _____ stage.
    a. sensorimotor

b. preoperational

c. concrete operational

d. formal operational

11. _____ During this cognitive stage, children progress from making judgments based on what they see (perceptual) to making judgments based on what they reason (conceptual). (true or false)

12. List the three concepts that children use to demonstrate their ability to conserve.

a.

b.

c.

13. Define the term *classification*.

14. _____ The most significant skill acquired during the school-age years is the ability to read. (true or false)

15. _____ is the statement that best describes the younger school-age child's perception of rules and judgment of actions.

a. Judges an act by its intentions rather than by the consequences alone

b. Believes that rules and judgments are not absolute

c. Understands the reason behind rules

d. Interprets accidents and misfortunes as punishments for misdeeds

16. _____ best describes the older school-age child's perception of rules and judgment of actions.

a. Does not understand the reasons for rules

b. Takes into account different points of view to make a judgment

c. Judges an act by its consequences

d. Believes that rules and judgments are absolute

17. Identification with _____ appears to be a strong influence in the child's attainment of independence from parents.

18. _____ During the early school years, there is considerable difference relative to sex in the play experiences of children. (true or false)

19. Identify three valuable lessons that children learn from daily interactions with age mates.

a.

b.

c.

20. One of the outstanding characteristics of middle childhood is the formation of _____ or _____.

21. A complex form of group play that evolves from group games is _____ or _____.

22. Identify the three significant characteristics of team membership that are relevant to child development.

a.

b.

c.

23. Until the child enters school, the primary sphere of influence is the _____.

24. List the four purposes of discipline.

a.

b.

c.

d.

25. _____ During middle childhood, it is common for children to engage in what is considered to be antisocial behavior. (true or false)

26. Identify three sources of stress during middle childhood.

a.

b.

c.

27. What three responses to stress may be observed?

a.

b.

c.

28. List the components of the yearly physical examination for the school-age child.

a.

b.

c.

d.

e.

29. _____ is a primary element in comprehensive health care.

30. Health education should allow the child to:

a.

b.

c.

31. Childhood _____ is an increasingly prevalent health problem of school-age children.

32. During middle childhood, the most common sleep disorders are _____ and _____.

33. _____ The eruption of permanent teeth in the school-age child begins with the eruption of the 6-year-molar. (true or false)

34. Prior to providing information on sexuality to parents and children, the nurse must first be knowledgeable about

a.

b.

35. Identify five routine health services provided by most schools.

a.

b.

c.

d.

e.

36. _____ The most common cause of severe accidental injury and death in school-age children is motor vehicle accidents.

37. Match the following behavior with the ages at which they are exhibited.

a. _____ centers life around school

b. _____ enjoys group activities involving both sexes

c. _____ enjoys sports

d. _____ displays sudden, uncontrolled outbursts.

a. 6 years

b. 9 years

c. 12 years

IV. Application, Analysis, and Synthesis of Essential Concepts

A. **Clinical Situation:** Jimmy Douglas, age 9, is brought to the pediatrician's office by his mother for his annual physical examination. His height and weight are obtained. Jimmy's height is 52 in. (132.2 cm) and his weight is 62 lb (28.13 kg). Jimmy's vision is evaluated as 20/30 in both eyes.

1. Plot Jimmy's height and weight on a growth chart. How do his measurements compare to the norms for this age?
   a. Height—
   b. Weight—
2. Mrs. Douglas is concerned because Jimmy does not have 20/20 vision. What response would be most appropriate?

3. Mrs. Douglas tells the nurse that Jimmy likes to help his father with the yard work. However, Jimmy's work is not always up to his father's expectations. What advice could be given?

4. In the area of personal care and responsibility, what tasks would Jimmy be able to perform?
   a.
   b.
   c.
5. Mrs. Douglas expresses concern because she is having a problem with dishonesty in her 6-year-old daughter.

What information could the nurse provide to assist Mrs. Douglas in dealing with this concern?

6. Mrs. Douglas asks the nurse for suggestions that will foster Jimmy's development. What should her response be?
   a.

   b.

   c.

   d.

   e.

   f.

B. **Experiential Exercise:** Interview a school-age child and his parents about changing interpersonal relationships and peer groups. Answer the following questions and include specific responses to illustrate the concepts.

1. Why do school-age children spend an increased amount of time away from their homes and families?

2. Why are relationships with age mates an important social interaction in the life of the school-age child?

3. What is the function of gang membership for the school-age child?

4. Briefly describe the characteristics of gangs in each of the following age groups.
   a. Early school-age—

   b. Middle school-age—

   c. Later school-age—

5. What is evident in the activities and games of school-age children?

6. What are some of the inherent dangers in strong peer-group attachment?

7. Why is it often difficult for parents to accept the child's membership in a peer group?
   a.
   b.
   c.
   d.
   e.

C. **Experiential Exercise:** Interview a school nurse about health education programs for the school-age child. Answer the following questions and include specific responses that illustrate these concepts.

1. What are the three roles of the school nurse?
   a.
   b.
   c.
2. Identify the components that should be included in a school health program.
   a.
   b.
   c.
   d.
   e.
3. A school nurse in an elementary school must teach a class on health promotion to a group of third graders. Prior to developing this program, what does the nurse need to know about the target audience?

a.
b.
c.
4. For each of the following goals of the teaching plan for this class, identify at least two specific nursing interventions.
   a. Promote adequate nutritional intake—

   b. Promote adequate sleep and rest—

   c. Provide for appropriate physical activity—

   d. Promote optimal dental hygiene—

5. When developing a sex education program for elementary school children, the nurse should include the following components:
   a.
   b.
   c.
   d.
   e.
   f.

V. Suggested Readings

1. Czupryna, L.: Primary prevention in a camp setting, Am. J. Maternal Child Nurs. **9**(3):197–199, 1984.
   This article examines the role of the camp nurse in anticipating specific health problems and taking the necessary actions to prevent them. It describes an assessment of the camp's environment which includes the areas of housing, water quality, nutrition, flora, fauna, climate, and camp program. It presents a camp population profile based on age, sex, ethnic and racial background, religion, social class, and special needs. These tools are explored as the means of identifying risk factors and actual health hazards.
2. Oda, D.S.: A viewpoint on school nursing, Am. J. Nurs. **81**:1677–1678, 1981.
   The historical background of school nursing is described and the role of the school nurse is defined. A framework which incorporates three areas and levels of service—health supervision, health counseling, and health education—is introduced. Two pathways, a health service provider approach and a health guidance approach, are explored as having potential utility for translating the problem-solving framework into an evaluation model.
3. Oda, D.S., DeAngelis, C., Meeker, R., and others: Nurse practitioners and primary care in schools, Am. J. Maternal Child Nurs. **10**(2):127–131, 1985.
   The controversy surrounding the employment of school nurse

practitioners to deliver primary health care services is introduced in this selection. A study that provided an opportunity to develop and study school nurse practitioner roles is presented. It analyzes three nurse practitioner role patterns: expanded provider, enhanced school nurse, and coordinator-provider. The coordinator-provider is identified as the most productive and viable.

4. Robinson, T.: School nurse practitioners on the job, Am. J. Nurs. **81**:1674–1676, 1981.

This article identifies the expansion of the traditional school nurse role to that of a school nurse practitioner as an essential step in increasing the availability and accessibility of health care for children. A project that demonstrates a way in which this concept is utilized to deliver care to school children is described.

5. Switzer, K.H., and Kelly, J.T.: The nurse: a member of the school team, Am. J. Maternal Child Nurs. **6**(3):189–193, 1981.

In this article, the challenge of fusing trends in the nursing profession with developments in the educational setting is described. A tool consisting of the Pediatric Data Base and Guidelines for parent Interview is presented as a means to establish and fulfill nursing role responsibilities. Two cases are presented that illustrate the application of the tool. It is seen to establish the school nurse's assessment as a unique and vital contribution to the child's special education evaluation.

6. Seybold, S.A., and Klisch, M.L.: Preparing grade school faculty to teach family life education, Am. J. Maternal Child Nurs. **7**(1):50–54, 1982.

The authors describe a workshop on family life and sex education conducted for the faculty of an elementary school. It included a needs assessment, a warm-up exercise, the presentation of the concept of sexuality throughout life, an activity of sharing early memories about sexuality, a name game involving sexual terminology, role playing of questions and answers, and a workshop evaluation. A follow-up survey of participating teachers who subsequently taught family life identified helpful aspects of the workshop and suggestions for future sessions.

Health Problems of Middle Childhood

I. Chapter Overview

Chapter 18 deals with the health problems most commonly seen during the middle childhood years. While this is a relatively healthy time for children, students need to be aware of the health problems that can result from the child's age-related outdoor activities and proximity to other children. At the completion of this chapter, the student will know the common physical and emotional problems of middle childhood and will be able to develop nursing goals and interventions directed at returning the child and family to optimal health.

II. Learning Objectives

Upon completion of this chapter, it is expected that the student will be able to:

1. Identify the factors that predispose the child to the development of dental caries.

2. Describe the distribution and configuration of the various skin lesions.

3. Discuss the nursing care associated with the various therapies for skin disorders.

4. Contrast the manifestations of the therapies for bacterial, viral, and fungal infections of the skin.

5. Develop a teaching plan for a child with a skin disorder related to a chemical or physical contact.

6. Discuss the nursing care of the child and family with a skin infestation.

7. Discuss the manifestations and nursing management of a selected emotional or behavioral problem.

III. Review of Essential Concepts

1. List the four most prevalent types of childhood dental health problems.

a.

b.

c.

d.

2. _____ The principal oral problem in children and adolescents is malocclusion. (true or false)

3. Identify the four factors that must be present in the right combination for dental caries to occur.

a.

b.

c.

d.

4. Identify six measures that are used to control dental caries

a.

b.

c.

d.

e.

f.

5. Define *periodontal disease*.

6. The two most common periodontal problems are
   _____ and _____.
7. Define the term *malocclusion*.

8. The two most important aspects in the treatment of
   malocclusion are:
   a.
   b.
9. List three ways in which a tooth may be prepared or
   maintained for reimplantation.
   a.
   b.
   c.
10. _____ The skin is the largest organ in the body. (true
    or false)
11. Identify the four functions of the skin.
    a.
    b.
    c.
    d.
12. Match the layers of the skin with their defining char-
    acteristics. (More than one answer may apply.)

a. _____ epidermis
b. _____ dermis
c. _____ subcutaneous tissue

a. constitutes the bulk of the
   skin

b. largely determines body
   contours

c. the outermost layer of the
   skin

d. focus of diseases of the
   skin

e. composed mainly of connective tissues

f. acts as depot for the storage of fat

g. often requires biopsy for
   diagnosis

13. List the four general etiologic factors related to skin
    lesions.
    a.
    b.
    c.
    d.
14. Match the following terms used to describe skin le-
    sions with their correct definitions.

a. _____ erythema
b. _____ ecchymoses
c. _____ petechiae
d. _____ primary lesions
e. _____ secondary lesions

a. pinpoint tiny and sharply
   circumscribed spots in the
   superficial layers of the epidermis

b. localized red or purple dis-
   colorations caused by extravasation of blood into
   the dermis and subcutaneous tissues

c. changes that result from
   alteration in a lesion, such
   as those caused by rubbing

d. a reddened area caused by
   increased amounts of oxy-
   genated blood in the der-
   mal vasculature

e. skin changes produced by
   some causative factor

15. The topical therapeutic agents used most widely for
    skin disorders are _____.
16. The nurse should teach parents that hydrocortisone
    preparations _____.
    a. can be used for all skin disorders
    b. should be applied as a heavy coating
    c. should be massaged into the skin
    d. can be used only for short periods.
17. _____ The incidence of staphylococcal infections in
    children increases with advancing age. (true or false)
18. The two major nursing goals related to bacterial skin
    infections are:
    a.
    b.
19. When a child is admitted to the hospital with celluli-
    tis, nursing interventions include:
    a.
    b.
    c.
20. In what two ways do epidermal cells react in viral in-
    fection?
    a.
    b.
21. When ringworm is suspected, the organism is identi-
    fied by means of a _____.
    a. culture
    b. Wood light
    c. skin biopsy
    d. patch test
22. When teaching families to care for children with
    ringworm, it is important to emphasize good
    _____ and _____.
23. The dermatophytoses (ringworm) are treated with the
    drug _____ for a period of weeks or
    months.

24. Define *contact dermatitis*.

25. The major nursing goal in the care of the child with contact dermatitis is
_____.

26. The most common contact dermatitis in infants occurs on the convex surfaces of the diaper area as a result of chemical irritation from _____,
_____, or
_____.

27. _____ A nursing intervention following known contact with a poisonous plant is to immediately help the child scrub the affected area with hot, soapy water. (true or false)

28. The organ in which adverse drug reactions are most often seen is the _____.
    a. liver
    b. kidney
    c. bone marrow
    d. skin

29. Describe the nurse's responsibility when it is suspected that a rash represents a drug reaction.

30. List three nursing goals in the care of the child with sunburn.
    a.
    b.
    c.

31. In assessing minor trauma in a child, what types of cuts should the nurse recommend be evaluated for suturing?
    a.
    b.
    c.

32. List four instances in which insect bites assume major significance in children.
    a.
    b.
    c.
    d.

33. The skin infestations encountered most frequently in childhood are _____ and
_____.

34. List the four areas of the child's body that the nurse should be particularly careful to assess for scabies lesions.
    a.
    b.
    c.
    d.

35. Scabies is treated by the application of
_____.

36. In teaching parents about pediculosis capitis, the nurse should emphasize that _____
    a. Head lice are carried by household pets
    b. Lice can be transmitted on personal items
    c. Cleanliness is the best protection against lice
    d. Cutting the child's hair prevents reinfestation

37. Define *attention deficit disorder*.

38. List the components of the multiple approach to the management of attention deficit disorder.
    a.
    b.
    c.
    d.
    e.

39. Define *enuresis*.

40. Match each of the following goals with the type of therapy for enuresis which is most likely to achieve it.

    a. _____ Develop a conditioned reflex.
    b. _____ Inhibit urination.
    c. _____ Increase bladder capacity.
    d. _____ Decrease nighttime output.
    e. _____ Reinforce positive behavior.

    a. drug therapy
    b. bladder training
    c. electrical devices
    d. sleep interruption
    e. restrict evening fluid intake

41. Define *encopresis*.

42. One of the most common causes of encopresis is
_____, often precipitated by
_____.

43. What is the primary goal of the nurse in the management of school phobia?

44. What four areas should the nurse assess in the child with recurrent abdominal pain?
    a.
    b.
    c.
    d.

45. What are the most valuable nursing interventions when dealing with the child with intermittent abdominal pain?

c. Prevent the development and/or complications of malocclusion—

IV. Application, Analysis, and Synthesis of Essential Concepts

A. **Experiential Exercise:** Spend a day in a pedodontist's office. Answer the following questions and include specific examples to illustrate these concepts.

d. Prevent complications from dental trauma—

1. Why is dental health especially important during middle childhood?

B. **Experiential Exercise:** Care for a hospitalized child with a skin disorder. Answer the following questions and include specific examples that illustrate these concepts.

1. What areas are considered in selecting a program for the therapeutic management of skin disorders?

2. What are the most common causes of malocclusion in childhood?
   a.
   b.
   c.
3. Why is orthodontic therapy most successful when started in the later school-age or early adolescent years?

   a.

   b.

   c.

4. For each of the following periods, identify the most frequent causes of dental trauma.
   a. Preschool (1-3 years)—

   d.

   b. School age (7-10 years)—

   e.

2. Develop five nursing diagnoses that would be appropriate for a child with a skin disorder.

   c. Adolescence (16-18 years)—

   a.

5. For each of the following nursing goals realted to dental health, develop at least two nursing interventions.
   a. Prevent the development of dental caries—

   b.

   c.

   b. Prevent the development of periodontal disease—

   d.

3. Provide the rationale for each of the following nursing
interventions which may be utilized in the care of the
child with a skin disorder.
a. Administer emollient soaks, baths, or lotions—

b. Apply topical corticosteroids to affected area—

c. Employ restraint devices and scrupulous hygiene—

d. Apply intermittent wet dresssings—

e. Apply occlusive dressings—

f. Apply powders—

g. Explain procedures and their rationale to parents—

4. What area of development may be affected by chronic
skin disorders in children?

C. **Clinical Situation:** Lester Robitaille, age 9, is
brought to the pediatric health center by his mother.
She states that Lester has been scratching his head and
she has found small white specks in his hair. Mrs. Robitaille brings a note from the school stating that head lice
have been found in several children in Lester's class-
room.

1. Why are school children highly susceptible to communicable diseases, including infestations?

2. What causes the characteristic itching seen with pediculosis?

3. _____ is the drug of choice in the treatment of pediculosis.

4. What two types of programs must accompany the
treatment of pediculosis in order for it to be effective?
a.
b.

5. What is the rationale for reapplying the pediculocide 7
to 10 days after the initial treatment?

. What instructions should the nurse provide to Mrs.
Robitaille regarding the application of Kwell (lindane)
and the eradication of the infestation?
a.
b.
c.

===COLUMN2===

scribed in terms of presentation, diagnosis, prognosis, and nursing implications.

3. McLaury, P.: Head lice: pediatric social disease, Am. J. Nurs. **83**:1300–1303, 1983.

This article provides a detailed description of head lice and the reasons for their prevalence in school populations. Methods of prevention, detection, and treatment are discussed. Guidelines to prevent reinfestation are included, along with tips drawn from the author's personal experience.

4. Thompson, S.: Summertime and ticks, Am. J. Nurs. **83**:768–769, 1983.

This entry discusses the major diseases transmitted by ticks, Rocky Mountain spotted fever and tick paralysis. The mode of infection is described and methods of prevention are presented. A step-by-step procedure for the removal of ticks is pictured and explained.

5. White, Judy E.: Special nursing needs of hospitalized children with learning disabilities, Am. J. Maternal Child Nurs. **8**(3):209–212, 1983.

This article presents a summary of the behavioral characteristics of children with learning disabilities and relates these to problems encountered with communication, structure, and play. Difficulties that these disabilities cause when health problems arise are explored. Suggestions are made for dealing with these problems and providing effective health teaching.

6. Ruble, J.A.: Childhood nocturnal enuresis, Am. J. Maternal Child Nurs. **6**(1):26–31, 1982.

This article summarizes the factual information about enuresis and critiques previous studies in this area. Theories of etiology are discussed and critically appraised. Approaches to management of the problem and a method for choosing the specific treatment modality in individual cases are presented.

7. Johns, C.: Encopresis, Am. J. Nurs. **85**:153–156, 1985.

This article presents an overview of the problem of childhood encopresis. A detailed chart compares the types of constipation and encopresis in terms of etiology, clinical findings, and management. Relevant diagnostic studies are described. The nurse's role in dealing with the encopretic child and his parents is discussed thoroughly.

8. Ryan, N.M.: Recurrent abdominal pain among school-aged children, Am. J. Maternal Child Nurs. **11**(2):102–106, 1986.

This article offers a review of the literature regarding recurrent abdominal pain. It compares the findings in abdominal pain resulting from a variety of organic causes with those in abdominal pain of psychosomatic origin. The role of stress is explained, and methods of assessing environmental stress are explored. The importance of a well coordinated interdisciplinary plan to improve stress management and effectively deal with recurrences is emphasized.

Chapter 19

Health Promotion of the Adolescent and Family

I. Chapter Overview

Chapter 19 examines the frequently perplexing adolescent period. Since this is often a time of difficult transition from childhood to adulthood, students need to be aware of problematic behavior that may occur. At the completion of this chapter, the student will understand the interplay of physical, psychosocial, and emotional factors in the adolescent's development and interpersonal relations. This knowledge will enable the student to provide anticipatory guidance to assist the child and family with the intricate developmental issues of the adolescence.

II. Learning Objectives

Upon completion of this chapter, it is expected that the reader will be able to:

1. Describe the physical changes that occur at puberty in the male and female.

2. Demonstrate an understanding of the processes by which the adolescent develops a sense of identity.

3. Discuss the reactions of the adolescent to physical changes that take place at puberty.

4. Discuss the significance of changing interpersonal relationships and the role of the peer group during adolescence.

5. Outline a health teaching plan for adolescents.

6. Plan a sex education session for a group of adolescents.

7. Identify the causes and discuss the preventive aspects of accidents in adolescence.

8. Discuss the major responsibilities of the parents in fostering development during adolescence.

II. Review of Essential Concepts

1. Adolescence is customarily viewed as beginning with the gradual appearance of _____ and ending with cessation of _____.

2. Differentiate between the following terms:
   a. Puberty—

   b. Adolescence—

3. The physical changes of puberty are primarily the result of _____ influenced by the central nervous system.

4. Identify the two most obvious physical changes that occur during adolescence.
   a.
   b.

5. Differentiate between the following two terms:
   a. Primary sex characteristics—

   b. Secondary sex characteristics—

6. _____ and _____ are the two types of sex hormones that are responsible for the variety of biologic changes observed during pubescence and puberty.

7. Most of the physical growth of adolescents occurs during a 24- to 36-month period known as the adolescent _____.

8. Puberty in girls usually begins between _____ and _____ years of age.

9. Puberty in boys usually begins between the ages of _____ and _____ years.

10. The normal age range of menarche is usually consid-

ered to be _____ to _____ years; the average age is _____ years.

11. The overt sign that indicates puberty in boys is the beginning of _____ of seminal fluid.

12. Skeletal growth differences between boys and girls are reflected in greater overall _____ and longer _____ in boys. There is also an increase in _____ width in boys and greater _____ in girls.

13. _____ Enlargement of the larynx and vocal cords occurs in both boys and girls to produce voice changes. (true or false)

14. _____ glands become extremely active during puberty contributing to the pathogenesis of _____.

15. _____ Adult values for the formed elements of the blood, respiratory rate, and basal metabolic rate are attained during adolescence. (true or false)

16. According to Erikson, the developmental crisis of adolescence is developing a sense of _____.
    a. industry
    b. identity
    c. initiative
    d. autonomy

17. A sense of _____ identity appears to be an essential precursor of the sense of _____ identity.

18. The group offers an identity to the young adolescent in terms of _____ and of the _____ it defines.

19. When does role diffusion occur?

20. Adolescents encounter expectations for mature sex-role behavior from both _____ and _____.

21. According to Freud, the adolescent is in the _____ stage.
    a. anal
    b. oedipal
    c. genital
    d. latent

22. According to Piaget, the adolescent is in the stage of _____.

23. Identify five characteristics that are typical of the adolescent's thought processes.
    a.
    b.
    c.
    d.
    e.

24. _____ It has been determined that the body image established during adolescence is temporary and subject to change. (true or false)

25. What is the principal characteristic of the change

from conventional to postconventional morality that takes place during late adolescence?

26. How are the adolescent's earliest attempts to achieve emancipation from parental controls manifested?

27. Identify ways in which the peer group serves as a source of support for the adolescent.
    a.
    b.
    c.

28. Why do adolescents turn increasingly toward the opposite sex?

29. Identify some of the emotional characteristics seen in adolescents.
    a.
    b.
    c.

30. At the end of the adolescent period, the child should be able to:
    a.
    b.
    c.
    d.
    e.
    f.

31. List five major areas of stress for the adolescent.
    a.
    b.
    c.
    d.
    e.

32. What are some of the health risks that can result from peer pressure?
    a.
    b.
    c.

33. Appropriate disciplinary strategies to be used with adolescents include:
    a.
    b.
    c.

34. _____ The increase in height, weight, muscle mass, and sexual maturity of adolescence is accompanied by greater nutritional requirements. (true or false)

35. List the mineral deficiencies that are most likely to characterize the adolescent diet.
    a.
    b.
    c.

36. How is an inadequate iron intake reflected in the adolescent population?

37. Adolescent involvement in sports contributes to:
    a.
    b.
    c.
38. What type of visual disturbance is most common during adolescence?
39. It is recommended that sex education should be presented from six aspects:
    a.
    b.
    c.
    d.
    e.
    f.
40. The greatest single cause of death in the adolescent age group is _____.
41. Almost half of the fatalities in the adolescent age group are related to _____.
42. What three factors contribute to the problem of motor vehicle injuries in adolescence?
    a.
    b.
    c.
43. What knowledge do parents need to support the growth and development of an adolescent?
    a.
    b.
    c.
    d.

J. Application, Analysis, and Synthesis of Essential Concepts

A. **Clinical Situation:** Alice Spears is a 14-year-old who comes to the pediatric clinic for a yearly check-up. She is accompanied by her mother. Although she has felt well recently, Alice is concerned because she is overweight and has recently developed acne. She also began menstruating 6 months ago.

Alice's height is 64 in. (162.7 cm) and her weight is 161 lb (73.08kg). How do her measurements compare to those of other girls her age?
a. Height—
b. Weight—
What principles of physical growth should be explained to Alice since she is concerned about her weight?

For each of the following reactions to the physical

changes of adolescence, identify the appropriate nursing interventions
a. Adopts a slouch or hunched posture to minimize increased height—

b. Stress related to the development of acne and body odors—

c. Stress related to reproductive changes—

B. **Experiential Exercise:** Interview the parents of an adolescent about the teenagers involvement in peer groups, relationship with parents, and sense of identity. Answer the following questions and include specific responses that illustrate these concepts.

1. How does the peer group contribute to the development of a sense of identity in the adolescent?

2. Identify some ways in which group identity is demonstrated by the adolescent.
   a.
   b.
   c.
   d.
3. Why are peer groups an important influence during the adolescent years?

4. During the interview, the parents state that their adolescent is very emotional, critical, and unpredictable. How does this reflect changing interpersonal relationships?

5. What parental guidance could the nurse offer for coping with the adolescent's behavior?

   a.

   b.

   c.

   d.

   e.

   C. **Experiential Exercise:** Interview an adolescent about his health promotion behavior. Answer the following questions and include specific responses to illustrate these concepts.

1. Why is an adequate intake of the following minerals necessary during adolescence.?

   a. Calcium—

   b. Iron—

   c. Zinc—

2. Why are eating disorders a common occurrence during adolescence?

3. Why is a fatigue a common complaint of adolescence?

4. Why should the nurse promote dental hygiene in the adolescent?

5. What are the most common types of accidents that occur during the adolescent years?

   a.

   b.

   c.

   d.

   e.

   f.

6. What developmental characteristics predispose the adolescent to accidents?

7. What elements should the nurse include in a sex education program for adolescents?

   a.

   b.

   c.

   d.

   e.

8. For each of the following nursing goals, develop nursing interventions that will promote optimal health in the adolescent.

   a. Promote adequate nutritional intake—

   b. Promote the development of proper sleep habits—

   c. Promote optimal physical activity—

   d. Promote good personal hygiene practices—

   e. Prevent physical injury—

V. Suggested Readings

1. Nelms, B.C.: What is a normal adolescent? Am. J. Matern. Child Nurs. **6**(6):402–406, 1981.

   This article presents guidelines for nurses and other health professionals who attempt to assess and interpret the behavior of adolescents. It is organized in three areas: the phases of adolescence; the method the adolescent uses to function within the family, school, and peer groups; and the progress in mastering developmental tasks. Each of these areas is related to expected outcomes, potential problems, and questions to be included in an assessment. A brief case history illustrates the application of the guidelines.

2. Adams, B.N.: Adolescent health care: needs, priorities, and services, Nurs. Clin. North Am. **18**(2):237–247, 1983.

This selection presents a developmental framework for professionals to utilize as a basis for providing health services for the child in early, middle and late adolescence. The health care setting, the manner in which interviews are conducted, the specific history to be obtained, the physical examination, and the characteristics of the care providers are discussed from the perspective of their reflection of the needs of adolescents. The problems and priorities of the delivery of adolescent health care services are identified.

3. Elkind, D.: Teenage thinking: implications for health care, Pediatr. Nurs. **10**:383–385, 1984.

This entry contrasts the reasoning abilities of children and adolescents. It labels the belief of adolescents that everyone is concerned with their thoughts and actions the ''imaginary audience'' and suggests that this construct provides insight into common adolescent health problems. It relates the adolescent ''personal fable'' of invulnerability to issues of noncompliance and risk taking. Finally, it offers approaches to health teaching and counseling based on these constructs.

4. Sheehan, M.K., Ostwald, S.K., and Rothenberger, J.: Perceptions of sexual responsibility: do young men and women agree? Pediatr. Nurs. **12**:17–21, 1986.

This study investigated the perception of responsibility for contraception among late adolescents to determine whether age, gender, or sexual activity influences perceptions of responsibility and to explore the relationship between this perceived responsibility and subsequent contraceptive choice. It found that older adolescents perceived contraception as a shared responsibility but that they were unlikely to use contraception during their first intercourse. The implications of the findings for sex education are discussed.

5. Kuhnen, K.K., Chewning, B., Day, T., and others: Barny: computer for teaching sex education, Am. J. Maternal Child Nurs. **8**(5):350–353, 1983.

This article reports the results of the Body Awareness Resource Network survey to measure adolescents' knowledge, attitudes, behaviors, and communication patterns regarding human sexuality. The findings suggest that many adolescents make decisions about their sex lives at very young ages without sufficient information to evaluate the consequences. Subsequently, a computer program was developed for use in schools, homes, and clinics to provide information and affirm the adolescent's role as an active decision-maker. It provides referrals to specific agencies for specific problems. While still in its implementation phase, the program seems an effective sex education tool that is both accepted and utilized by adolescents.

6. Josephson, S.: Scuba diving hazards: health counseling, Am. J. Nurs. **81**:1458–1461, 1981.

This article examines the stress of physiological changes which occur during a dive. It applies information related to the effects of pressure, temperature, and other stressors in the underwater environment to a health assessment directed toward predicting problems. It describes how the data base can be used in referral and teaching to reduce the potential hazards of this popular adolescent sport.

Chapter 20

Physical Health Problems of Adolescence

I. Chapter Overview

Chapter 20 introduces nursing considerations that are integral to the care of the adolescent experiencing physical health problems. While adolescents are usually healthy, students need to be aware of the common health problems related to their physical changes and of other potentially serious illnesses or injuries. At the completion of this chapter, the student will understand the commonly encountered physical health deviations of the adolescent and recognize the potential for secondary psychologic problems. This knowledge will provide a basis for the student to develop nursing goals and interventions to support and educate the adolescent and family.

II. Learning Objectives

Upon completion of this chapter, it is expected that the student will be able to:

1. Outline a plan of care for the adolescent with a health problem.

2. Demonstrate an understanding of health problems related to sports participation.

3. Describe the most common causes of growth or maturational failure in adolescence.

4. Demonstrate an understanding of common disorders of the male and female reproductive system.

5. Demonstrate an understanding of health problems related to sexuality.

6. Identify the most common types of sexually transmitted diseases.

III. Review of Essential Concepts

1. The skin disorder that appears predominantly during the adolescent period is _____.

2. List six specific factors that appear to be related to the development of acne.

a.

b.

c.

d.

e.

f.

3. The statement that correctly describes acne is _____.
   a. The peak incidence of acne is during the period of early adolescence.
   b. Lesions seen in acne may be either noninflamed comedones or inflamed lesions.
   c. The pathogenesis of acne is related to an abnormality of the sebaceous glands.
   d. Primary inflammation in acne is usually due to the presence of *Staphylococcus albus*.

4. Six goals in the care of the adolescent with acne are:
   a.
   b.
   c.
   d.
   e.
   f.

5. The most effective therapy for acne involves the use of _____ or _____, or a combination of the two drugs.

6. Two purposes for the nontraumatic removal of comedones are:
   a.
   b.

7. Provide two specific factors related to the onset of smoking during adolescence in each of the following categories.
   a. Social—

   b. Sociodemographic—

c. Psychosocial—

d. Biologic—

8. List the four stages of the process of becoming a smoker.
   a.
   b.
   c.
   d.
9. _____ The use of smokeless tobacco products is a safe substitute for cigarette smoking. (true or false)
10. Two recent areas of focus for smoking-prevention programs are:
   a.
   b.
11. The principal cause of infectious mononucleosis is the _____.
12. The insidious symptoms of mononucleosis are:
   a.
   b.
   c.
13. The _____, a slide test of high specificity, is utilized in the diagnosis of infectious mononucleosis.
14. The role of health professionals in relation to sports injuries is directed toward _____, _____, and _____. Of these, _____ is the most important.
15. _____ At least two thirds of sports injuries involve the bony skeleton. (true or false)
16. Match the following sports injuries with their definitions.

_____ contusion

_____ dislocation

_____ sprain

_____ strain

_____ overuse syndrome

a. Joint injury in which the normal position of the opposing bone ends or the bone end to its socket is displaced.

b. Microscopic tear to the musculotendinous unit.

c. Tearing of the soft tissue, muscle, subcutaneous structures, and small blood vessels resulting in hemorrhage, edema, and pain.

d. Repetitive microtrauma that occurs to a particular anatomic structure as a result of chronic overload.

e. Partial or complete tearing or stretching of a ligament, often accompanied by damaged blood vessels, tendons, and nerves.

17. List five components of the management of soft tissue injuries.
   a.
   b.
   c.
   d.
   e.
18. Management of overuse syndromes is directed toward:
   a.
   b.
   c.
19. Identify the three instances in which sudden death associated with sports activities may occur.
   a.
   b.
   c.
20. _____ Prevention of sports injuries is probably the most important aspect of any athletic program. (true or false)
21. What six criteria are utilized to assess delayed development?
   a.
   b.
   c.
   d.
   e.
   f.
22. Short stature is usually caused by either _____ or a simple _____.
23. Manifestations of sexual development before age _____ in boys and age _____ in girls are considered precocious.
24. Identify the three outstanding features of girls with Turner syndrome.
   a.
   b.
   c.
25. Characteristic features of boys with Klinefelter syndrome include:
   a.
   b.
   c.
   d.
   e.
26. _____ The majority of urethral infections in the male are the result of sexual contact. (true or false)
27. _____ cancer constitutes the most common solid tumor in males between ages 15 and 35.
28. The most common cause of secondary amenorrhea

during adolescence is inhibition of the secretion of _____ hormones.

29. _____ is the most common gynecologic complaint, affecting half of all female adolescents.

30. The treatment of choice for dysmenorrhea in adolescents is the administration of drugs that block the formation of _____.

31. The cause of pelvic inflammatory disease in adolescents is usually _____ or _____ infections.

32. All girls exposed to diethylstilbestrol (DES) during their mother's pregnancy should have annual screening exams beginning at age _____ which include a pelvic examination and a _____.

33. _____ Each year approximately 1 in 10 adolescent girls in the United States becomes pregnant. (true or false)

34. The most serious complication of adolescent pregnancy is _____.

35. Prolonged labor in younger adolescents is a reflection of the girl's _____ and _____.

36. Infants of adolescents have a higher incidence of _____ and _____.

37. _____ Children of adolescent mothers experience more developmental problems than children of adult mothers. (true or false)

38. Identify four reasons why adolescents use contraception inconsistently or ineffectively.
   a.
   b.
   c.
   d.

39. _____ More than half of rape victims are between 10 and 19 years of age. (true or false)

40. During the initial contact with the adolescent rape victim, it is important that she know that she is:
   a.
   b.

41. The two phases of the rape trauma syndrome are:
   a.
   b.

42. _____ ranks first in numbers of cases and is considered the most serious of the sexually transmitted diseases.

43. Match the following sexually transmitted diseases with their causative organisms and the drug of choice for treatment. (Answers may be used more than once.)

a. _____ gonorrhea   a. *C. trachomatis*

b. _____ chlamydial infection   b. herpesvirus hominis Type II

c. _____ herpes genitalis   c. *Trichomonas vaginalis*

d. _____ syphilis   d. *Neisseria gonorrhoeae*

e. _____ moniliasis   e. *Treponema pallidum*

f. _____ trichomoniasis   f. *Candida albicans*

g. metronidazole

h. tetracycline

i. acyclovir

j. nystatin

k. penicillin

IV. Application, Analysis, and Synthesis of Essential Concepts

A. **Clinical Situation:** Rosemary, age 16, is admitted to the adolescent unit with a severe sore throat, persistent fever, fatigue, and general malaise. A diagnosis of infectious mononucleosis is made.

1. How was the diagnosis of infectious mononucleosis established?

2. What might the nurse tell Rosemary about the usual course of infectious mononucleosis in the following areas:
   a. Acute symptoms—
   b. Persistent fatigue—
   c. Restricted activity—

3. What therapeutic measures may be used to relieve Rosemary's sore throat?

4. What are the nursing goals in caring for Rosemary?
   a.
   b.

5. What nursing interventions would be used in caring for Rosemary?
   a.
   b.
   c.
   d.
   e.
   f.

B. **Clinical Situation:** Derek, age 15, has been experiencing a deep, persistent, dull ache over the left tibia which progressed to pain with each heel strike during a cross-country meet. The coach refers Derek to the sport medicine team at University Medical Center for evaluation. A stress fracture of the left tibia is discovered.

1. What two general types of injury are related to sport
   a.
   b.

2. What factors may be related to overuse syndromes such as Derek's stress fracture?
   a.
   b.
   c.
   d.
   e.
   f.
3. Stress fractures such as Derek's are usually caused by _____.
   a. friction of one structure against another
   b. repeated tractional pull on a ligament or tendon
   c. cyclic loading of impact forces
4. What is the major goal of the therapeutic management of overuse syndromes such as Derek's stress fracture?

5. Rest is the primary therapy for overuse syndromes. How is this treatment modality likely to be interpreted in Derek's case?

6. Derek asks the nurse on the sports medicine team if she thinks running is a good sport for him. What should the nurse assess in order to answer this question?

. What nursing interventions might the nurse on the sports medicine team employ to prevent sports injuries?
   a.
   b.
   c.
   d.

C. **Experiential Exercise:** Spend a day in a gynecoloy clinic to oversee the management of sexually transmited diseases and other disorders affecting the female eproductive system. Answer the following questions and clude specific examples to illustrate these concepts.

. What two problems in the female adolescent most frequently require attention from health professionals?
   a.
   b.
. What are four advantages of undergoing the initial pelvic examination in early adolescence?
   a.

b.

c.

d.

3. Define the following terms to differentiate their meanings:
   a. Primary amenorrhea—

   b. Secondary amenorrhea—

4. Identify the most common causes of secondary dysmenorrhea in adolescents.
   a.
   b.
5. Formulate five nursing interventions to be utilized with an adolescent who has menstrual problems.
   a.
   b.
   c.
   d.
   e.
6. Why are adolescents particularly at risk of sexually transmitted diseases?

7. What are the nursing goals related to the prevention of sexually transmitted diseases?
   a.
   b.
   c.
   d.
8. Formulate four nursing diagnoses which could apply to the adolescent with a disorder of the female reproductive system.
   a.
   b.
   c.
   d.

D. **Experiential Exercise:** Interview a pregnant adolescent to identify her concerns and the psychologic, economic, and environmental impact of her pregnancy. Answer the following questions and include specific responses to illustrate these concepts.

1. What threat does pregnancy pose to the adolescent girl's normal development?

2. Briefly describe the differences in the ways that pregnancy is viewed by girls in the following age groups:
   a. Early adolescence—

   b. Middle adolescence—

   c. Late adolescence—

3. Identify four potential social consequences of adolescent pregnancy.
   a.
   b.
   c.
   d.

4. Formulate a nursing intervention to be utilized in each of the following situations:
   a. The adolescent decides to terminate her pregnancy—

   b. The adolescent decides to place her child for adoption—

   c. The adolescent decides to rear her child—

5. Identify four nursing goals in the care of the adolescent who is pregnant.
   a.
   b.
   c.
   d.

6. What information should the nurse include in a teaching plan for the pregnant adolescent regarding child care?
   a.
   b.
   c.
   d.
   e.
   f.

V. Suggested Readings

1. Stone, A.C.: Racing up to acne, Pediatr. Nurs. **8**(4):229–234, 1982.

   This article explores the role of the pediatric nurse in the management of adolescent acne. The pathophysiology of acne is described and related to the assessment of both subjective and objective data through an acne assessment questionnaire. Guides to patient teaching and to both over-the-counter and prescription acne preparations are provided.

2. MacVicar, M.G., Harlan, J.D., and Ouellette, M.: What do we know about the effects of sports training on the menstrual cycle? Am. J. Maternal Child Nurs. **7**(1):55–58, 1982.

   This article reviews the literature on stimuli that challenge normal physiological response to the menstrual cycle, particularly those that affect the female athlete. Variables include genetic predisposition, sociocultural attitudes and perceptions of menstruation, and body composition expressed as the ratio of fat to lean body weight. The needs for further research in this area, for counseling of parents, and for physical and emotional assessment of the young female athletes are discussed.

3. Thorne, B.P.: A nurse helps prevent sports injuries, Am. J. Maternal Child Nurs. **7**(4):236–239, 1982.

   This entry describes the role of the nurse in a preventive sports medicine program for a high school. It involved the education of the coaches and athletes about the purpose of the program, the use of a Sports Medical Questionnaire as a screening tool, individual interviews and physical examinations of the athletes, and advice to the athlete on conditioning and training techniques that will help avoid injury. These measures have identified a potential for injury in half of the students screened.

4. Stern, N., and Zaiken, H.: Assessing the child with short stature, Pediatr. Nurs. **11**(2):106–110, 1985.

   This selection reviews concepts related to normal growth and normal variants of growth before discussing conditions associated with short stature. It provides guidelines for screening for the need for a more thorough evaluation of short stature, including a history, physical examination, laboratory and x-ray studies, and referral to an endocrinologist. Management of the child according to the information provided by these measures is described.

5. Williams, H.A.: Screening for testicular cancer, Pediatr. Nurs. **7**(5):38–40, 1981.

   Testicular cancer is discussed in terms of symptoms, incidence, etiology, and prognosis as a basis for establishing the need for routine screening. The screening procedure is described in detail, and illustrations are provided. A case is made for the initiation of public education about testicular cancer with young children and adolescents. Resources for nurses involved in testicular cancer screening are suggested.

6. Sasso, S.C.: Prostaglandin inhibitors for primary dysmenorrhea, Am. J. Maternal Child Nurs. **9**(3):177, 1984.

   This MCN pharmacopoeia entry describes primary dysmenorrhea and the reason for the use of prostaglandin-inhibiting drugs in its treatment. The two most commonly used prostaglandin inhibitors, ibuprofen and naproxen, are discussed in terms of action, absorption, contraindications, adverse reactions, dosage, and nursing implications.

7. Frank, E.P.: What are nurses doing to help PMS patients? Am. J. Nurs. **86**:137–140, 1986.

   This article briefly reviews current knowledge about premenstrual syndrome and describes three PMS programs that maximize the role of the nurse. The three protocols include diagnosis by patient charting over 2 to 3 months; management that begins with self-help measures such as diet, exercise, and stress reduction; and the weeding out of a high proportion of patients who suffer from other disorders. A list of resources is provided.

8. Burke, P.J.: A community health model for pregnant teens, Am. J. Maternal Child Nurs. **8**(5):340–344, 1983.

This selection describes a state-funded community-based outreach program for pregnant adolescents which addresses social and health-related issues of pregnancy and parenting through an interdisciplinary team (nursing and social work) approach. Case studies are presented to illustrate means of overcoming adolescent resistance, delivering support and anticipatory guidance, and providing long-term follow-up.

9. Sewall K.S.: Peer-group reality therapy for the pregnant adolescent, Am. J. Maternal Child Nurs. **8**(1):67–69, 1983.

This article proposes the peer-group application of Glasser's model of reality therapy to help pregnant adolescents change irresponsible behavior and develop plans to deal with problems. The reality therapy group of pregnant adolescents is also seen as serving as a forum for teaching and as a support system. The steps of the protocol and the nurse's role in implementing it with pregnant adolescents are described.

10. Bahr, J.E.: *Herpesvirus hominis* Type II in women and newborns, Am. J. Maternal Child Nurs. **3**(1):16–21, 1978.

This entry provides detailed information about the history, pathophysiology, incidence, and diagnosis of herpes infections. The course of the disease in women, its transmission to the fetus or newborn, and the course of the infection in the newborn are described. The role of the nurse in the areas of observation, identification, prevention, treatment, teaching, and counseling is analyzed.

Chapter 21

Behavioral Health Problems of Adolescence

I. Chapter Overview

Chapter 21 explores health problems that are caused primarily by the psychologic responses to adolescence. Although these problems are not physical in origin, the student needs to be aware of their potential to dramatically affect the health and well-being of the adolescent. At the completion of this chapter, students should understand both the physical and psychologic aspects of the eating disorders and other destructive behavior prevalent in the adolescent population. This knowledge will enable students to formulate nursing interventions which will assist both the adolescent and family in dealing with the complex psychologic concerns of this developmental period.

II. Learning Objectives

Upon completion of this chapter, it is expected that the student will be able to:

1. Outline a plan of care for the child or adolescent with an eating disorder.

2. Differentiate between the characteristic behaviors associated with anorexia nervosa and bulimia.

3. Identify the behaviors which may precede a suicide attempt by an adolescent.

4. Identify the nursing considerations used in caring for the adolescent substance abuser.

III. Review of Essential Concepts

1. List six factors which influence the amount and distribution of body fat.
   a.
   b.
   c.
   d.
   e.
   f.

2. _____ is an increase in body weight resulting from an excessive accumulation of fat or, simply, the state of being too fat.

3. _____ is the state of weighing more than average for height and body build, which may or may not include an increased amount of fat.

4. What is the cause of obesity?

5. List the common emotional sequelae of obesity in adolescence.
   a.
   b.
   c.
   d.

6. _____ Adolescent-onset obesity appears to be closely related to the child's inability to master the developmental tasks of adolescence. (true or false)

7. What three factors contribute to the development of a disturbed body image in the obese adolescent?
   a.
   b.
   c.

8. Identify four complications of childhood obesity.
   a.
   b.
   c.
   d.

9. _____ As a rule, children who are 10% over normal for their height and weight should be further evaluated. (true or false)

10. The two essential components of any weight-reduction program are _____ and _____

1. In the management of obesity, it has been observed that _____.
   a. A diet containing 800 to 1200 kcal per day achieves a desirable weight loss for adolescents.
   b. There is little correlation between motivation to lose weight and the success of the weight-reduction program.
   c. The most successful diets are those that require the avoidance of specific foods.
   d. The alteration of eating behavior has little effect in maintaining long-term weight control.
2. What five factors may be predictive of potential for the success of a weight-reduction program in adolescence?
   a.
   b.
   c.
   d.
   e.
3. _____ is a disorder characterized by severe weight loss in the absence of obvious physical cause in which emaciation occurs as a result of self-inflicted starvation.
4. The onset of anorexia nervosa generally takes place at or near _____.
5. Identify the characteristics frequently displayed by young women with anorexia nervosa.
   a.
   b.
   c.
   d.
6. The two dominant psychologic aspects of anorexia nervosa are:
   a.
   b.
7. What three major areas of disordered psychologic functioning do these dominant aspects reflect in the syndrome of anorexia nervosa?
   a.
   b.
   c.
8. Identify two characteristics that are common in families with an anorectic child.
   a.
   b.
9. List the clinical manifestations of anorexia nervosa.
   a.
   b.
   c.
   d.
   e.
   f.
   g.
10. Identify the three major aims of the management of anorexia nervosa.
    a.

b.
c.
21. _____ is an eating disorder characterized by binge eating and purging.
22. Purging methods employed by bulimics include _____, _____, _____, and rigorous exercise.
23. It is characteristic that bulimics _____.
    a. Have been successful dieters in the past.
    b. Usually represent the lower socioeconomic groups.
    c. Were of normal weight or underweight in childhood.
    d. May consume 20,000 to 30,000 calories per day.
24. Briefly describe the two categories of bulimics.
    a.

    b.

25. _____ Medical complications occur in bulimics primarily as a result of their frequent vomiting. (true or false)
26. Identify two nursing interventions that are important during the acute phase of treatment of bulimia.
    a.
    b.
27. Identify the three factors that render adolescents vulnerable to superimposed stresses.
    a.
    b.
    c.
28. _____ Suicide is the third leading cause of death during the adolescent years. (true or false)
29. Distinguish between the following terms:
    a. Suicide gesture—

    b. Suicide attempt—

    c. Impulsive act—

30. The statement that most accurately reflects the incidence of adolescent suicide is _____.
    a. Black adolescents have a higher incidence of suicide than do white teenagers.

b. Boys account for a greater percentage of successful suicides.

c. Girls make fewer suicidal gestures or attempts than do boys.

d. Depression is seldom diagnosed in adolescents who attempt suicide.

31. List three general factors associated with teenage suicide.

    a.

    b.

    c.

32. _____ is the method of choice for most adolescents who attempt suicide.

33. _____ Most adolescents' suicidal gestures are impulsive acts committed to force parents or other significant persons to pay attention to their need for help. (true or false)

34. Identify three motivations for suicide in adolescents.

    a.

    b.

    c.

35. _____ Severely depressed adolescents usually make several suicidal gestures as signals of their need for help prior to making a serious suicide attempt. (true or false)

36. What characteristics of depression indicate that the condition is serious and the child needs special intervention?

    a.

    b.

    c.

37. In the therapeutic management of suicide threats or attempts, _____.

    a. Long-term intervention is needed for response.

    b. Hospitalization is usually avoided.

    c. Antidepressant medication is used routinely.

    d. Attachment to a caring adult may be sufficient.

38. List seven guidelines designed to help the nurse assess the seriousness of a suicide gesture or attempt.

    a.

    b.

    c.

    d.

    e.

    f.

    g.

39. Match the following terms related to substance abuse to their correct definitions.

a. _____ drug abuse

b. _____ drug misuse

c. _____ narcotic addiction

d. _____ drug tolerance

e. _____ physical dependence

a. the overzealous use of drugs or the exercise of bad judgment in their use

b. an adaptive physiologic state that occurs when a drug is taken in increasing amounts and that is manifest by the development of physiologic symptoms when the drug is withdrawn

c. behavioral pattern of overwhelming involvement with obtaining and using a narcotic for its psychotropic effects rather than for medical reasons, thereby eliciting social disapproval

d. the regular use of drugs for other than the accepted medical purposes and to the extent that it results in physical or psychologic harm to the user or is used in a way that is detrimental to society

e. the clinical need to increase the dosage of a drug in order to attain the same desired effect, caused by an increased capacity to metabolize and eliminate the drug or the ability of the individual's tissues to adapt to the drug

40. Problems that involve the use of drugs can be classified as _____, _____, _____, and _____.

41. What factors might the nurse assess in determining the severity of an adolescent's drug problem?

    a.

    b.

    c.

    d.

    e.

42. The two broad categories of adolescents who use drugs are _____ and _____.

43. During early and middle adolescence, what four groups designate the motivation for drug use?

    a.

    b.

    c.

    d.

44. What three factors influence the individual reaction to drug use?

    a.

    b.

    c.

45. _____ is now considered the adolescent drug of choice.

46. _____ are gaining in popularity as agents of abuse in school-age children and economically disadvantaged groups.

47. _____ The hallucinogens produce physical dependence. (true or false)
48. Heroin and related narcotics produce both _____ and _____ dependence.
49. _____ is the most powerful antifatigue agent.
50. Rehabilitation of the hard drug user may require withdrawing the adolescent from both the _____ and the chemical agent.
51. Careful assessment in the nonacute stage helps the nurse to determine the _____ in the adolescent's life.

IV. Application, Analysis, and Synthesis of Essential Concepts

A. **Experiential Exercise:** Interview an obese adolescent to assess eating patterns. Answer the following questions and include specific responses that illustrate these concepts.

1. Why is obesity considered a major problem of adolescence?

2. Why may obese adolescents tend to be taller than average and also have somewhat greater than average lean body mass?

. Identify six factors that may contribute to the development of obesity.
a.
b.
c.
d.
e.
f.
. Identify six behaviors that are characteristic of the eating patterns of obese adolescents.
a.
b.
c.
d.
e.
f.
. What are the essential components of a nursing assessment directed toward the evaluation of obesity?
a.
b.
c.

d.
e.
f.
g.
h.

6. Formulate four nursing diagnoses that could apply to the obese adolescent.
a.
b.
c.
d.

7. For each of the following nursing goals utilized in the care of the obese adolescent, provide at least two nursing interventions which are directed toward meeting the goal.
a. Reduce the quantity eaten—

b. Alter the quality of food eaten—

c. Alter the eating situation—

B. **Experiential Exercise:** Role-play an interaction between a nurse and an anorexic or bulimic adolescent to demonstrate the adolescent's perception of her disorder and how the nurse would counsel her.

1. What usually precedes the onset of anorexia nervosa?

2. What contemporary trend is considered a factor in the greatly increased incidence of anorexia and bulimia?

3. Formulate a nursing diagnosis that is appropriate for each of the following areas of disordered psychologic functioning in the anorexic.
a. Disturbed body image and body concept of delusional proportions—

b. Inaccurate and confused perception and interpretation of inner stimuli—

c. Paralyzing sense of ineffectiveness that pervades all aspects of daily life—

4. The following are characteristics associated with anorexia nervosa and/or bulimia. Mark A if the item is

related to anorexia, B if it applies to bulimia, and A,B if it may be associated with both disorders.

a. _____ binge-eating
b. _____ self-induced vomiting
c. _____ self-imposed starvation
d. _____ awareness of abnormality of eating pattern
e. _____ denial of existence of hunger
f. _____ cold intolerance
g. _____ normal or slightly above normal weight
h. _____ emaciated appearance
i. _____ increased incidence of dental caries
j. _____ distinctive hand lesions
k. _____ control is major issue
l. _____ secondary amenorrhea

5. Behavior modification may be utilized in the treatment of both anorexia nervosa and bulimia. Identify the essential aspects of such a program.
a.
b.
c.
d.
e.

6. Develop seven nursing goals to be utilized in the care of an anorexic or bulimic adolescent.
a.

b.

c.

d.

e.

f.

g.

C. **Clinical Situation:** Michelle is a 16-year-old girl who is admitted to the adolescent unit following the ingestion of 10 of her mother's barbiturates with an un-known quantity of alcohol. She is known to be a "problem drinker." When she recovers consciousness after gastric lavage, Michelle sobs that she wishes she were dead because she has broken up with her boyfriend.

1. In what category might this suicide attempt be classified?

2. In what ways was Michelle's suicide attempt a typical one for an adolescent girl?

3. In assessing Michelle's family status, what factors is the nurse likely to discover?

4. What five purposes might hospitalization serve in Michelle's care?
a.
b.
c.
d.
e.

5. In each of the following areas, describe what the nurse should assess to evaluate the seriousness of Michelle's suicide attempt.
a. Social set—

b. Intent—

c. Method—

d. History—

e. Stress—

f. Mental status—

g. Support—

6. Beyond the immediate care, follow-up of the adolescent who has made a suicide attempt is most important. Michelle has a history of being a "problem drinker." What characteristic behaviors of adolescent alcoholics should the nurse be alert for in following Michelle after her discharge?

7. What nursing intervention is a factor in alcohol management?

V. Suggested Readings

1. White, J.H.: An overview of obesity: its significance to nursing, Nurs. Clin. North Am. **17**(2):191–197, 1982.

This article provides a summary of current knowledge and theories concerning obesity. It argues that obesity is a complex problem caused by the interaction of several factors—environmental, physiologic, and psychological—and that, consequently, a combination of strategies is needed to treat it. The various forms of treatment which may be combined are explored.

2. Hagenbuch, E.G.: Obesity and the school-age child, Nurs. Clin. North Am. **17**(2):207–215, 1982.

This entry presents a holistic approach to the problem of obesity in children, utilizing the nursing process. The assessment involves the complete family field as well as fields interacting with the obese child and the family. Nursing interventions discussed include teaching, advocacy, direct nursing care, coordination, collaboration, referral, anticipatory guidance, counseling, and continuing professional development. Concurrent evaluation is stressed.

3. Ciseaux, A.: Anorexia nervosa: a view from the mirror, Am. J. Nurs. **80**:1468–1470, 1980.

This is a personal account of the experience of anorexia nervosa written by a nurse who has been anorexic for 17 years. It provides insight into the thought processes, motivations, and behaviors of the anorexic.

4. Richardson, T.F.: Anorexia nervosa: an overview, Am. J. Nurs. **80**:1470–1471, 1980.

This article describes the historical development of anorexia nervosa and lists its generally accepted diagnostic criteria. It briefly explores possible etiologies of the condition in six general theoretical categories: psychodynamics, family interactions, behavioral, medical, distortions of perception, and cultural.

5. Claggett, M. S.: Anorexia nervosa: a behavioral approach, Am. J. Nurs. **80**:1471–1472, 1980.

This entry briefly reviews traditional therapeutic approaches to the management of anorexia nervosa and some of the problems encountered in their implementation. It then examines behavior modification as a possible alternative. The question of what disciplines should be involved in the therapeutic management plan is raised.

6. Hoff, L. A., and Resing, M.: Was this suicide preventable? Am. J. Nurs. **82**:1106–1111, 1982.

This article employs a case study of a young man who committed suicide within hours of being assessed by mental health professionals as a vehicle for the discussion of theory related to suicide. A parallel scenario illustrates how things might have gone if recommended assessment techniques had been followed. A sample plan of crisis intervention and follow-up service is presented.

7. Rice, M.A., and Kibbee, P.E.: Review: identifying the adolescent substance abuser, Am. J. Maternal Child Nurs. **8**(2):139–142, 1983.

Alcohol and drug abuse are discussed in this article from the perspective of their interference with the achievement of adolescent developmental tasks. A case study presents a typical example of the development of substance abuse in the adolescent. A table of biophysical clues to substance abuse links symptoms to specific drug groups. Several innovative programs for treating adolescent substance abusers are briefly described.

8. Michael, M.M., and Sewall, K.S.: Use of the adolescent peer group to increase the self-care agency of adolescent alcohol abusers, Nurs. Clin. North Am. **15**(1):157–176, 1980.

This article describes the use of the peer group to change the behavior of alcoholic adolescents in a program based on reality therapy. Theory related to adolescent development, alcohol abuse, and reality is presented. The program is correlated with the phases of the nursing process and is proposed as an instrument for teaching, a support system, and an agent of change.

Chapter 22

Impact of Chronic Illness or Disability on the Child and Family

I. Chapter Overview

Chapter 22 introduces nursing considerations essential to the care of the child with a chronic illness or disability. Since nursing students will be required to care for children with special needs, it is important that they understand the family's reaction to the loss of a "perfect" child and become familiar with the process of adjusting to a disability. At the completion of this chapter, the student should understand the impact that a diagnosis of a chronic illness or disability has on both the child and family and be able to develop appropriate nursing interventions to assist each family member to adjust and develop to his fullest potential despite the disability.

II. Learning Objectives

Upon completion of this chapter, it is expected that the student will be able to:

1. Identify the scope of and changing trends in the care of the child with a chronic illness or disability.

2. Define the stages of adjustment to the diagnosis of a chronic illness or disability.

3. Describe the reactions of and effects on the family of a child with a chronic illness or disability.

4. Identify the factors that affect the family's adjustment to a diagnosis of a disability.

5. Outline nursing interventions that will promote a family's optimal adjustment to the diagnosis of a chronic illness or disability.

III. Review of Essential Concepts

1. Match each of the following terms with the appropriate definition.

a. _____ chronic illness

b. _____ disability

c. _____ developmental disability

d. _____ handicap

a. broadly refers to a loss of function

b. refers to environmental barriers preventing or making it difficult for full participation or integration

c. a condition that interferes with daily functioning for more than 3 months in a year, causes hospitalization of more than 1 month in a year, or is likely to do either of these

d. any severe, chronic disability attributable to a mental or physical impairment or a combination of both that is manifested before age 22 years, is likely to continue indefinitely and will result in substantial limitation of function

2. _____ Two thirds of all cases of chronic illness are attributable to asthma and congenital heart defects. (true or false)

3. Define normalization.

4. Identify the three major goals of home care for the child with special needs.

a.

b.

c.

5. _____ refers to the integration of children with special needs into regular classrooms.

6. The family of the child with special needs is faced with the crisis of:
   a.
   b.

7. List the sequence of stages that a family progresses through following the diagnosis of a chronic illness or disability.
   a.
   b.
   c.
   d.

8. The two most common responses manifested during the adjustment stage are:
   a.
   b.

9. Describe the four types of parental reactions to the child that may occur during the period of adjustment.
   a. Overprotection—

   b. Rejection—

   c. Denial—

   d. Gradual acceptance—

10. _____ The main concerns of fathers of chronically ill children often involve the child's future and the unpredictable nature of the illness. (true or false)

11. List three variables that influence the resolution of a crisis following the diagnosis of a serious health problem.
    a.
    b.
    c.

12. _____ are those behaviors aimed at reducing the tension caused by a crisis.

13. Identify four variables which influence a child's reaction to chronic illness or disability.
    a.
    b.
    c.
    d.

14. _____ The impact of a chronic illness or disability is influenced by the age of onset. (true or false)

15. List five individual factors that influence the child's ability to cope with stress.
    a.
    b.
    c.
    d.
    e.

16. The three most common responses of families to the diagnosis of a disability are:
    a.
    b.
    c.

17. The three factors which should be considered when attempting to foster a reality adjustment are:
    a.
    b.
    c.

IV. Application, Analysis, and Synthesis of Essential Concepts

A. **Experiential Exercise:** Spend a morning at a clinic or school for children with disabilities to observe various treatment modalities and programs. Answer the following questions and include specific examples that illustrate these concepts.

1. Identify four ways in which the nurse can prevent the occurrence of disabling disorders.
   a.
   b.
   c.
   d.

2. Describe the four major changes that have occurred in the provision of services to children with special needs.
   a.

   b.

   c.

   d.

3. How have the above changes served to improve the care of children with special needs?

a.

b.

c.

d.

B. **Experiential Exercise:** Care for a child who has recently been diagnosed as having a chronic illness or disability.

1. Why is it important for the nurse to understand the responses of family members to a diagnosis of a chronic illness or disability?
   a.
   b.
   c.

2. Briefly describe the stages that a family progresses through following the diagnosis of a chronic illness or disability.
   a. Shock and denial—

   b. Adjustment—

c. Reintegration and acceptance—

d. Freezing-out phase—

3. List nine examples of behavior that should alert the nurse to the presence of denial.
   a.
   b.
   c.
   d.
   e.
   f.
   g.
   h.
   i.

4. Why is it important for the nurse to allow denial to occur for a reasonable period of time?
   a.

   b.

5. Briefly describe the reactions and effects of a diagnosis of chronic illness or disability on each of the following family members:
   a. Parents—

   b. Child—

c. Siblings—

e.

5. What is the major nursing goal when dealing with a family who has a child with special needs

6. A major nursing goal that should be used to deal with families following the diagnosis of a serious health problem is:

6. Why is the mutual participation model an effective method when developing nursing interventions for a child with special needs and his family?
   a.

   b.

C. **Experiential Exercise:** Interview the parents of a child with a disability to determine the family's adjustment. Answer the following questions and include specific responses to illustrate these concepts.

1. Identify the three areas which the nurse should assess when determining the adequacy of a family's support systems.
   a.
   b.
   c.

   c.

2. Why is it necessary for the nurse to assess the family's specific perceptions concerning the illness or disability?

7. What areas must the nurse assess prior to developing a plan of care for a disabled child and his family?
   a.
   b.
   c.
   d.
   e.

3. Why is it important for the nurse to assess how a family reacted to previous crises?

8. Identify two nursing interventions that should be utilized to provide support to parents at the time of diagnosis.
   a.
   b.

4. Briefly describe some of the behaviors that might be observed in a child who has adjusted well to his disability.
   a.

9. Identify at least three appropriate nursing interventions to be utilized when helping each of the following family members to cope:
   a. Parents—

   b.

   c.

   b. Child—

   d.

c. Siblings—

10. For each of the following nursing goals, identify at least three appropriate nursing interventions that can be used to promote reality adjustment.
    a. Supply information—

    b. Promote normal development—

    c. Establish realistic future goals—

V. Suggested Readings

1. Levenson, P.M., and Signer, B.: Using computers to help children cope with chronic illness, Child. Health Care 14(2):76–82, 1985.

    This article focuses on some of the educational and psychosocial needs of chronically ill and disabled children that may be provided through computer-related technologies. It describes technologies that might be utilized and provides examples of how these may be incorporated into the care and education of chronically ill children. It emphasizes the potential of such technology for expanding existing services and allowing health professionals to use the limited time they have for patient contact more effectively.

2. Rodgers, B.M., Hillemeier, M.M., O'Neill, E., and others: Depression in the chronically ill or handicapped school-aged child, Am. J. Maternal Child Nurs. 6(4):266–273, 1981.

    The authors address three predisposing factors believed to contribute to depression in the chronically ill school-aged child: the chronic illness itself, latency-age developmental characteristics, and the family setting. Clinical manifestations of depression are identified. Guidelines are provided for nursing intervention in the areas of prevention, early detection, and management of depression in chronically ill children.

3. McKeever P.T.: Fathering the chronically ill child, Am. J. Maternal Child Nurs. 6(2):124–128, 1981.

    This selection is a study conducted to gain an understanding of what it is like to be the father of a chronically ill child. Interviews were conducted to elicit information on communication with health professionals, the effects of the child's illness on the father, the father's involvement with his chronically ill child, coping mechanisms, and fathers' main concerns. The implications for delivery of family-centered nursing care are discussed.

4. Craft, M.J.: Help for the family's neglected "other" child, Am. J. Maternal Child Nurs. 4(5):297–300, 1979.

    This article discusses the need for anticipatory guidance about sibling adjustment for the family with a chronically ill child. Symptoms of a sibling's adjustment difficulty are described. Facilitating honest communication, encouraging sibling participation in care, dealing with fear and guilt, recognizing the inevitability of sibling rivalry, and promoting family unity are identified as components of the anticipatory guidance process.

5. Oremland, E.K.: Communicating over chronic illness: dilemma of affected school-aged children, Child. Health Care 14(4):218–223, 1986.

    This article describes a participant-observation study of eight school-age boys with hemophilia. It describes chronic illness in childhood as posing a dilemma for the child who is forced to choose between normal participation in peer group activities and efforts to maintain physical stability as dictated by the medical condition. Suggestions are made for team efforts by parents, health care professionals, teachers, and the child to enable social interactions and group participation.

6. McLane, M.B.: Lekotek: a unique play library for families with handicapped children, Child. Health Care 14(3):178–182, 1986.

    This article describes the Lekotek program, a library of toys and other materials designed to facilitate the integration of the handicapped child into the family. By focusing on what the child can enjoy doing, Lekotek helps parents establish playful ways of relating to their handicapped child. The placing of the handicapped child in a normal context allows family members to gain new perspectives as the child gains an increased sense of competence.

7. Frauman, A.C., and Sypert, N.S.: Sexuality in adolescents with chronic illness, Am. J. Maternal Child Nurs. 4(6):317–375, 1979.

    This article addresses the necessity of incorporating issues of sexuality into the plan of care for the adolescent with a chronic illness in order to help the young person and his family lead as normal a life as possible. Suggestions are made for interventions to minimize both physical and psychological problems. The promotion of normal socializing and activity to alleviate isolation is stressed.

Impact of Life-Threatening Illness on the Child and Family

I. Chapter Overview

Chapter 23 introduces nursing considerations essential to the care of the child with a life-threatening illness. Since nursing students will be required to care for children with fatal illnesses, it is important that they gain an understanding of the family's reaction to the impending loss of a child and become familiar with the process of adjusting to this outcome. At the completion of this chapter, the student should know the impact of a life-threatening illness on the child and the reactions of and effects on family members. This knowledge will enable the student to develop nursing goals and interventions that will support the child with a life-threatening illness and his family.

II. Learning Objectives

Upon completion of this chapter, it is expected that the student will be able to:

1. Describe how death is interpreted by children of various ages.

2. Discuss the issues involved in informing the fatally ill child of his condition.

3. Define the stages of the grief process that may be experienced when the death of a child is anticipated.

4. List the phases of adjustment through which families progress following the diagnosis of a fatal illness in a child.

5. Describe the role of the nurse when caring for the fatally ill child and his family.

III. Review of Essential Concepts

1. _____ The concept of death is acquired through the sequential development of cognitive abilities and follows closely with Piaget's stages. (true or false)

2. The abstract adult meaning of death as irreversible, inevitable, and universal is not understood by most children until _____.

3. For the preschool child, the greatest fear concerning death is _____.

4. _____ One of the initial reactions of parents to the discovery of a life-threatening illness is to protect the child from the impact of the diagnosis. (true or false)

5. The initial reaction of parents following diagnosis of a potentially terminal illness is _____ and _____.

6. Identify three arguments for protecting the child from a knowledge of his disease.
   a.
   b.
   c.

7. List the three guidelines that should be used when explaining death to children.
   a.
   b.
   c.

8. Differentiate between the following terms:
   a. Acute grief—

   b. Grief work or mourning—

9. Identify the five stages that terminally ill people experience.
   a.
   b.
   c.
   d.
   e.

10. Briefly describe the characteristics that Lindemann has associated with acute grief.

    a.

    b.

    c.

    d.

11. List the four phases of the grief process according to Parkes' theory.

    a.
    b.
    c.
    d.

12. _____ is holistic care for the patient and family that is intended to maximize the present quality of life when there is no reasonable expectation of cure.

13. Identify the concepts that set hospice care apart from hospital care.

    a.

    b.

    c.

    d.

14. List the phases of adjustment through which families progress following the diagnosis of a life-threatening illness in their child.

    a. Phase I—
    b. Phase II—
    c. Phase III—
    d. Phase IV—
    e. Phase V—

15. _____ One of the most common manifestations of

overprotectiveness is parents' inability to set appropriate limits. (true or false)

16. One of the hazards of caring for dying children is the risk of _____.

IV. Application, Analysis, and Synthesis of Essential Concepts

A. **Experiential Exercise:** Interview children in various age groups to determine their perceptions of death. Answer the following questions and include specific responses to illustrate these concepts.

1. How do children between the ages of 3 and 5 years of age view death?

    a.
    b.
    c.

2. If a preschooler becomes seriously ill, how is he likely to perceive the illness?

3. By age _____ or _____ years of age, most children have an adult concept of death.

4. What factor greatly influences the school-age child's attitude toward death?

5. Why do adolescents have the most difficulty in coping with death, especially their own?

6. Identify at least eight nursing interventions that could be utilized when caring for a terminally ill adolescent in the hospital.

    a.

    b.

    c.

    d.

    e.

f.

g.

h.

7. List at least four ways in which the nurse can help
   children to develop positive attitudes toward death.
   a.

   b.

   c.

   d.

B. **Experiential Exercise:** Role-play the interaction
between a nurse and family regarding whether or not to
inform a fatally ill child of his condition.

1. Why is it often difficult for the nurse to determine
   whether or not a child is aware of his potentially fatal
   diagnosis?

2. Briefly describe the advantages of not telling a child
   that he has a terminal illness.
   a.

   b.

   c.

3. Briefly describe the disadvantages of not telling a
   child that he has a terminal illness.
   a.

   b.

4. What effect does the decision not to tell have on the
   following family members:
   a. Terminally ill child—

   b. Siblings—

   C. Parents—

C. **Experiential Exercise:** Care for a child who is hospitalized with a life-threatening illness.

1. Briefly describe the following five stages that a family
   proceeds through when there is an anticipated loss of a
   child and identify at least one nursing intervention that
   will support the family during these stages.
   a. Denial—

   b. Anger—

c. Bargaining—

c. Phase III, recovery: cessation of therapy and possible cure—

d. Depression—

d. Phase IV, recurrence: relapse and death—

e. Acceptance—

e. Phase V, the beginning: postdeath—

2. How does the grief process in the surviving family members differ when the child's death is expected as opposed to unexpected?
   a. Expected—

4. Why is it important for the nurse to understand and analyze her reactions when caring for a dying child and his family?

   b. Unexpected—

5. The following are the most common reactions the nurse may experience when caring for fatally ill children. Why are these likely to occur?
   a. Denial—

3. Briefly describe the following phases of adjustment through which families progress following the diagnosis of a life-threatening illness in their child. Develop at least two appropriate nursing interventions to be utilized in each phase.
   a. Phase I, revelation: diagnosis and treatment—

   b. Anger and depression—

   c. Guilt—

   d. Ambivalence—

   b. Phase II, reprieve: remission and maintenance therapy—

6. Why is burnout a hazard for the nurse who cares for dying children?

7. Briefly describe the four ways in which the nurse can learn to cope constructively with the stress of this role.
   a. Self-awareness and consciousness raising—

   b. Knowledge and practice—

   c. Support systems—

   d. Other strategies—

V. Suggested Readings

1. Martocchio, B.C.: Grief and bereavement: healing through hurt, Nurs. Clin. North Am. **20**(2):327–339, 1985.

   This selection examines the reactions of adults to bereavement, focusing on grief responses, factors that affect the responses of survivors, and facilitation of healthy grieving in family and staff. Some variables which may help to identify families in need of more intensive bereavement follow-up are presented.

2. Wong, D.L.: Bereavement: the empty-mother syndrome, Am. J. Maternal Child Nurs. **5**(6):385–389, 1980.

   This selection identifies the reaction of the mother whose chronically ill child has died: grief for the loss of the child and for the loss of the mothering role. The stages of the grieving process are discussed in relation to this syndrome. Specific nursing interventions are suggested to help these mothers resolve their grief.

3. Yoak, M., Chesneym B.K., and Schwartz, N.H.: Active roles in self-help groups for parents of children with cancer, Child. Health Care **14**(1):38–45, 1985.

   Self-help and support group involvement are presented as active coping approaches that parents can use when childhood cancer occurs. Such groups are seen as giving parents an opportunity to share themselves interpersonally, their skills and energies organizationally, and their efforts to improve the care of their child institutionally. It is suggested that health care professionals can play the most constructive role by providing active support and assistance to parental leadership.

4. Williams, H.A., Rivara, F.P., and Rothenberg, M.B.: The child is dying: who helps the family? Am. J. Maternal Child Nurs. **6**(4):261–265, 1981.

   This entry describes a family-centered approach to the care of a family with a dying child which includes the participation of siblings and members of the extended families. It offers guidelines which emphasize the unique skills and roles of each member of the health care team. The care process outlined includes the initial assessment, identification of high-risk situations, assistance at the time of death, and follow-up care.

5. Moldow, D.G., and Martinson, I.M.: From research to reality—home care for the dying child, Am. J. Maternal Child Nurs. **5**(3):159–166, 1980.

   This article describes the process by which the authors developed a pilot program and facilitated the development of community-based home care programs for children dying of cancer. The importance of educating both parents and professionals to new roles and attitudes is emphasized. The support of health professionals and lay consumers is identified as contributing to the project's success. Suggestions are offered for the development of similar projects.

6. Ross-Alaolmolki, K.: Supportive care for families of dying children, Nurs. Clin. North Am. **20**(2):457–466, 1985.

   This article reviews the effect on various family members of living with a dying child. The importance of facilitating communication among the child, parents, and care givers is discussed. Examples illustrate children's concerns and questions about the dying process, and the various ways in which the parents experienced and coped with their impending loss.

Chapter 24

The Child with Cognitive Impairment

I. Chapter Overview

Chapter 24 introduces nursing considerations essential to the care of the child with cognitive impairment. Since this disorder poses a special threat to the child's developmental potential, it is important for students to understand the care of children with this type of deficit. At the completion of this chapter, the student should know the factors that contribute to cognitive impairment, and be familiar with management. This knowledge will enable the student to develop nursing strategies that promote optimal realization of the child's potential.

II. Learning Objectives

Upon completion of this chapter, it is expected that the student will be able to:

1. Describe the major classifications of mental retardation.

2. Identify nursing interventions to promote optimal development of the retarded child.

3. List nursing interventions appropriate for caring for a cognitively impaired child who is hospitalized.

4. Identify the major biologic and cognitive characteristics of the child with Down syndrome.

5. Identify nursing interventions that will promote optimal development for the child with Down syndrome.

III. Review of Essential Concepts

1. _____ is the most common developmental disability in the United States.

2. Define *mental retardation*.

3. Why is the term *adaptive behavior* a critical component of the definition of mental retardation?

4. When is a diagnosis of cognitive impairment usually made?

5. The diagnosis and classification of mental retardation is based on _____.

6. Identify the four causes of severe mental retardation.
   a.
   b.
   c.
   d.

7. Identify nine prenatal, perinatal, and postnatal causes of mental retardation.
   a.
   b.
   c.
   d.
   e.
   f.
   g.
   h.
   i.

8. Differentiate among the following types of strategies used to prevent mental retardation.
   a. Primary prevention strategies—

   b. Secondary prevention strategies—

c. Tertiary prevention strategies—

9. Describe the Education for All Handicapped Children Act.

10. Why should the skill of independent toileting be taught after self-feeding skills?

11. The cognitively impaired child is considered mentally ready for dressing training if he can:
a.
b.
c.
d.
e.

12. _____ is a major consideration in the selection of toys.

13. _____ is the most common chromosomal abnormality of a generalized syndrome.

14. Approximately 92 to 95% of all cases of Down syndrome are attributable to an extra _____ chromosome.

15. How is the presence of Down syndrome confirmed?

16. _____ Children with Down syndrome usually have a normal intelligence level. (true or false)

17. What factors contribute to the development of respiratory difficulties in children with Down syndrome?
a.
b.
c.

18. Why do children with Down syndrome often experience feeding difficulties?

IV. Application, Analysis, and Synthesis of Essential Concepts

A. **Experiential Exercise:** Spend a day in an early intervention unit to observe the various methods used in the management of the child with cognitive impairment.

1. The major intervention for the prevention of mental retardation is _____ for the small premature infant and other high-risk newborns.

2. Identify at least two strategies in each of the following prevention areas that are directed toward eliminating or minimizing the effects of mental retardation:
a. Primary prevention—

b. Secondary prevention—

c. Tertiary prevention—

3. What is the major nursing goal of caring for children with mental retardation?

4. What must the nurse assess prior to teaching a child with subnormal intelligence?

5. Briefly describe the following models on which many early intervention programs are based:
a. Parent training/infant curriculum model—

b. Parent/therapy model—

c. Parent-infant interaction model—

6. Identify at least three nursing interventions that will promote the development of independent self-help skills in the cognitively impaired child.
a. Feeding—

b. Toileting—

c. Dressing skills—

d. Grooming—

7. For each of the following areas, identify at least two nursing interventions that will assist families in providing an environment that fosters optimal development.
   a. Play—

   b. Communication—

   c. Discipline—

   d. Socialization—

8. What areas should the nurse assess when a child with cognitive impairment is hospitalized?
   a.
   b.
   c.
9. Identify five nursing interventions that should be utilized when caring for a hospitalized child who is cognitively impaired.
   a.
   b.

c.
d.
e.

B. **Experiential Exercise:** Interview the parents of a child with Down syndrome to identify the major management problems related to this disorder. Answer the following questions and include specific responses that illustrate these concepts.

1. Briefly describe the following outstanding features of Down syndrome:
   a. Intelligence—

   b. Social development—

   c. Congenital anomalies—

   d. Sensory problems—

   e. Other physical disorders—

   f. Growth and sexual development—

2. Based on the above listed features, formulate at least three nursing diagnoses related to the care of the child with Down syndrome.
   a.
   b.
   c.

3. What are the three major objectives of therapeutic management of the child with Down syndrome?
   a.
   b.
   c.

4. What is the nurse's role when parents are informed of a diagnosis of Down syndrome in their child?
   a.

   b.

   c.

   d.

   e.

5. Identify at least four nursing interventions for each of the following nursing goals related to the care of the child with Down syndrome:
   a. Help parents prevent physical problems—

   b. Promote the child's developmental progress—

6. How can the nurse aid in the prevention of Down syndrome?

7. Suggested Readings

Brady, M.A.: Fragile-X syndrome: an overview, Pediatr. Nurs. **10**(3):210–211, 1984.

This article discusses a recently discovered syndrome that accounts for a substantial number of previously unexplained cases of varying degrees of mental retardation in males. Cytogenetic findings and clinical manifestations are described. The implications of the identification of this condition for research and practice are outlined.

2. Lepler, M.: Having a handicapped child, Am. J. Maternal Child Nurs. **3**(1):32–33, 1978.

The author, a pediatric nurse, describes her reactions during the period when she began to realize that her infant son was developmentally delayed. From the vantage point of personal experience, she identifies pitfalls to be avoided by professionals who deal with the parents of a handicapped child and suggests specific interventions to support the parents.

3. Tudor, M.: Nursing intervention with developmentally disabled children, Am. J. Maternal Child Nurs. **3**(1):25–31, 1978.

This selection identifies the need to provide a holistic continuum of care for the developmentally disabled child and his family with interventions based on the child's abilities and development. The primary goals of early intervention and some potential problems with this type of program are discussed. Specific roles of the nurse in prevention, case-finding, supporting programs, acting in the community, assessing families, providing health care for the infant, and assessing and promoting development are explored.

4. Silva, M.C.: Assessing competency for informed consent with mentally retarded minors, Pediatr. Nurs. **10**(4):261–265, 1984.

This article examines the complex issues involved in balancing respect for the self-determination of mentally retarded minors with the promotion of their well-being. It defines three elements of decision-making competency, describes five tests of competency, and presents a tool for the assessment of competency. The implications of both outcomes are discussed.

5. Roberts, M.J., and Canfield, M.: Behavior modification with a mentally retarded child, Am. J. Nurs. **80**:679, 1980.

This entry describes how behavior modification was used to modify the eating behavior of a child hospitalized with Down syndrome and tetralogy of Fallot. The effectiveness of withholding procedures in response to uncooperative behaviors is documented. The gains the child made over a 16-month period are offered as proof of the program's value.

6. Veach, S.A.: Down's syndrome: helping the special parents of a special infant, Nursing 83 **13**(9):42–43, 1983.

This article provides a brief overview of the factual information about Down syndrome as a basis for formulating interventions for the support of new parents. The elements of physical care, emotional care, and support which such parents need are identified.

7. Williams, J.K.: Reproductive decisions: adolescents with Down syndrome, Pediatr. Nurs. **9**(1):43–44, 1983.

This article identifies the potential problems associated with the fertility of adolescent girls with Down syndrome. The need for simple, appropriate sex education and the teaching of socially acceptable sexual behavior is stressed. Methods of contraception and issues related to sterilization are explored. The responsibilities of health professionals in this area are detailed.

Chapter 25

The Child with Sensory or Communication Impairment

I. Chapter Overview

Chapter 25 introduces nursing considerations essential to the care of the child with a sensory or communication disorder. Since these deficits pose a special threat to the child's developmental potential, it is important for students to understand the care of children with these types of disorders. At the completion of this chapter, the student should know the etiologies, detection methods, and management of sensory and communication impairments. This will enable them to develop nursing strategies that will promote rehabilitation and the realization of optimal potential in the impaired child.

II. Learning Objectives

Upon completion of this chapter, it is expected that the student will be able to:

1. Describe the general classifications of hearing impairment and their effect on speech.

2. Identify nursing interventions to be utilized when dealing with a child with a hearing impairment.

3. Describe the nursing interventions that are appropriate when caring for the hearing-impaired child who is hospitalized.

4. List the major types of visual impairment that are common in childhood.

5. Identify nursing interventions to be utilized in dealing with a child who has a visual impairment.

6. Describe nursing interventions that are appropriate when caring for the hospitalized child with a temporary loss of vision.

7. Describe the major types of communication disorders and their causes.

8. Identify the methods of assessment that can be utilized to detect communication disorders in children.

III. Review of Essential Concepts

1. Differentiate among the following terms:
   a. Hearing impairment—

   b. Deaf—

   c. Hard-of-hearing—

2. List five significant causes of hearing impairment.
   a.
   b.
   c.
   d.
   e.

3. In adults, the maximum sound intensity that does not produce sensorineural hearing loss is _____.

4. Match the following types of hearing losses with their defining characteristics. (Answers may be used more than once.)

a. _____ conductive

b. _____ sensorineural

c. _____ mixed conductive-sensorineural

d. _____ central auditory imperception

a. most frequently occurs as the result of recurrent otiti media

b. involves damage to the inner ear structures and/or the auditory nerve

c. results from interference with transmission of soun in the middle ear and alon neural pathways

d. most common of all types of hearing loss

e. deficits are divided into organic or functional losses

f. hearing is improved with the use of a hearing aid

g. most common causes of this are congenital defects of inner ear structures, or consequences of acquired conditions

h. refers to all hearing losses that do not demonstrate defects in the conductive or sensorineural structures

i. results in distortion of sound and problems of discrimination

j. results from interference in transmission of sound to the middle ear

k. also referred to as perceptive loss or nerve deafness

5. Differentiate among the following terms used to describe receptive-expressive disorders:
   a. Aphasia—

   b. Agnosia—

   c. Dysacusis—

6. How is hearing impairment described?

7. _____ Infants with hearing loss conpensate for the deficient auditory input with increased visual alertness by as early as 3 months of age. (true or false)
8. How does an infant learn speech?
   a.
   b.
   c.
9. The most common cause of impaired hearing is chronic _____.
10. One of the most common problems with hearing aids is _____, an annoying whistling sound usually caused by improper fit of the ear mold.
11. When is an individual considered to be legally blind?

12. Briefly describe the following classifications for the etiologies of visual impairment:
    a. Familial factors—

    b. Prenatal/intrauterine factors—

c. Perinatal factors—

d. Postnatal factors—

13. _____ are the most common causes of visual impairment.
14. Define the term *refractive errors*.

15. _____ Refractive errors are evaluated by testing visual acuity. (true or false)
16. Match the following types of refractive errors with their defining characteristics.

a. _____ myopia
b. _____ hyperopia
c. _____ anisometropia
d. _____ astigmatism

a. also referred to as far-sightedness

b. also referred to as near-sightedness

c. refers to unequal curvatures in the cornea or lens so that light rays are bent in different directions, producing a blurred image

d. refers to the ability to see objects clearly at close range but not at a distance

e. refers to a difference of refractive strength in each eye

f. correction involves the use of specially ground lenses

g. refers to the ability to see objects clearly at a distance, but the continued muscular effort to see things at close range produces eye strain

h. correction involves the use of biconcave lenses

i. treated with corrective lenses to improve vision in each eye so they work as a unit

j. correction involves the use of convex lenses

k. child often squints in an attempt to try and correct the defect

17. Define *amblyopia*.

18. What is the most effective method for treating amblyopia?

19. _____ refers to malalignment of the eyes.
20. What occurs when there is a malalignment of the eyes?

21. The most common type of strabismus is _____, an inward deviation of the eye.
22. Identify the three goals in treating strabismus.
    a.
    b.
    c.
23. Define the following terms.
    a. Cataract—

    b. Glaucoma—

24. The most common eye disease in children is _____.

25. Why are mobility and locomotion skills typically delayed in blind children?

26. What is the most traumatic sensory impairment?

27. Describe the effects that auditory and visual impairments have on the child's development.

28. Define the term *communication impairment*.

29. _____ are the most prevalent type of communication impairments.
30. Differentiate among the following impairments:
    a. Language impairment—

b. Speech impairment—

c. Nonspeech communication—

31. Identify some of the most common causes of communication impairment.
    a.
    b.
    c.
    d.
    e.

IV. Application, Analysis, and Synthesis of Essential Concepts

A. **Experiential Exercise:** Spend a day in a hearing clinic to observe testing, evaluation, and treatment modalities for the child with a hearing impairment. Answer the following questions and include specific examples which illustrate these concepts.

1. Why is the hearing-impaired child at a great disadvantage for developing social relationships?

2. For each of the following nursing goals, list at least three nursing interventions that would be utilized when caring for a child with a hearing impairment and his family.
    a. Prevention of hearing loss—

    b. Detection of hearing loss—

    c. Rehabilitation—

. What areas should the nurse assess when evaluating a child for a possible hearing loss?

a. Infancy—

b. Childhood—

. What type of speech is seen most often in children with a hearing impairment?

. Briefly describe how speech difficulties are manifested in children with the following types of hearing losses:

a. Mild conductive hearing loss—

b. Sensorineural hearing loss—

c. Central auditory hearing loss—

Why is it especially difficult to teach a deaf child to speak?

Formulate at least four nursing goals directed toward the care of the deaf child who is hospitalized.

a.
b.
c.
d.

For each of the above nursing goals, identify at least two nursing interventions to be utilized when caring for the deaf child and his family.

a.

b.

c.

d.

B. **Experiential Exercise:** Spend a morning in a vision clinic to observe testing, evaluation, and treatment modalities for the child with a visual impairment. Answer the following questions and include specific examples that illustrate these concepts.

1. For each of the following nursing goals, list at least three nursing interventions that would be utilized when caring for a child with a visual impairment and his family.

a. Prevention—

b. Detection—

c. Rehabilitation—

2. How can the nurse increase an older child's compliance with vision treatment regimes?

a.

b.

c.

3. What instructions regarding preservation of sight should be incorporated into a preventive health teaching plan for parents?

a.

b.

c.

d.

a. Prevention—

b. Detection—

4. Identify the five major nursing goals in the rehabilitation of the visually impaired child and his family.
   a.
   b.
   c.
   d.
   e.

c. Education—

5. Formulate at least four nursing goals directed toward the care of the hospitalized child with a temporary loss of vision.
   a.
   b.
   c.
   d.

3. Why is the preschool period considered to be a prime age for the detection of communication disorders?

6. For each of the above nursing goals, identify at least two nursing interventions to be utilized when caring for the child with a temporary loss of vision.
   a.

   b.

4. What knowledge must the nurse have in order to detect communication disorders in a child?
   a.
   b.
5. Identify the three methods that are available for assessing speech and language development.
   a.
   b.
   c.
6. Briefly describe the Denver Articulation Screening Examination.

   c.

   d.

V. Suggested Readings

1. Sataloff, R.T.: Pediatric hearing loss, Pediatr. Nurs. **6**(5):1 18, 1980.
   This selection emphasizes the relationship between good hearing and normal psychologic development. It defines the various classifications of hearing loss and provides a detailed discussion of the causes of hearing loss in children. Methods c detection and prevention of hearing loss in children are identified.
2. Campbell, S.L.: Some sound advice for managing a hearing impaired patient, Nursing 84, **14**(12):46, 1984.
   While this article addresses communicating with an adult patient who is hearing impaired, it provides several tips that are applicable for dealing with a child with a hearing loss.

   C. **Experiential Exercise:** Spend a morning in a speech clinic to observe testing, evaluation, and treatment modalities for the child with a communication impairment. Answer the following questions and include specific examples which illustrate these concepts.

1. Develop three nursing goals directed toward the care of the child with a communication impairment.
   a.
   b.
   c.
2. For each of the above listed nursing goals, identify at least two nursing interventions.

. Steffee, D.R., Suty, K.A., and Delcalzo, P.V.: More than a touch: communicating with a blind and deaf patient, Nursing 85 **15**(8):36–39, 1985.

This article utilizes a case study of a deaf and blind elderly atient to solicit suggestions for communication techniques to be mployed when such patients are hospitalized. Nurses, doctors, nd speech pathologists offered ideas from the perspective of eir specific professions. The importance of coordinated effort nong professionals in such a situation is stressed. Many of the ggestions are applicable to communicating with hospitalized af and blind patients of all ages.

Wassenberg, C.: Common visual disorders in children, Nurs. Clin. North Am. **16**(3):479–485, 1981.

This entry reviews the general characteristics of the normal e in children and traces normal visual development as the ba- s for understanding visual disorders. It discusses refractive ates, strabismus, glaucoma, and infection and inflammation as e prevalent visual disorders of childhood.

Tumulty, G., and Resler, M.M.: Eye trauma, Am. J. Nurs. **84**:740–744, 1984.

Short case studies illustrate various concepts related to eye auma. Vulnerable eye structures are identified and linked to e most common types of injuries. Emergency treatment, as-

sessment, and inflammatory complications are discussed. Interventions to alleviate the psychologic effects of a temporary loss of sight are outlined. The responsibility of professionals in prevention of eye trauma is explored.

6. Goldberg, R.: Identifying speech and language delays in children, Ped. Nurs. **10**(4):252–259, 1984.

This article divides communication disorders into language, articulation, fluency, and voice disorders as the basis for screening and for speech and language referral evaluations. A parent history instrument and guidelines for an open conversation with the child are presented as additional components of the tool. The use of the tool, its scoring, and value in screening are described in detail.

7. Biro, P., and Thompson, M.: Screening young children for communication disorders, Am. J. Maternal Child Nurs. **9**(6):410–413, 1984.

In this selection, communication disorders are defined as speech disorders, language disorders, and hearing disorders. The importance of isolating the specific problem is stressed. A table presents the name, format, administration, and cost of several language-screening instruments. Major language development milestones are also summarized in table form. The importance of early identification and treatment is discussed.

Chapter 26

Reaction of Child and Family to Illness and Hospitalization

I. Chapter Overview

Chapter 26 provides an overview of how children of various ages react to illness and hospitalization. Since children are extremely vulnerable to the stress of such experiences, it is important to understand their reactions. Children respond to these stressors in a manner consistent with their developmental level. A child's illness and hospitalization also have a profound effect on the family unit. At the completion of this chapter, the student will be aware of how the child and his family react to the stress of illness and hospitalization and will be able to intervene to lessen the trauma of these experiences.

II. Learning Objectives

Upon completion of this chapter, it is expected that the student will be able to:

1. Identify the stressors of illness and hospitalization most common in children at each developmental stage.

2. Identify the reactions of parents and siblings to the hospitalization of a child in the family.

3. Outline nursing interventions to prevent or minimize the stress of separation during hospitalization.

4. Outline nursing interventions to minimize the stress of loss of control during hospitalization.

5. Outline nursing interventions to minimize the fear of bodily injury during hospitalization.

6. Describe methods of assessing and managing pain in children.

7. Identify the role of the nurse in maximizing the growth potential of the experience of illness and hospitalization.

8. Outline nursing interventions to support parents and siblings during a child's illness and hospitalization.

9. List the admission procedures for a child upon arriv at the hospital.

10. Identify the goals of discharge planning and home care.

III. Review of Essential Concepts

1. What five factors affect the child's reaction to the stress of hospitalization?
   a.
   b.
   c.
   d.
   e.

2. From middle infancy through preschool years _____ is the major stressor related to ho pitalization.

3. The three phases in the crisis of separation are: _____, _____, and _____.

4. Adolescents experience the stress of separation primarily from their _____ rather than their family.

5. The three major areas in which children experience loss of control are: _____, _____ or _____, and _____.

6. The needs of children vary with age. Identify which age group the following responses to loss of control exemplify by placing the appropriate letter in the pr ceding blank.

   a. toddler

   b. preschooler

   c. school-age

   d. adolescent

   _____ They strive for autonomy, react with n gativism to any physical restriction.

   _____ The same feelings th make them feel omni potent also make them feel out of control.

_____ Explanations are understood only in terms of real events.

_____ The initial reaction to dependency is negativism and aggression.

_____ Respond with depression, hostility, and frustration to physical restriction.

_____ They often voluntarily isolate themselves from age-mates until they can compete on an equal basis.

_____ When routine and rituals are altered, it results in regression.

_____ Any threat to their sense of identity results in a loss of control.

_____ Particularly vulnerable to feelings of loss of control because they are striving for independence and productivity.

_____ Perceive illness or hospitalization as punishment for real or imagined misdeeds.

7. Parents respond to the illness and hospitalization of their child in a fairly consistent manner. What are the stages of reaction?
   a.
   b.
   c.
   d.

8. The defense mechanisms used by parents to cope with the stress of the illness and hospitalization of their child are:

9. Match the following defense mechanisms in the left column with the definitions in the right column.

_____ intellectualization

_____ projection

_____ displacement

a. transference of emotion or concern from one object or event to another

_____ introjection

b. parents turn all their blame, anger, and guilt inward

c. placing responsibility outside oneself

d. use of knowledge to control the intense emotional impact of illness

10. The siblings of the hospitalized child may react with feelings of:

11. With continued pain the body adapts and there is a _____ (increase, decrease) in physiologic responses.

12. The six scales that are appropriate to assess pain in children are:
    a.
    b.
    c.
    d.
    e.
    f.

13. Identify which of the following nursing goals are appropriate to decrease the effects of bodily injury and pain in children. (Mark C before correct goals and X before incorrect goals).
    _____. Preparation for painful procedures decreases fear.
    _____. Children should be encouraged to express pain.
    _____. Procedures should be explained at the child's cognitive level.
    _____. Insure pain relief by administering medication on a p.r.n. basis.

14. Programs to prepare the child and his family for the hospitalization experience are based on what principle?

15. Identify each of the following statements regarding bodily injury and pain in children as true or false.
    _____ Neonates' general reaction to painful stimuli is body movement associated with brief loud crying.
    _____ Toddlers are able to describe the type or intensity of the pain.

_____ Preschoolers' primary reaction to the stress of pain and fear is aggression.

_____ Distraction is an effective intervention for pain in infants.

_____ School-age children use passive methods of dealing with pain.

_____ Behaviors indicating pain in the toddler are: grimacing, clenching teeth or lips, opening eyes wide, rocking, rubbing, and aggressiveness.

_____ Adolescents react to pain with resistance and aggression.

16. Children's tolerance to pain _____ (increases, decreases) with age.

17. The three primary actions involved in pain assessment are: _____, _____, and _____.

18. The nurse assesses pain by observing _____ and _____.

19 The nurse should intervene on behalf of the siblings of the hospitalized child by teaching the parents to share _____ about the ill child with the siblings.

20. Play is the _____ of children.

21. Nursing interventions should focus on maximizing the potential benefits of the hospitalization experience by: fostering _____; providing _____; promoting _____; and providing _____.

22. Children may demonstrate temporary behavioral changes following discharge. Identify at least three of these behaviors.

23. List the usual admission procedures for a child.
    a.
    b.
    c.

IV. Application, Analysis, and Synthesis of Essential Concepts

A. **Clinical Situation:** Ronik, age 2 years, was admitted to the pediatric unit with a diagnosis of meningitis. When Ronik's parents briefly left the room, Ronik began to shake the bars of the crib, to scream and cry loudly, and refuse attention from the nurse.

1. When the nurse assesses Ronik's behavior she knows it is characteristic of the _____ stage of separation.

2. List at least one appropriate intervention to deal with Ronik's behavior.

B. **Clinical Situation:** Amy, 2 years old, was admitted to the pediatric unit for evaluation and treatment of a urinary tract infection. Both Amy and her parents appear anxious.

1. Identify at least three nursing interventions to accomplish the nursing goal of minimizing the effects of separation for Amy.
    a.

    b.

    c.

2. Identify at least two nursing interventions to accomplish the nursing goal of minimizing the effects of loss of control.
    a.

    b.

C. **Clinical Situation:** Roberto, age 4 years, is admitted to the pediatric unit with a diagnosis of gastroenteritis.

1. List at least three nursing interventions to accomplish the nursing goal of supporting the parents of the hospitalized child.
    a.

    b.

    c.

2. List at least three nursing interventions to accomplish the nursing goal of supporting the siblings of the hospitalized child.

a.

b.

c.

3. Roberto's mother asks you, the nurse, for advice on what toys she should bring to her child. With consideration for developmental needs and for safety, what types of toys would you recommend?

D. **Clinical Situation:** Manuel, age 6 years, is being admitted to the pediatric unit with a complaint of abdominal pain.

. What steps (interventions) should the nurse follow when admitting Manuel to the unit?

a.

b.

c.

. What steps (interventions) should the nurse follow when discharging Manuel?

a.

b.

c.

d.

e.

f.

V. Suggested Readings

1. Calkin, J.D.: Are hospitalized toddlers adapting to the experience as well as we think? Am. J. Maternal Child Nurs. **4**(1):18–23, 1979.

The author describes several scales based on Erikson's psychosocial growth that may be used to assess the responses of toddlers to specific situations related to their hospitalization. Areas assessed include toileting, eating, resting and sleeping, separation from and return of a familiar person, and indications of independence or emotional dependence on adults. The use of the scales to develop interventions that promote adaptive skills is discussed.

2. Riffee, D.M.: Self-esteem changes in hospitalized school-age children, Nurs. Res. **30**(2):94–97, 1981.

This study compares changes in self-esteem in groups of children aged 9 through 12 who were hospitalized for surgery, hospitalized for non-surgical reasons, and not hospitalized. Using the Coopersmith Self-Esteem Inventory, it was found that total self-esteem scores of children undergoing surgery dropped more than those of the other groups. Significant drops in scores were also noted in the peer-social and school subscales. Possible interventions to prevent these drops in self-esteem are discussed.

3. Denholm, C.J.: Hospitalization and the adolescent patient: a review and some critical questions, Child. Health Care, **13**(3):109–116, 1985.

This article reviews the literature over 30 years on the effects of hospitalization on the ''non-psychiatric'' adolescent patient. It provides information on patient self-reports, effects of illness, visitor preference, sex and age differences, methods of caring for the adolescent, and evidence of posthospitalization behavior. Questions related to each of these areas are raised for further study.

4. Beckemeyer, P., and Gahr, J.E.: Helping toddlers and preschoolers cope while suturing their minor lacerations, Am. J. Maternal Child Nurs. **5**(5):326–330, 1980.

This article addresses two nursing goals related to the fears of young children who have wounds needing sutures, reduction of anxiety and reduction of pain. Specific interventions and their rationales are supplied in the form of a detailed care plan.

5. Broome, M.E.: The relationship between children's fears and behavior during a painful event, Child. Health Care **14**(3):142–145, 1986.

This study examines the relationship between the level of fear of medical experiences reported by preschool children during an interview, their behavior during that interview, and their subsequent behavior in a highly threatening medical situation. The study confirmed that individual children differ in their degree of fear of bodily harm and that there is some relationship between these fears and the child's behavior. Further questions for research are raised.

6. Fore, C.V., and Holmes, S.S.: A care-by-parent unit revisited, Am. J. Maternal Child Nurs. **8**(6):408–410, 1983.

This entry describes a care-by-parent unit which provides cost-effective hospital services to children while promoting positive parent-child interactions, decreasing the emotional trauma of separation, and enhancing health care education. The way in which the nurse contributes to parental learning and parent-child interaction is noted.

7. Franck, L.S.: A new method to quantitatively describe pain behavior in infants, Nurs. Res. **35**(1):28–31, 1986.

This is the report of a pilot study conducted to demonstrate a method by which quantitative data regarding pain responses in infants can be obtained and evaluated. A video recorder was used to record the responses of normal newborns to a routine heel-stick procedure. The time of the observed responses and the time required to return to the behavioral state displayed prior to the procedure were noted.

8. Sheredy, C.: Factors to consider when assessing responses to pain, Am. J. Maternal Child Nurs. **9**(4): 250–252, 1984.

This article reviews the physiology of pain and outlines several variables that may affect pain in the hospitalized child. It describes the reactions to pain of children at the different developmental levels, exploring appropriate nursing interventions to evaluate, reduce, and manage these reactions.

9. Clements, D.B.: Reminiscence: a tool for aiding families under stress, Am. J. Maternal Child Nurs. **11**(2):114–117, 1986.

This article explores how reliving the traumatic events leading up to a child's hospitalization may help parents to deal with their guilt and anger. It suggests that, with proper support from the nurse or another health professional, the act of talking about an event helps to create personal distance from the event and growth and adaptation in all family members. Specific situations in which this technique may be used effectively are suggested.

10. Zweig, C.D.: Reducing stress when a child is admitted to the hospital, Am. J. Maternal Child Nurs. **11**(1):24–26, 1986.

This selection identifies the factors that contribute to the fears that children and their families may experience during the admission process. Components to be included in hospital orientation booklets are described. Helpful practices which nurses may use during admission procedures, from the admitting office through the diagnostic departments and arrival in the child's room, are explored.

11. Miles, M.S., and Carter, M.C.: Assessing parental stress in intensive care units, Am. J. Maternal Child Nurs. **8**(5):354–359, 1983.

This article describes a conceptual framework designed to assist the nurse in assessing parental stress in the Intensive Care Unit and in formulating clinical nursing interventions in this situation. Stressors are presented as arising from personal and family background factors, situational conditions, and environmental stimuli. Parental responses are viewed as resulting from interactions between these stressors mediated by parental cognitive appraisal of the situation, their coping responses, and available resources. Intervention strategies based on this model are outlined.

12. Kruger, S., and Rawlins, P.: Pediatric dismissal protocol to aid the transition from hospital care to home care, Image **16**(4):120–125, 1984.

This study examines the effectiveness of a written Home Care Instruction Sheet being utilized with parents of children being dismissed from a pediatric unit. It was found that the written tool increased the accuracy of understanding and follow-through of home care instructions, particularly in instructions related to physician's visits and diet. A higher level of problems associated with home care was reported by parents who received only verbal instructions.

13. Stein, R.E.: Home care: a challenging opportunity, Child. Health Care **14**(2):90–95, 1985.

This article examines the issue of home care for children with serious chronic health problems as an alternative to hospital care. The factors to be considered in selecting candidates for home care are identified. The essential components of a successful home care program are described, and potential pitfalls of such programs are presented.

Chapter 27

Pediatric Variations of Nursing Interventions

I. Chapter Overview

Chapter 27 provides an overview of the common variations of nursing procedures that must be implemented when working with children. Since children differ from adults in the areas of biologic, cognitive, and emotional function and response, it is important for the student to understand how nursing practice must be altered to meet the special needs of the pediatric patient. Small children who are hospitalized are separated from their usual environment and do not possess the capacity for abstract thinking and reasoning, which has ramifications both for compliance and for safety. At the completion of this chapter the student should have the theoretical basis to be able to safely implement nursing procedures specific to the pediatric population.

II. Learning Objectives

Upon completion of this chapter, it is expected that the student will be able to:

1. Identify those instances in which consent is required and those in which minors may be considered emancipated.

2. Describe the general guidelines for preparing children for procedures.

3. Describe how play may be incorporated into therapeutic procedures.

4. Identify strategies to enhance compliance of the child.

5. Outline general care and hygiene procedures for hospitalized children.

6. Describe feeding techniques that encourage food and fluid intake.

7. Describe the methods of reducing the body temperature of a febrile child.

8. Identify the factors that must be considered to reduce safety hazards to the hospitalized child.

9. Outline the problems encountered in the collection of 24-hour urine specimens in infants and children.

10. Describe correct procedures for the administration of oral, parenteral, rectal, optic, otic, and nasal medications.

11. Describe the procedures involved in providing nutrition via gavage or gastrostomy.

12. Describe the procedures involved in administering an enema or performing ostomy care for children.

13. Describe the preoperative, perioperative, and postoperative nursing goals and interventions for the child undergoing surgery.

III. Review of Essential Concepts

1. What is informed consent?

2. Three conditions must be met for an informed consent to be valid. What are they?
   a.

   b.

   c.

3. In relation to informed consent the nurse should know the state law regarding an emancipated or mature minor, and the age of majority. Define the following:

a. Emancipated minor—

b. Mature minor—

c. Age of majority—

4. Children, regardless of their age, require _____ to minimize the fear and discomfort experienced during procedures.

5. The nurse should plan an approach best suited to the individual child. What five principles should guide the nurse in developing her plan to prepare the child?

a.

b.

c.

d.

e.

6. What eleven nursing considerations apply when describing a procedure to a child.

7. Play can be utilized as part of nursing care. Play can be used to:

a.

b.

c.

8. The definition of compliance is:

9. When assessing compliance the nurse would utilize a combination of two measurement techniques. List the techniques used to measure compliance.

a.

b.

c.

d.

e.

f.

g.

10. Strategies to enhance compliance are grouped into three categories, they are:

a.

b.

c.

11. In order to care for their hair properly, black children need to have a comb with _____ and a jar of _____.

12. A nursing intervention to prevent dehydration and enhance fluid intake in the young child is to offer:

a.

b.

c.

13. One of the most common symptoms of illness in children is _____.

14. Match the following terms regarding body temperature with their definitions.

_____ set point

_____ fever

_____ hyperthermia

a. an elevation in set point such that body temperature regulated at higher level

b. body temperature exceeds set point

c. the temperature around which body temperature is regulated

15. In treating fever, the most effective intervention is the use of _____ to lower the set point.
16. Shivering will _____ (increase, decrease) the body temperature.
17. Discipline is necessary to insure a child's safety in the hospital. A useful discipline technique is the _____.
18. The method of transporting children safely is determined by their:
    a.
    b.
    c.
19. The mid-stream urine specimen procedure must be modified for the child who cannot void on command. What modification is necessary?

20. _____ may be utilized to increase the adhesion of the 24-hour collecting bag.
21. The method most used to determine accurate drug dosage for a child is?
22. The only safe method for identifying a child is to _____.
23. What are the preferred sites for injections in infants and small children?
    a.
    b.
24. There are several gastric feeding techniques; to differentiate between these techniques complete the following chart.

Inserted nasally or orally to the stomach _____

Inserted nasally or orally into the jejunum _____

Inserted directly into the stomach _____

Inserted directly into the jejunum _____

25. To prevent a gastrostomy tube from rotating and causing erosion and enlargement of the skin opening the nurse would:

26. Plain water is not used in an enema for children because, being hypotonic, it can cause _____.

27. Fleet's enema is not recommended for children.

What are the possible complications of this form of enema?
a.

b.

28. When attempting to measure eliminated fluid the nurse weighs the diaper dry and then weighs it wet. The difference in the weight is calculated as fluid. The formula used in this calculation is:

29. Tincture of benzoin or karaya powder or -gum is used around an ostomy to _____.

30. List the six stressful events for the child undergoing surgery.
    a.
    b.
    c.
    d.
    e.
    f.
31. One special fear associated with surgery is fear of anesthesia. Match the following:

_____ Fear of what will happen when they wake up

_____ Fear of possible death, change in body image, and loss of control

_____ Fear of anesthesis, operation itself, and possible death

a. Children under 5 years old

b. School-age

c. Adolescent

32. When explaining an impending surgical procedure to a 5-year-old, the nurse must choose her words carefully. Each of the words below should be avoided. Replace each word with a more suitable word or phrase.
    a. Pain—
    b. Cut, fix—
    c. Put to sleep—
    d. Incision—
    e. Organ, tissue—

IV. Application, Analysis, and Synthesis of Essential Concepts

A. **Clinical Situation:** Murray, 5 years old, is scheduled to have a lumbar puncture performed.

1. What interventions would the nurse institute to accom-

plish the nursing goal of completing needed procedures safely and with a minimum of stress for the child. List them.

a.

b.

c.

d.

e.

B. **Clinical Situation:** Ralph, age 13, is admitted for treatment of a fractured femur and is noncompliant of the medical regime.

1. Identify one nursing intervention to enhance compliance when the obstacles to compliance with the medical regime are: confusion, denial of illness, or lack of skills.

   a. Confusion—

   b. Denial of illness—

   c. Lack of skills—

C. **Clinical Situation:** Juan is admitted with a diagnosis of meningitis, and has a fever of 103 degrees.

1. How and when would you evaluate whether your intervention of administration of an antipyretic is effective?

2. What interventions upon the environment will help to reduce Juan's fever?

3. To insure Juan's safety you would always make sure the _____ are in the "up" position.

D. **Clinical Situation:** Jonathan, age 1 year, needed to have both legs restrained to protect the surgical site and the catheter in his penis.

1. What is the rationale for each of the following interventions?

   a. Applying a clove hitch restraint to Jonathan's extremities.

   b. Removing Jonathan's restraints every 2 hours—

E. **Experiential Exercise:** Spend a morning on a pediatric floor and survey the type, route, amount, and method of administration of the medications being administered to the children.

1. When administering an oral medication the nurse should try to avoid mixing it with food or liquid. If she must mix it, what guidelines (interventions) should she follow? Give a rationale for each guideline.

   a.

   b.

F. **Clinical Situation:** Debra, 1 day old, is admitted to the pediatric floor for medical evaluation. She has a weak suck reflex and cannot drink from a bottle adequately. She is being fed 1 ounce of Enfamil via gavage every 3 hours.

1. Give a rationale for each of the following interventions the nurse would perform when feeding Debra via gavage.

   a. Insert the feeding tube through the mouth—

   b. Place Debra's head in a hyperflexed position—

   c. When checking placement of the feeding tube, return aspirated contents to stomach—

   d. Secure the feeding tube to the cheek, not the forehead—

   e. Flow should not exceed 5 ml every 5 to 10 minutes—

   f. Flush an indwelling feeding tube with 1 ml sterile water—

   g. Position Debra on right side or abdomen after feedings—

2. Before inserting formula in feeding tube the nurse assesses whether the tube is correctly positioned in the stomach by:

   a.

b.

 . What interventions regarding gavage feeding are vali-
dated by these rationales:
a. Refed to prevent electrolyte imbalance—

b. So that sucking is associated with feeding—

G. **Clinical Situation:** Franklin, age 6 weeks, is admitted for surgical repair of a pyloric stenosis.

 . State at least two appropriate nursing diagnoses related
to Franklin's surgery.
a.

b.

 . Avoid keeping infant npo for more than 3 hours prior
to surgery. What is the rationale for this nursing goal?

 . What would the evaluation criteria be for the following postoperative intervention?
Turn infant every 2 hours and allow him to cry for at
least 3 minutes frequently to encourage deep breathing.

 . **Suggested Readings**

 . Silva, M.C.: Assessing competency for informed consent
with mentally retarded minors, Pediatr. Nurs. **10**(4):261–
265, 1984.
This article examines the complex issues involved in balanc-
ng respect for the self-determination of mentally retarded mi-
rs with the promotion of their well being. It defines three
ements of decision-making competency, describes five tests of
mpetency, and presents a tool for the assessment of compe-
ncy. The implications of both possible assessment outcomes
e discussed.

 . Rae, W.A., and Fournier, C.J.: Ethical issues in pediatric
research: preserving psychosocial care in scientific inquiry,
Child. Health Care **14**(4):242–248, 1986.
This article reviews the ethical considerations associated with
diatric psychosocial research. Concepts examined include
es of risk, risk versus benefit, informed consent of the parts, and assent of the child. The implications of each of these
ncepts for the pediatric researcher are identified. Five ethical
idelines for pediatric psychosocial research are presented.

 . Dininny, J.B.: Food rummy, the game of nutrition, Am. J.
Maternal Child Nurs. **2**(2):90–91, 1977.
A card game which colorfully depicts and labels various in-
vidual food items is described. The object of the game is to
ther in one's hand cards showing a well-balanced meal. It is
ggested as a useful approach to teaching and encouraging the

choice of both normal and special diets to children and adolescents.

4. Farrell, S.E., and Kiernan, B.S.: A positive approach to
nutrition for hospitalized children, Am. J. Maternal Child
Nurs. **2**(2):113–117, 1977.
This article presents a general guideline to intervention with
children from infancy through adolescence whose care may require some form of dietary alteration. Areas covered include the
diet history to be obtained upon admission, nutritional requirements in standard hospital diets and in children of different age
levels, criteria for assessing diet tolerance, fostering good nutrition practices, and education of the parents and other family
members.

5. Hansen, B.D., and Evans, M.L.: Preparing a child for
procedures, Am. J. Maternal Child Nurs. **6**(6):392–397,
1981.
This selection suggests that preparation for surgery and other
procedures should be based upon two factors: the developmental
norms for the child's age and the individual child's ability to
cope with problems. Children's observable strategies for coping
with problems are identified. Guidelines are presented which relate specific nursing interventions to characteristics of the child's
developmental stage.

6. Strohbach, M.E., and Kratina, S.H.: Diaper versus bag
specimens: a comparison of urine specific gravity values,
Am. J. Maternal Child Nurs. **7**(3):198–201, 1982.
This study compares urine specific gravity values obtained
from diaper specimens with those obtained from urine collected
in bags. There was no significant difference in the specific
gravity of the specimens collected by these two methods. The
study confirms the cost- and time-effective practice of diaper aspiration as accurate, and obviates irritating specimen bags to determine specific gravity.

7. Evans, J.L., and Hansen, B.D.: Administering injections to
different-aged children, Am. J. Maternal Child Nurs.
6(3):194–199, 1981.
This article discusses an approach to administering injections
which incorporates correct technique, principles of preparing
children for painful procedures, and principles of development.
Guidelines are presented for site selection and for administering
an injection to an infant, toddler, preschooler, school-age child,
and adolescent. When to tell a child about an injection, when to
administer a prn injection, and how to deal with the parents are
discussed.

8. Weitsching, J.H.: Reconstituting parenteral antibiotics for
children, Am. J. Maternal Child Nurs. **7**(2):128–133, 1982.
This entry provides guidelines for the preparation of antibiotics to be administered to children by way of intramuscular injection, direct intravenous injection, and auxiliary intravenous unit
infusion. Taking into account that children often receive doses
that are only a portion of the drug available in the vial, preparation directions give a final concentration once the vial is reconstituted. Eighteen specific antibiotics are presented in the
accompanying table.

9. Rimar, J.M.SS: Guidelines for the intravenous administration of medications used in pediatrics, Am. J. Maternal
Child Nurs. **7**(3):184–197, 1982.
This selection presents an extensive chart for the administration of intravenous pediatric medications. For each drug information is included regarding IV push administration,
intermittent infusion, continuous drip infusion, pediatric dosage,

the compatible infusion solution, compatibility with other drugs, and special instructions.

10. Perez, R.C., Becom, L., Jebara, L., Patenaude, Y. and others: Care of the child with a gastrostomy tube: common and practical concerns, Issues Compr. Pediatr. Nurs. 7:107–119, 1984.

This entry identifies the most common pediatric conditions requiring gastrostomy tube placement and describes the care of the child with a gastrostomy tube, including illustrated techniques for tube feeding, changing, and maintenance. In addition, it addresses issues related to growth and development, parent teaching, and emotional support.

11. Perry, S.E., Johnson, S.K., and Trump, D.S.: Gastrostomy and the neonate, Am. J. Nurs. 83(7):1030–1033, 1983.

This article describes the surgical procedure for the insertion of a gastrostomy tube in a neonate, as well as the postoperative management of the infant. Guidelines for a gastrostomy feeding schedule related to the weight of the child are provided. Care of the stoma and surrounding skin is discussed. Concerns related to removing the tube and complications related to the tube's placement are explored.

12. Bishop, W.S., and Head, J.J.: Care of the infant with a stoma, Am. J. Maternal Child Nurs. 1(5):315–319, 1976.

This article addresses the differences between the adult and infant stoma and the implications for nursing care. Care of the stoma is described in the immediate postoperative period, and dressing techniques are suggested for the convalescent period. The later use of a collection device is discussed. Issues related to the parent adjustment and education are explored.

13. Smith, D.B.: The ostomy: how is it managed? Am. J. Nurs. 85(11):1246–1249, 1985.

This selection provides a comprehensive review of the care of both colostomies and ileostomies. Photographs are used to illustrate techniques of stoma management. Factors to consider when deciding whether to irrigate the colostomy are outlined, and a detailed procedure for irrigation is presented. A table of *dos* and *don'ts* for postoperative care is provided as a general reference.

Balance and Imbalance of Body Fluids

I. Chapter Overview

Chapter 28 introduces the basic principles of fluid and electrolyte balance and the nurse's role in maintaining and restoring fluid balance. These principles are important because infants and children are more susceptible to fluid imbalances, and many of the common problems seen in this age group are associated with disturbances in fluid and electrolyte balance. At the completion of this chapter the student should have a basic understanding of the pathologic processes that produce fluid and electrolyte disturbances, the principles of fluid therapy and the role of the nurse in restoring equilibrium. This will enable the student to formulate nursing interventions when caring for a child with a fluid and electrolyte imbalance based on correct interpretation of clincial observations.

I. Learning Objectives

Upon completion of this chapter, it is expected that the student will be able to:

Describe the characteristics of infants that affect their ability to adapt to fluid loss or gain.

Differentiate between the various types of dehydration.

Identify factors that may produce an acid-base imbalance.

Identify nursing reponsibilities in maintaining fluid balance.

Describe the procedure involved in providing nutrition via hyperalimentation.

I. Review of Essential Concepts

1. _____ Extracellular fluid volume increases during childhood. (true or false)

2. _____ Infants are prone to disturbances in fluid and electrolytes because they have

a. decreased amount of surface area
b. a slower metabolic rate
c. decreased ability to handle solutes and water
d. decreased amounts trancellular fluid

3. The 6-month-old infant requires approximately _____ water in 24 hours.

4. Dehydration results _____.

5. _____ Sodium is the major osmotic force controlling fluid movement. (true or false)

6. _____ A sign or symptom of isotonic dehydration is:
a. seizures
b. serum sodium below 130 meq/l
c. signs of shock
d. increased urine output

7. _____ The most reliable indicator of the magnitude of fluid loss is
a. comparing the intake with the output
b. assessment of blood pressure
c. assessment of skin turgor
d. comparing preillness weight with current weight

8. The therapeutic management of dehydration is based on:

9. Acidosis results _____.

10. The normal value for the P_{CO_2} in the infant is _____.

11. Match the acid-base imbalance with its associated laboratory value change.

_____ respiratory acidosis	a. decreased CO_2
_____ respiratory alkalosis	b. increased T_{CO_2}
_____ metabolic acidosis	c. increased CO_2
_____ metabolic alkalosis	d. decreased T_{CO_2}

12. The etiologic factors that lead to respiratory acidosis are usually the result of _____.

13. _____ A condition that may lead to respiratory alkalosis is fever. (true or false)
14. List six etiologic factors in the development of metabolic acidosis
    a.
    b.
    c.
    d.
    e.
    f.
15. _____ is a common cause of metabolic alkalosis in infants.
16 An important nursing responsibility when caring for a child at risk for fluid and electrolyte imbalances is the _____ of the signs and symtoms.
17. _____ Careful intake and ouput records should be kept when the patient is receiving steroid therapy. (true or false)
18. _____ Specific gravity is a measurement of;
    a. sodium concentration
    b. osmolarity
    c. output
    d. active transport
19. _____ The presence of sunken fontanels may indicate fluid volume deficits. (true or false)
20. Cold extremities are the result of _____ peripheral blood flow.
21 _____ A hypertonic parenteral fluid solution has a solute concentration less than that of plasma. (true or false)
22. Modifications in equipment used for the intravenous infusion of children include the use of

_____.

23. List the conditions for which total parenteral nutrition is indicated.
    a.
    b.
    c.
    d.
    e.
24. Hyperalimentation involves the infusion of

_____.

25 The most common vessels used in hyperalimentation include the _____.
26. The major complication of TPN associated with the catheter is _____

IV. Application, Analysis, and Synthesis of Essential Concepts

A. **Clinical Situation:** Michael, age 3 years, was admitted to the pediatric unit with a diagnosis of 10% isotonic dehydration secondary to diarrhea:

1. What physiologic factors predisposed Michael to the development of dehydration?
   a.
   b.
   c.
2. How is the diagnosis of 10% isotonic dehydration made?

3. What is the first priority in the therapeutic management of dehydration and how is it usually accomplished?

4. Michael is going to have parenteral therapy to treat his dehydration. What nursing interventions could be utilized to prepare Michael and his parents? Appropiate nursing interventions would include:
   a.
   b.
   c.
   d.
   e.
5. What is the rationale for the use of a volume control chamber for parenteral therapy in children?

6. What assessments are made in Michael's general appearance that alerted the nurse to the presence of fluid and electrolyte disturbances?

7. What is the rationale for taking Michael's vital sign and weight immediately upon his admission to the unit?

8. What assessments should be made on Michael in the areas of neurologic and sensory status

9. List the nursing interventions that are utilized to monitor and maintain the intravenous site:
   a.
   b.
   c.
   d.
   e.
10. How can the nurse evaluate whether interventions aimed at preventing infection at the infusion site were effective?

B. **Experiential Exercise:** Care for a child who has an acid-base disturbance.

1. What laboratory tests are used to assess whether an acid-base disturbance is present?

2. Your patient's arterial blood gas is pH 7.25; P_{CO_2} is 50; T_{CO_2} is 21. What acid-base imbalance does this probably indicate?

3. What areas should you assess when caring for this patient?

4. What is the rationale for not administering intravenous potassium to your patient until he voids?

5. The patient is receiving parenteral therapy to correct the acid-base imbalance and the site is immobilized. What interventions should you institute to prevent complications from immobilization?
   a.
   b.
   c.
   d.
   e.

C. **Experiential Exercise:** Care for a child who is receiving total parenteral nutrition.

1. What is the rationale for infusing TPN solutions into a large blood vessel only?

2. List the metabolic complications that you should assess for in your patient.
   a.
   b.
   c.
   d.
   e.
   f.

3. List the nursing interventions you perform when caring for this patient.
   a.
   b.
   c.
   d.

e.
f.

4. What is the rationale for monitoring the child's blood glucose levels?

5. Care of the TPN line is an important responsibility. How would you evaluate whether your interventions concerning the care of the line are effective?

6. What is the rationale for not compensating for a decreased flow rate of the TPN solution?

V. Suggested Readings

1. Lander, J.D: Nursing care of children with fluid and electrolyte disorders, Iss. Comp. Ped. Nurs. **2**(2): 41–52,1980

   The major principles governing fluid and electrolyte balance are reviewed as well as a discussion of the characteristics peculiar to children that make them more vulnerable to these disturbances. A discussion of dehydration is presented. the nurses role in parenteral and oral therapy is presented.

2. Urrows, S.T: Physiology of body fluids, Nurs. Clin. North Am. **15**: 537–547, 1980

   Although this article is not directed toward the pediatric patient, the discussion of physiology of body fluids provides the student with an excellent base for understanding disorders that are frequently encountered. It addresses the basic principles of water balance, factors governing the movement of water, and the electrolyte composition of the body fluids. An excellent supplement to the text.

3. Menzel, L.K.: Clinical problems of electrolyte balance, Nurs. Clin. North Am. **15**: 559–576, 1980.

   An excellent review article on the causes of electrolyte balance, the signs and symptoms of electrolyte balance, and the laboratory studies used to diagnose the specific disturbance. A discussion of the treatment is also presented.

4. Mentzel, L.K: Clinical problems of fluid balance, Nurs. Clin. North Am. **15**: 549–558, 1980.

   The responsibility of the nurse in the detection of these conditions is addressed. The two types of fluid disturbances are presented in general terms. The laboratory data that aid in the assessment process are discussed. The clinical signs of hypo- and hypervolemia are presented.

5. McGrath, B.J.: Fluids, electrolytes and replacement therapy in pediatric nursing, MCN **5**:58–62, 1980.

A discussion of dehydration is presented. The aims of therapy for dehydration are discussed as well as the formulas used to calculate replacement therapy. Parenteral therapy and the importance of careful monitoring of IV administration are discussed. An example of an IV flow sheet is presented.

6. Birdsall, C.: When is TPN safe? Am. J. Nurs. **85**:73, 1985.

The compatibility of TPN with other drugs is presented. The use of other intravenous medications, such as albumin, and plasma, is discussed. How to prevent sepsis and what to do about air emboli are also addressed.

7. Doran, E.: Care of the Hickman catheter in children, Nurs. Clin. North Am. **18**(3);579–81, 1983.

The Hickman catheter is used for intravenous hyperalimentation. A discussion of what the catheter is, where it is placed, and how it is inserted is presented. The care of children who have this type of catheter is explored.

8. Neilson, L.: Interpreting blood gases, Am. J. Nurs. **80**: 2197–2201, 1980.

An excellent review of acid-base balance. The major principles are presented. Renal and pulmonary regulation of acid-base balance is addressed. The primary effects and compensating mechanisms are discussed as well as how to analyze blood gases. Clinical situations are presented to illustrate the content.

Conditions That Produce Fluid and Electrolyte Imbalance

I. Chapter Overview

Chapter 29 introduces the various conditions that can produce fluid and electrolyte disturbances. It builds upon the principles of fluid balance and imbalance that were addressed in Chapter 28. Students need to be aware of these alterations in health, because many of these conditions are extremely common in childhood. They are often a result of the anatomic and physiolgic structure of the child, and often the disturbances of body fluids that result are more threatening than the primary disorder. The more serious imbalances involve the gastrointestinal tract, cardiovascular system, and losses from burns. The knowledge gained from this chapter will help the student formulate effective goals and interventions when caring for children who have alterations in health owing to fluid and electrolyte imbalance.

II. Learning Objectives

Upon completion of this chapter, it is expected that the reader will be able to:

1. Differentiate between acute and chronic diarrhea.
2. Outline a plan of care for an infant with acute diarrhea.
3. Discuss the etiologic agents and modes of transmission in acute infectious gastroenteritis.
4. Describe the pathophysiology of vomiting.
5. Outline a plan of care for the child with hypertrophic pyloric stenosis.
6. Describe the nursing responsibilities when caring for a child in shock.
7. Discuss the pathophysiology of anaphylaxis.
8. Describe how a diagnosis of toxic shock syndrome is established.
9. Describe the methods used to assess a burn wound.
10. Discuss the physical and emotional care of a child with a severe burn.

III. Review of Essential Concepts

1. How is diarrhea defined?

2. List the four etiologic mechanisms that produce diarrhea in infants and children.
   a.
   b.
   c.
   d.
3. _____ Chronic diarrhea is often a result of an infectious process. (true or false)
4. _____ A common clinical manifestation of diarrhea is:
   a. shock
   b. overhydration
   c. metabolic alkalosis
   d. diuresis
5. _____ The most common causative agent of diarrhea in infancy is:
   a. meningococcus
   b. *E. coli*
   c. salmonella
   d. shigella
6. List the ways in which the diagnosis of diarrhea is established.
   a.
   b.
   c.
   d.
   e.
   f.
7. The usual approach for oral rehydration in mild diarrhea is to administer _____ within 4 hours and _____ over 6 hours in moderate diarrhea.

8. Why are antidiarrheal medications such as opiates and absorbents usually not given to children?

9. Intravenous fluid therapy in severe diarrhea is directed toward

10. Management of the child with mild diarrhea involves

11. _____ Intractible diarrhea of infancy usually is caused by an infectious agent. (true or false)

12. Most organisms that cause gastroenteritis are spread by the _____ or by _____.

13. _____ Rhinoviruses are the most common causes of winter diarrhea in children under the age of two. (true or false)

14. List the three sources that stimulate the vomiting center.
   a.
   b.
   c.

15. Why is vomiting common in hypertrophic pyloric stenosis?

16. _____ A clinical manifestation of pyloric stenosis is:
   a. the presence of bile-stained vomitus
   b. metabolic acidosis
   c. increased frequency of stools
   d. decreased urine output

17. Diagnosis is made on the basis of _____.

18. _____ Surgical relief of the pyloric obstruction is accomplished by a pyloromyotomy. (true or false)

19. The goals of the preoperative nursing care of the child with pyloric stenosis include _____.

20. The physiologic consequences of shock are _____.

21. List the three stages of shock
   a.
   b.
   c.

22. _____ The most common type of shock in children is cardiogenic shock. (true or false)

23. Why is metabolic acidosis a common occurrence in the child with shock?

24. _____ A clinical manifestation seen in shock is
   a. tachycardia
   b. widening pulse pressure

   c. increased urine output
   d. erythema

25. List the three major emphases of the treatment of shock:
   a.
   b.
   c.

26. _____ A drug used to improve cardiac output and circulation is:
   a. atropine
   b. aldactone
   c. dopamine
   d. indomethacin

27. The initial nursing goal in the care of the child in shock is _____.

28. Anaphylaxis results from _____.

29. Why is shock seen in anaphylaxis?

30. _____ A criterion used to establish the diagnosis of toxic shock syndrome is a diffuse macular rash. (true or false)

31. List the three methods that are used to assess the severity of a burn.
   a.
   b.
   c.

32. Why is the rule of nines not used to estimate the size of the burn in children?

33. A characteristic of a partial-thickness burn is:
   a. minimal tissue damage
   b. absence of pain
   c. involvement of a portion of the corium
   d. presence of visible thrombosed veins

34. _____ Blister formation is a characteristic sign of full-thickness burns. (true or false)

35. _____ A systemic response to a thermal injury would include:
   a. decreased metabolic rate
   b. decreased urine output
   c. hypoglycemia
   d. hypertension

36. Why is anemia often seen in patients with a burn injury?

37. The immediate threat to life following a thermal injury is _____.

38. The aims of the immediate treatment of a thermal injury are:

39. List the major complications associated with a thermal injury:

    a.

    b.

    c.

    d.

    e.

40. List the seven aims in the therapeutic management of major burns.

    a.

    b.

    c.

    d.

    e.

    f.

    g.

41. Match the type of permanent graft with its definition

    _____ autograft

    _____ isograft

    _____ allograft

    _____ xenograft

    a. tissue obtained from genetically different members of the same species

    b. tissue obtained from the patient's twin

    c. tissue obtained from the patient's own body

    d. tissue obtained from a different species

IV. Application, Analysis, and Synthesis of Essential Concepts

A. **Clinical Situation:** Leah, age 6 months, was admitted to the hospital. Leah's mother reported that Leah has been having frequent watery stools for the past 3 days. Leah's physician had placed Leah on an electrolyte solution to treat the mild acute diarrhea. Leah's condition does not improve and she exhibits signs of dehydration. Her admitting diagnosis is gastroenteritis. Upon admission, stool cultures were obtained for rotoviruses.

1. Why did Leah's physician believe that Leah's diarrhea was acute?

2. What factors might lead you to believe that Leah's gastroenteritis is caused be a rotovirus?

3. Develop three nursing goals to prevent injury (infection trauma) in Leah:

    a.

    b.

    c.

4. List at least three nursing interventions that can be used to assess the progress of hydration.

    a.

    b.

    c.

    d.

5. Leah was made npo upon admission. What would be an appropriate nursing diagnosis for Leah now that she is npo?

6. How would you evaluate whether the interventions were effective at preventing skin breakdown?

7. What is the rationale for monitoring Leah's blood pressure, and why does this complication occur in patients with diarrhea?

8. List six nursing interventions for the nursing goal of providing comfort:

    a.

    b.

    c.

    d.

    e.

    f.

9. Leah will be placed on a lactose-free diet when she goes home. How will you evaluate whether Leah's mother understands the dietary instructions?

B. **Experiential Exercise:** Care for a child who has hypertrophic pyloric stenosis.

1. List two nursing goals that you developed for the nursing diagnosis of fluid volume deficit.

    a.

    b.

2. What nursing interventions do you use to achieve the nursing goal of preventing vomiting?
   a.
   b.
   c.
   d.
3. What is the rationale for placing the patient in a high Fowler's position after the feeding?

4. What nursing diagnosis reflects the effects of hospitalization on the patient?

5. The patient is going home tomorrow, and the parents have been taught the home care for the infant. How would you evaluate whether your interventions were effective in teaching the parents home care?

6. The patient is weighed daily; the urine output is monitored closely, and vital signs, especially blood pressure are monitored closely. What is the rationale for these actions and what complication occurs in patients with pyloric stenosis?

C. **Clinical Situation:** Tina, age 17, was rushed to the emergency room. She developed a sudden high fever, a red macular rash, and low blood pressure. She has had her menstrual period for 2 days and has been using superabsorbent tampons. She was admitted to the pediatric floor with a diagnosis of toxic shock syndrome.

1. What factors in Tina's history are indicative of toxic shock syndrome?

2. List at least three nursing interventions aimed at the presence of shock when caring for Tina.
   a.
   b.
   c.
   d.
   e.
3. What is the rationale for placing Tina in a flat position with her lower extremities slightly elevated rather than in the Trendelenberg position?

4. What interventions could you develop to teach Tina to

prevent the recurrence of toxic shock syndrome? Tina should be taught:
   a.
   b.
   c.
   d.
   e.
5. Tina was placed on intravenous penicillin to treat the TSS. While on the penicillin she developed tachycardia, difficulty in breathing, dizziness, and angioedema. It was believed that Tina was exhibiting an anaphylactic reaction to the penicillin. Why do anaphylactic reactions occur.?

6. What is the most important drug used in the therapeutic management of anaphylaxis?

7. What nursing intervention could have prevented the occurrence in Tina?

D. **Experiential Exercise:** Care for a child who has sustained a thermal injury.

1. List at least ten nursing goals for the nursing diagnosis, injury, potential for infection, tissue damage.
   a.
   b.
   c.
   d.
   e.
   f.
   g.
   h.
   i.
   j.
2. What interventions prevent fluid overload?
   a.
   b.
   c.
3. How do you evaluate the success of the interventions in maintaining your patient's renal function?

4. What is the rationale for wearing sterile gowns, masks, and gloves while in the patient's room?

5. You notice that your patient is not eating all of the food on the plate. Formulate one nursing diagnosis that reflects this observation.

6. List at least four interventions aimed at promoting optimal functioning:
   a.
   b.
   c.
   d.

7. What is the rationale for monitoring the patient's bowel function?

8. What interventions do you use to meet the emotional needs of your patient?
   a.
   b.
   c.
   d.
   e.

9. How do you evaluate whether the nursing goal of preparing the family for discharge is accomplished?

10. The Cardex orders state that you should monitor the patient's output, blood pressure, and vital signs; if blood pressure falls, notify the physician. What is the rationale for these actions?

V. Suggested Readings

1. De Benham, J.J. and others: Initial assessment and management of chronic diarrhea in toddlers. Ped. Nurs. **11**(4):281–285, 1985

   The definitions of acute and chronic diarrhea are presented. The causes of chronic diarrhea are presented in chart form as well as narrative. A nursing assessment is provided that will assist students when they are in primary-care facilities. Management strategies are also addressed.

2. Morgan, S.R. and Parks, B.: What is the role of oral electrolyte solutions in diarrheal dehydration in children? Ped. Nurs. **11**(3):215–227, 1985.

   A review of diarrheal dehydration, addresses principles of mangement in mild dehydration. The purpose of oral rehydration solutions is discussed as well as their nutritional and electrolyte composition. An excellent supplement to text material.

3. Brown, L.K.: Toxic shock syndrome. MCN.**6**:57–60, 1981.

   A clinical example is used to illustrate the signs and symptoms. A table listing the signs and symptoms used in the diagnosis is presented as well as the possible causative factors. The nurse's role in the prevention of toxic shock syndrome is discussed.

4. Lushbaugh, M.A.: Critical care of the child with burns. Nurs. Clin. North Am. **16**:635–646, 1981.

   A comprehensive article that discusses all aspects of burn care. The initial management of the child with severe thermal injury, the care of the wound, rehabilitation, nutrition and psychosocial aspects of care are presented. Nursing interventions are integrated throughout this excellent article.

5. Dittmore, I.L.: Behavioral responses in the early recovery of a severely burned 4-year-old. Maternal Child Nurs. J. **12**(1):21–34.

   A case study of a four-year-old is presented as the vehicle for the exploration of the psychologic repercussions of a thermal injury. Common behavioral responses are illustrated throughout.

Chapter 30

The Child with Renal Dysfunction

I. Chapter Overview

Chapter 30 introduces the nursing considerations essential to the care of the child who is experiencing renal dysfunction. Students need to understand these illnesses, because diseases of the kidney are relatively common in children. Disturbances in renal function often are the most difficult to master because the complex anatomy and physiology of the kidney are essential to understanding how the pathologic process progresses. This chapter builds upon the principles of fluid and electrolyte balance that were presented in Chapter 28, because illnesses involving the kidney usually produce disturbances in the composition and volume of body fluids. At the completion of this chapter the student will understand the tests used to assess renal function, the more common disorders of renal function, the various types of dialysis, and renal transplantation. The student will be able to care for the child who is experiencing renal dysfunction in the practicum setting.

II. Learning Objectives

Upon completion of this chapter, it is expected that the student will be able to:

1. Discuss renal function in early infancy.

2. Identify the signs and symptoms that could indicate renal or urinary tract disease in children at different ages.

3. Discuss the various factors that contribute to urinary tract infections in infants and children.

4. Demonstrate an understanding of the etiologies and the mechanism of edema formation in nephrotic syndrome.

5. Outline a nursing care plan for a child with nephrotic syndrome.

6. Compare the manifestations and nursing care of the child with minimal-change nephrotic syndrome and a child with acute glomerulonephritis.

7. Differentiate between glomerular diseases and renal tubular disorders.

8. Discuss the clinical manifestations of obstructive uropathy.

9. Relate the pathophysiology to the clinical manifestations seen in hemolytic uremic syndrome.

10. Contrast the causes, complications, and management of acute and chronic renal failure.

III. Review of Essential Concepts

1. _____ Newborn infants are more likely to develop severe alkalosis. (true or false)

2. The kidney of the infant is less able to adapt to deficits and excesses of _____.

3. List at least five signs and symptoms of renal or urinary tract disease in children ages 1 to 24 months.

4. _____ The purpose of an intravenous pyelogram (IVP) is to:
   a. yield microscopic information about the glomeruli
   b. give detailed pictures of excretory function
   c. visualize the renal vascular system
   d. provide information about the integrity of the kidneys, ureters, and bladder

5. _____ is a reliable indicator of glomerular function.

6. The single most important host factor influencing the occurrence of a urinary tract infection is

   _____.

7. List at least five extrinsic factors that can lead to a urinary tract infection:

8. _____ The presence of alkaline urine inhibits the growth of bacteria. (true or false)

9. The three objectives of the therapeutic management of the child with a urinary tract infection are:
   a.
   b.
   c.

10. _____ The massive edema seen in nephrotic syndrome is a result of:
    a. inability to excrete excess sodium
    b. hypoalbumenemia leading to decreases in osmotic pressure
    c. narrowing of the renal afferent arterioles
    d. decreased urine output leading to increased intravascular volume

11. _____ A clincial manifestation of nephrotic syndrome is:
    a. hypertension
    b. coffee-colored urine
    c. proteinuria
    d. low specific gravity

12. _____ are the primary therapeutic agents used to treat nephrotic syndrome.

13. _____ A common side effect of steroid therapy is:
    a. growth retardation
    b. hypotension
    c. renal calculi
    d. constipation

14. _____ is a common immunosuppressive drug used in the treatment of steroid-resistant nephrotic syndrome.

15. _____ A high-protein diet is recommended for children with nephrotic syndrome. (true or false)

16. Match the clinical manifestation on the left with the renal disease on the right in which it is seen.

    _____ hypertension   a. nephrotic syndrome

    _____ hematuria   b. acute glomerulonephritis

    _____ anasarca

    _____ azotemia

    _____ increased serum lipid
          levels

17. List the three complications of acute glomerulonephritis that may occur in the acute phase of the illness
    a.
    b.
    c.

18. List the methods used in the diagnostic evaluation of acute glomerulonephritis.
    a.
    b.
    c.
    d.
    e.

19. _____ Water intake is restricted in all children with acute glomerulonephritis. (true or false)

20. _____ A drug utilized to treat the acute hypertension of acute glomerulonephritis is:
    a. digitalis   c. aterax
    b. apressoline   d. atropine

21. The function of the _____ is the reabsorption of substances and the function of the _____ is filtration.

22. Match the clinical manifestation on the left with the disease on the right in which it is seen

    _____ proteinuria   a. proximal Type II acidosis

    _____ massive hematuria   b. nephrotic syndrome

    _____ urine pH above 6.0   c. distal Type I acidosis
          with metabolic aci-
          dosis   d. acute glomerulonephritis

    _____ hypercloremic meta-
          bolic acidosis

23. Nephrogenic diabetes insipidus results from

24. List the clinical manifestations of nephrogenic diabetes insipidus
    a.
    b.
    c.
    d.
    e.

25. _____ A clinical manifestation of a chronic obstruction in the urinary system is:
    a. polycythemia
    b. anuria
    c. hematuria
    d. daytime or nocturnal enuresis

26. _____ Urinary tract infections are commonly seen in patients with obstructive uropathy. (true or false)

27. _____ represents one of the most frequent causes of acute renal failure in childhood.

28. The primary site of injury in hemolytic uremic syndrome is _____.

29. List the clinical manifestations of hemolytic uremic syndrome.
    a.
    b.
    c.
    d.
    e.
    f.
    g.
    h.

30. The anemia seen in hemolytic uremic syndrome results from

31. _____ A prerenal cause of acute renal failure is:
    a. renal hypoplasia
    b. Alport's syndrome
    c. dehydration
    d. obstructive uropathy
32. _____ Cortical necrosis resulting in acute renal failure can be caused by severe hypoxia. (true or false)
33. The prime clinical manifestation of acute renal failure is _____.
34. _____ Metabolic alkalosis is commonly seen in patients with acute renal failure. (true or false)
35. Treatment of acute renal failure is directed toward

36. The purpose of administering 50% glucose and 1 U/kg of insulin to the patient with acute renal failure is to _____
37. List at least five causes of chronic renal failure in children:
    a.
    b.
    c.
    d.
    e.
    f.
38. List the clinical manifestations of chronic renal failure
    a.
    b.
    c.
    d.
    e.
    f.
    g.
    h.
39. _____ Children with chronic renal failure are placed on high-protein, high-calorie diets. (true or false)
40. Treatment of renal osteodystrophy is aimed at

IV. Application, Analysis, and Synthesis of Essential Concepts

A. **Clinical Situation:** Barry, age 3 months, is brought to the pediatrician by his mother, who says that for the past few days Barry has been eating poorly, is running a high temperature, is sleeping much more than usual, and seems to be voiding large amounts. A urine culture is obtained. The pediatrician believes that Barry may have a urinary tract infection secondary to an obstruction and has him admitted to the hospital.

1. The nursing assessment yielded several signs and symptoms of renal disease in Barry. List them:
   a.
   b.
   c.
   d.
   e.
2. Why did the pediatrician suspect that Barry may have obstructive uropathy?

3. The most important nursing goal when caring for children with urinary tract infections is _____.
4. Formulate two nursing diagnoses for the child with a urinary tract infection.
   a.
   b.
5. List the nursing interventions used to care for Barry.
   a.
   b.
   c.
   d.
   e.
   f.
   g.
6. How would you evaluate whether the interventions were successful in teaching Barry's parents how to prevent recurrences.

B. **Experiential Exercise:** Care for a child who has minimal-change nephrotic syndrome.

1. Formulate one nursing diagnosis that is related to the presence of edema in this child.

2. List one nursing goal related to the susceptibility of this child to infection:

3. List the nursing interventions used to provide good nutrition to this patient:
   a.
   b.
   c.
   d.
   e.
4. What is the rationale for providing meticulous skin care?

5. List four nursing interventions aimed at conserving the child's energy.
   a.
   b.
   c.
   d.
6. What interventions should be developed to prepare the child for discharge?

7. How do you evaluate whether the interventions were successful in preparing the parents for discharge of the child?

C. **Clinical Situation:** Tina, age 6, was admitted to the pediatric unit. Tina's history reveals that she had a severe sore throat and had been on antibiotics. Her mother stopped giving them when Tina felt better. Her admitting diagnosis is acute glomerulonephritis. She is anuric and has severe hypertension. It is believed that she has acute renal failure, secondary to the nephritis.

. What nursing intervention might have prevented the occurrence of acute glomerulonephritis in Tina?

. What items should the nurse assess in Tina to detect complications?
   a.
   b.
   c.
   d.
. Formulate one nursing goal related to the alteration of fluid balance in Tina.

. List four nursing interventions to provide diversion in Tina.
   a.
   b.
   c.
   d.
List the nursing interventions necessary to maintain fluid balance in Tina while she has acute renal failure:
   a.
   b.
   c.
   d.
   e.
   f.

6. What is the rationale for placing Tina on a low-protein diet while she has acute renal failure?

7. How would you evaluate whether the nurse was successful at supporting the family?

D. **Clinical Situation:** Brad was admitted to the pediatric unit. He is severely dehydrated, tachypneic, weak, and has been vomiting. Laboratory examination reveals that he is experiencing a severe metabolic acidosis, decreased serum potassium levels, and has a urine pH of 7. A diagnosis of renal tubular acidosis is suspected.

1. Nursing goals for Brad are aimed at

2. List several interventions to be used when caring for Brad:
   a.
   b.
   c.
   d.
   e.
3. What is the rationale for stressing to Brad's parents the importance of continuing the citrate solution even when Brad feels better?

E. **Clinical Situation:** Betsy is a patient on the pediatric unit. She was first admitted to the unit with hemolytic uremic syndrome. She has recovered from the primary disease but now appears to have chronic renal failure. she is to be taught how to perform home peritoneal dialysis.

1. What were the signs and symptoms of hemolytic uremic syndrome that Betsy probably exhibited?

2. Formulate one nursing diagnosis related to the susceptibility of Betsy to infection:

3. List the three nursing goals aimed at Betsy's possible self-concept problem:
   a.
   b.
   c.
4. List the nursing interventions to be developed to promote optimal home care for Betsy:
   a.
   b.

c.

d.

e.

g.

g.

5. What is the rationale for Betsy's taking supplemental vitamin D?

6. List the nursing interventions aimed at treating Betsy's hypertension:

a.

b.

c.

d.

7. How would you evaluate whether nursing interventions were successful in assisting the child with the stresses of chronic renal failure?

a.

b.

c.

V. Suggested Readings

1. Thomas, C.K.: Childhood urinary tract infection. Ped. Nurs. **8**:114–119, 1982.

This comprehensive article defines the occurrence of urinary tract infection, addressess the signs and symptoms, presents the tests used in the diagnosis, and discusses the medications used in the treatment. The need for follow-up and prevention is stressed.

2. Stark, J.L. How to succeed against acute renal failure. Nursing 82 **12**:26–33, 1982.

A review of the function of the kidney is presented as well as the interpretation of laboratory data. The three major classifications that lead to acute renal failure are dissussed in detail, as well as the clinical manifestations that would be seen in each area. The treatment and nursing care are explored in detail.

3. Pickering, L., and Robbins, D.: Fluid electrolyte and acid/base in the renal patient. Nurs. Clin. North Am. **15**: 577–592, 1980.

A review of the anatomy and physiology of the kidney is explored as well as the role of the kidney in acid-base balance. The causes, clinical manifestations and treatment of acute and chronic renal failure are discussed.

4. Lopes, G.S.: A dietary approach to chronic renal failure. Issues Comp. Ped. Nurs. **6**:23–62,1983.

A review of kidney function and definitions of acute and chronic renal failure are presented. the dietary management of these patients is disscussed in detail. Plans are included for teaching clients about the dietary management of renal failure.

5. Dracopoulos, D.T, and Weatherly, J.B.: Chronic renal failure the effects on the entire family. Issues Comp. Ped. Nurs. **6**:613–629, 1983

The article was written by two mothers whose children have renal failure. It discusses the problems they faced and the effects of the disease on the whole family. Both the positive and negative aspects are explored. An excellent resource to assist families in the coping process.

6. Topor, M.: Chronic renal failure in children. Nurs. Clin. North Am. **16**:587–597, 1981.

The incidence and etiology of chronic renal disease in children is addressed as well as the clinical manifestations of the disease. The various treatment modalities are discussed with respect to all age groups. The effects of renal disease on growth i explored.. A discussion of transplantation in children is presented. The psychosocial responses of children at various developmental stages is addressed.

The Child with Disturbance of Oxygen and Carbon-Dioxide Exchange

I. Chapter Overview

Chapter 31 presents the theoretical basis of the care of the child with problems related to the transfer of oxygen and carbon dioxide. Interference with respiratory function may be a life-threatening disorder, because the body is unable to survive without a constant source of oxygen. Students need to have an understanding of these concepts since an alteration in the ability to supply oxygen is one of the more common problems encountered in childhood. Very young children are extremely susceptible to respiratory dysfunction, and often the effects are more serious. This chapter provides students with a foundation that will help them understand the nurse's role in facilitating adequate oxygenation.

II. Learning Objectives

Upon completion of this chapter, it is expected that the student will be able to:

1. Identify the significant differences between the respiratory tract of the infant or young child and that of the adult.

2. Identify the various diagnostic tools that are used to assess respiratory function or disorders.

3. Identify the correct procedures for postural drainage.

4. List the major signs of respiratory distress in infants and children.

II. Review of Essential Concepts

1. _____ A factor that facilitates respiration is the presence of surfactant.

2. List at least seven differences between the respiratory tract of the adult and that of the infant.

a.

b.

c.

d.

e.

f.

g.

3. Lung volume is _____ in the upright position.

4. The upper airways are less subject to constriction because

5. _____ Infants are more vulnerable to respiratory distress because:
   a. they have more alveolar surface area
   b. of narrow branching of peripheral pathways
   c. of presence of collateral pathways
   d. of diaphragmatic breathing

6. List seven items that would be included in a physical examination of the chest:

7. _____ The presence of intercostal retractions always signifies a disease state. (true or false)

8. _____ Wheezing in the older child usually indicates:
   a. upper airway obstruction
   b. large airway obstruction
   c. small bronchiolar narrowing
   d. presence of secretions in the alveoli

9. List the criteria used to assess a cough:
   a.
   b.
   c.
   d.
   e.

10. _____ Pulmonary function tests are used to assess tidal volume. (true or false)
11. _____ The purpose of angiography is to:
    a. visualize the chest
    b. detect bronchiolar obstruction
    c. locate aspirated foreign body
    d. investigate pulmonary hypertension
12. The purpose of a lung puncture is

13. The mode of delivery of oxygen is based

14. _____ Bronchial drainage is more effective immediately after aerosol therapy. (true or false)
15. Bronchial drainage is indicated whenever

    _____

16. Match the physical therapy maneuvers with their correct definitions

    _____ squeezing
    _____ vibration
    _____ percussion
    _____ clapping

    a. hands in cupped position and repeated strikes to the chest wall
    b. firm pressure is applied to sides of the chest during expiration
    c. a vibratory impulse over lung segment during expiration

17. List the goals of breathing exercises:
    a.
    b.
    c.
18. _____ Respiratory insufficiency is said to occur if the child has increased work of breathing and preserves gas exchange function. (true or false)
19. A pressure cycled ventilator produces

20. The nurse promotes effectiveness of ventilation by

21. List the indications for tracheostomy:
    a.
    b.
    c.
    d.
    e.
    f.
22. _____ Placement of the fingers for chest compression in infants is now determined to be at the middle portion of the sternum. (true or false)
23. _____ The use of the Heimlich maneuver is the recommended procedure for airway obstruction in the infant. (true or false)
24. List the cardinal, early, and severe signs of respiratory distress in infants and children.

IV. Application, Analysis, and Synthesis of Essential Concepts

A. **Clinical Situation:** Meghan, age 6 months, is a patient on the pediatric unit. She was admitted to the unit in severe respiratory distress. She was placed in a mist tent in 30% oxygen.

1. List 10 items that were assessed in Meghan to monitor the respiratory status:

2. Meghan is having her blood gases monitored. List the nursing interventions that are associated with this diagnostic procedure:
   a.
   b.
3. What is the rationale for warming the oxygen that is being administered to Meghan?

4. List the interventions that can be used to lessen Meghan's fear of the mist tent:
   a.
   b.
   c.
   d.
5. What is the rationale for making sure that Meghan's diaper is not too tight?

6. List the nursing interventions used to assure that the tent is functioning correctly:
   a.
   b.
   c.
   d.
   e.
7. What is the rationale for performing postural drainage before meals or 1 to 2 hours after feeding?

8. How would you evaluate whether the postural drainage was succesful in removing excess fluid?

B. **Clinical Situation:** Ramon, age 11 months, is a patient on the pediatric unit. He was admitted to the unit 1 week ago in respiratory failure as a result of having swallowed a small piece of a toy. A tracheostomy was performed.

1. What signs of respiratory distress did the nurse probably assess in Ramon?

2. Ramon had a bronchoscopy. What was the rationale for this procedure?

3. List the nursing interventions that are used to care for Ramon's tracheostomy:
   a.
   b.
   c.
   d.
   e.
   f.

4. What would you assess in Ramon to determine that he needed to be suctioned?

5. What is the rationale for inserting saline into the tracheostomy tube prior to suctioning?

6. List three nursing goals regarding the routine care of Ramon.
   a.
   b.
   c.

7. What procedure should have been used to attempt to remove the foreign body?

V. Suggested Readings

Cardin, S.: Acid-base balance in the patient with respiratory disease. Nursing Clin. North Am. **15**:593–601, 1980.

The role of the lungs in the maintenance of acid-base balance is presented as well as the values one would see on an arterial blood gas report in a patient with an acid-base disturbance.

Nursing implications in the care of patients with respiratory acidosis or alkalosis are discussed.

2. McFadden, R.: Decreasing respiratory compromise during infant suctioning. Am. J. Nurs. **81**:2158–2161, 1981.

An excellent article, which reviews the procedure of suctioning in the infant. The article provides excellent illustrations as a companion to the text material. This article is useful as a preparation for clinical experiences.

3. Neilson, L.: Pulmonary O_2 toxicity and other hazards of oxygen therapy. Am. J. Nurs. **80**:2213–2215, 1980.

This article defines pulmonary oxygen toxicity and discusses the etiology. It explores other hazards of oxygen toxicity, such as RLF and hypoventilation. Methods are discussed to prevent these problems

4. Neilson, L.: Ventilators and how they work. Am. J. Nurs. **80**:2201–2205, 1980.

A comprehensive article that addresses the various types of ventilators, the functions of the dials, settings, and the alarms. A case situation is presented to illustrate the material that was presented.

5. Neilson, L.: Potential problems of mechanical ventilation. Am. J. Nurs. **80**:2206–2213, 1980.

The problems associated with mechanical ventilation are presented in three areas: problems related to artificial control, problems related to pressure, and problems related to artifical air. The signs and symptoms are addressed. A review of breath sounds is also disscussed.

6. Lichtenstein, M.A.: Pediatric home tracheostomy care; a parent's guide. Ped. Nurs. **12**:41–48, 69, 1986.

This superb article can be used to teach parents how to care for their child with a tracheostomy. The contents of this article, along with the pictures and checklists, can be used by students in the clinical area as a teaching tool. All aspects of care are discussed in detail.

7. Hoops, E. J.: Cardiopulmonary resuscitation in children. Nurs. Clin. North Am. **16**:623–634, 1981.

A review of the prearrest preparation and the necessary equipment. The causes of arrest as well as the early signs are explored. The procedures, medications used, and the postarrest care are discussed in detail.

Chapter 32

The Child with Respiratory Dysfunction

I. Chapter Overview

Chapter 32 introduces nursing considerations essential to the care of the child experiencing respiratory dysfunction. Because some of the most common problems in the pediatric age group are related to disturbed respiratory function, and respiratory failure is the chief cause of morbidity in the newborn period, it is important for the student to gain an understanding of the care of children with these types of disorders. The conditions discussed in this chapter impair the exchange of oxygen and/or carbon dioxide and are often more serious in young children. At the completion of this chapter, the student will be able to formulate nursing goals and identify nursing responsibilities to assist the child and his family to effectively cope with the physical, emotional, and psychosocial stressors imposed by an alteration in respiratory function.

II. Learning Objectives

Upon completion of this chapter, it is expected that the reader will be able to:

1. Describe the clinical manifestations of a respiratory infection in children.

2. Outline a nursing care plan for a child with an upper respiratory tract infection.

3. Describe the postoperative nursing care of the child who has a tonsillectomy.

4. Describe the nursing care of the child who has otitis media.

5. Outline a nursing care plan for a child who has a lower respiratory tract infection.

6. Differentiate among the various types of pneumonia in terms of etiology, clinical manifestations, and therapeutic management.

7. Identify the infectious respiratory disorders that are capable of causing significant morbidity.

8. Demonstrate an understanding of the ways in which inhalation of noninfectious irritants produces pulmonary dysfunction.

9. Describe the various modalities used to treat asthma.

10. Outline a plan for teaching home care of the child with bronchial asthma.

11. Describe the physiologic effects of cystic fibrosis on the gastrointestinal and pulmonary systems.

12. Outline a plan of care for a child who has cystic fibrosis.

III. Review of Essential Concepts

1. _____ is the chief cause of morbidity in the neonatal period.

2. What are the factors that influence the incidence and severity of respiratory infections?
   a.
   b.
   c.

3. The largest percentage of infections is caused by _____.

4. What is the factor that causes an increased incidence of respiratory tract infections in infants and young children?

5. Explain why size is a significant variable in respiratory infection of the child.
   a.

b.

c.

VIRAL	BACTERIAL
a.	b.
c.	d.
e.	f.
g.	h.
i.	j.
k.	l.

6. Infants and young children develop generalized signs and symptoms as well as local symptoms within respiratory infection. Identify the following statements as true or false.

_____ Newborns may not develop a fever even with severe infections.

_____ The 6-month to 3-year-old will develop fever even with a mild respiratory illness.

_____ Febrile convulsions occur with a gradual rise in temperature.

_____ Menigeal signs without infection of the meninges may be present in small children who present with an abrupt onset of fever.

_____ Vomiting is uncommon with respiratory infection.

_____ Diarrhea may accompany respiratory infection.

_____ Abdominal pain is an uncommon complaint in small children with a respiratory infection.

_____ Respiratory illness causes difficulty with feeding owing to nasal blockage.

_____ Children with a respiratory infection often complain of a sore throat.

_____ Penicillin is the drug of choice for a viral respiratory infection.

7. _____ may be instilled to clear nasal passages and promote feeding.

8. What is the rationale for use of warm or cool mist?

9. What is a quick method of producing humidification?

10. The therapy for nasopharyngitis is primarily _____.

11. If a child is coughing but has a profuse nasal discharge, potent antitussives are avoided. Why?

12. _____ are ineffective in treating nasopharyngitis and tend, as a side effect, to _____ children.

13. Acute pharyngitis of bacterial origin is usually caused by _____.

14. Compare the signs and symptoms of viral vs bacterial pharyngitis by completing the following chart.

15. A _____ must be done to differentiate between a viral and hemolytic streptococcal infection.

16. The recommended treatment for a streptococcal sore throat is:

17. If a child is sensitive to penicillin, the drug of choice for streptococcal sore throat is _____.

18. Children with streptococcal infection are noninfectious to others within a _____ _____.

19. The function of the tonsils is:

20. The _____ are those removed during a tonsillectomy.

21. The pharyngeal tonsils are also known as the _____.

22. The clinical manifestations of tonsillitis are chiefly caused by _____. Because of swelling, the child has difficulty _____ and _____.

23. Because of the proximity of the adenoids to the eustachian tubes, adenoids cause:

24. The indication for the tonsillectomy and adenoidectomy procedure is controversial. A tonsillectomy is recommended when:

An adenoidectomy is recommended when.

25. Tonsils should not be removed until after 3 or 4 years of age. Why?
    a.
    b.

26. The major complication of a T and A is _____.

27. The terminology regarding otitis media is confusing. List the accepted definitions for the following terms:
    a. Otitis media—

b. Acute otitis media—

c. Otitis media with effusion—

d. Subacute otitis media—

e. Chronic otitis media with effusion—

28. Acute otitis media is most frequently caused by

29. The etiology of the noninfectious type of otitis media is unknown, although it is a frequent result of _____ from the edema of allergic rhinitis or hypertrophic adenoids.
30. What factors predispose infants and young children to development of otitis media.
   a.

   b.

   c.

   d.

   e.

31. The principal functional consequence of prolonged middle ear pathology is _____.
32. In acute otitis media otoscopy reveals an

33. The antimicrobial of choice for initial treatment of acute otitis media is _____ or _____.

34. Following antibiotic therapy, the child should be evaluated for the effectiveness of the treatment to identify the potential complication of _____.
35. _____ are often utilized to treat otitis media with effusion.
36. Croup is usually described according to
37. The most serious complication of croup is
38. The major objective in medical management of laryngotracheobronchitis (LTB) is maintaining an _____ and providing for _____
39. Why is the child with LTB placed in an atmosphere of high humidity with cool mist? State the rationale.

40. Acute epiglottitis is
41. Epiglottitis presents with a _____ epiglottis.
42. The nurse should not examine the throat of a child with suspected epiglottitis with a tongue depressor because:
43. The _____ is the causative agent of 50 to 75% of the cases of bronchiolitis.
44. The primary pathophysiological process in bronchiolitis that causes difficulty is:

45. Asthma is differentiated from bronchiolitis when:

46. Pneumonia is caused by four etiologic processes: _____, _____, _____, and _____.

47. The etiologic agent of pneumonia is identified from:

48. Pertussis, also known as _____, is an acute respiratory infection caused by _____
49. The causative organism in tuberculosis is _____
50. In the absence of positive evidence, diagnosis of tu-

berculosis (TB) is based on information derived from the

1. The single most important therapeutic modality for TB is _____.
2. What are the three most commonly used drugs to treat TB?
   a.
   b.
   c.
3. The only certain means to prevent tuberculosis is to _____ with the tubercle bacillus. Limited immunity can be produced by administration of the _____ vaccine.
4. Small children are particularly vulnerable to aspiration of foreign bodies because

5. Initially, a foreign body in the air passages produces

6. Foreign bodies are usually removed by direct _____ and _____.

7. It is the obligation of nurses to learn two simple procedures to treat aspiration of a foreign body. The nurse should learn and teach the following techniques: _____ and the _____.

8. It is important to use these techniques only when a child is truly in distress. A child who is in distress _____, _____, and _____.

9. Aspiration rarely causes death from asphyxia. The irritated mucous membrane becomes a site for

10. The most serious complication of ingesting hydrocarbons is _____.

11. What is the rationale for not inducing vomiting in the child who has ingested a hydrocarbon?

12. The major nursing goal regarding aspiration is aimed at _____.

13. Smoke inhalation causes three different types of injury:
    a.
    b.
    c.
Gases that are nontoxic to the airways can cause injury and death by interfering with or inhibiting cellular respiration. _____ is responsible for more than half of the fatal poisonings in the United States.
The symptoms of carbon monoxide are secondary to tissue hypoxia and vary with the level of carboxyhemoglobin. The treatment for a suspected poisoning is the administration of _____.

66. _____ during childhood may well be the most important precursor of chronic lung disease in the adult.
67. Therapy for allergic rhinitis is directed toward avoidance of offending _____.
68. Allergens are identified through_____.
69. Treatment of allergic rhinitis is by:
    a.
    b.
    c.
70. Bronchial asthma is defined as:

71. The usual cause of asthmatic manifestations is an

72. Identify three mechanisms that are responsible for the obstructive symptoms of asthma.
    a.

    b.

    c.

73. _____ is the central physiologic feature in the clinical manifestations of asthma. This forces the individual to breathe at a _____ _____.
74. The most prominent complications associated with asthma are:

75. A characteristic substance in the sputum of the asthmatic child is the presence of _____ and _____.
76. The overall goal of asthma management is to _____ and to _____ and _____ and to help the child to live as normal and happy a life as possible.
77. _____ control is basic to any therapeutic plan.
78. The goal of drug therapy is to _____.
Early recognition and treatment at the onset are most important for _____ effect.
79. _____ are the major therapeutic agents for the relief of bronchospasm.
80. What are the two types of bronchodilator drugs?
    a.
    b.

81. The most effective and versatile asthmatic drugs are the _____ drugs.
82. What is the role of exercise in the management of asthma?

83. What components of physical therapy are essential to the management of the asthmatic child?
    a.
    b.
    c.
    d.
84. The most frequently prescribed drug is _____. _____ must be monitored when this drug is being administered.
85. Define *status asthmaticus*.

86. The drug of choice for status asthmaticus is _____. What are the side effects of this drug?

87. When aminophylline is being administered intravenously the nurse must monitor the child for side effects. What are they?

88. Parental responses to the asthmatic child with emotional disturbances range from _____ to _____.
89. Cystic fibrosis is a _____.
90. Cystic fibrosis is inherited as an _____.
91. The primary pathologic factor in cystic fibrosis is

92. _____ are present in almost all children with cystic fibrosis and constitute the most serious threat to life.
93. Describe the effects of thickened secretions on the gastrointestinal tract of the child with cystic fibrosis.

94. Excessive stool fat is termed _____ and excessive stool protein is termed _____.

95. The earliest manifestation of cystic fibrosis is _____ in the newborn.
96. Owing to the large amount of undigested food excreted, the stools of the child with cystic fibrosis become _____.
97. The diagnosis of cystic fibrosis is based on four findings; list them.
    a.
    b.
    c.
    d.
98. The presence of a positive _____ is characteristic of cystic fibrosis.
99. The child with cystic fibrosis should be placed on a diet that is _____.
100. Pancreatic enzyme replacement is given, in conjunction with meals and snacks, to the child with cystic fibrosis. The most commonly used drug is _____.
101. The goal of pulmonary therapy is:

102. What three techniques are utilized to improve ventilation in the child with cystic fibrosis?
    a.
    b.
    c.
103. The ultimate prognosis for the child with cystic fibrosis is determined by the degree of _____.

IV. Application, Analysis, and Synthesis of Essential Concepts

A. **Clinical Situation:** Theodore, age 6 months, is hospitalized with an acute upper respiratory infection. Theodore has a fever (104°), rhinitis, nasal congestion, difficulty feeding, and diarrhea.

1. List the possible nursing diagnoses for Theodore.
    a.

    b.

    c.

    d.

e.

f.

g.

h.

i.

B. Clinical Situation: Kara, age 7 years, has returned
to the recovery unit from the operating room after having
tonsillectomy and adenoidectomy.

. There are two nursing goals for the postop complication of hemorrhage.
a. List the interventions that would accomplish the
   nursing goal of detecting bleeding.

b. List the interventions that would accomplish the
   nursing goal of preventing bleeding.

What evaluation data would indicate that the above
nursing goals have been accomplished?

List the types of fluids that you would offer to Kara to
promote adequate hydration?

C. Clinical Situation: Karen, age 11 months, is seen
the pediatrician's office for a complaint of ear pain and
ever of 102°. A diagnosis of otitis media is made:

You would intervene with Karen's parents by teaching
them the signs of otitis media. List the signs.

2. What interventions regarding drug therapy will accomplish the nursing goal of "prevention of complications"?

D. Clinical Situation: Peter, age 20 months, is admitted to the pediatric unit with a diagnosis of acute laryngotracheobronchitis. His symptoms on admission included
fever, horseness, a brassy cough, pallor, rales and rhonchi, and restlessness.

1. What would you assess to establish Peter's respiratory
status and detect any impending airway obstruction?

2. Identify the nursing goals appropriate for Peter.
a.
b.
c.
d.
e.
f.
3. What is the rationale for the use of high humidity with
cool mist?

E. Experiential Exercise: Spend a day on a pediatric
unit and observe the children admitted for treatment of
pneumonia. Differentiate among the various types of
pneumonia by completing the following chart.

	VIRAL	PRIMARY ATYPICAL	BACTERIA
Etiology	1.	2.	3.
Clinical Manifestations	4.	5.	6.
Therapeutic Management	7.	8.	9.

F. **Experiential Exercise:** Observe small children at play.

1. List at least two of the nursing measures necessary to prevent aspiration of foreign bodies and liquids by children.
   a.

   b.

G. **Clinical Situation:** Alice, a 6-year-old white female, came to the emergency room with acute respiratory distress. Her mother noted that she was well until an hour before, when she began to cough without production and "couldn't catch her breath." There is a family history of asthma (her father) and hay fever (her mother).

1. When you take a nursing history from Alice and her mother, what are the pertinent findings that you know predispose her to asthma?

2. What signs and symptoms of an acute asthmatic attack did you assess in Alice?

3. As the attack progessses, what additional symptoms would you expect to assess.

4. Alice will be treated with epinephrine. Before administering this drug, the nurse should know the intended effects and side effects of the drug.
   a. Intended effect—
   b. Side effects—

5. What parameters would you use to assess Alice's condition?

H. **Experiential Exercise:** You are assigned to a pulmonary clinic where you will teach self-care to an asthmatic child. What are the three main objectives of self-management?

a.
b.

c.

I. **Clinical Situation:** Dennis, age 3 years, is hospitalized for treatment of cystic fibrosis.

1. List the possible nursing diagnoses that are essential to planning the nursing care of Dennis.
   a.

   b.

   c.

   d.

   e.

   f.

   g.

   h.

   i.

   j.

2. What are the evaluative data that would give evidence of the attainment of the nursing goal, "assist the patient to expectorate sputum"?

3. Give a rationale for each of the following clinical manifestations that Dennis displays.
   a. Respiratory symptoms—

   b. Large, bulky, frothy, foul smelling stools—

   c. Voracious appetite—

   d. Weight loss—

   e. Anemia and bruising—

4. Dennis will be going home soon and his mother must be taught the pulmonary therapy necessary for Dennis's care. You would intervene by teaching what two procedures?
   a.
   b.

Suggested Readings

1. Adams, J.L., Evans, G.A., and Roberts, J.E.: Diagnosing and treating otitis media with effusion, Am. J. Maternal Child Nurs. 9(1):22–28, 1984.
This selection reviews the distinguishing features and pathophysiology of otitis media with effusion. The various courses the condition may follow are discussed. Examination techniques and treatment protocols and their possible ramifications are presented in considerable detail.

2. Sataloff, R.T., and Colton C.M.: Otitis media: a common childhood infection, Am. J. Nurs. 81(8):1480–1483, 1981.
This article provides a comparison of the most common types of childhood otitis media in terms of their etiology, pathophysiology, and treatment. The commonly used diagnostic procedures are described. Nursing considerations for the particular problems associated with each type of the disorder are emphasized.

3. Simpkins, R.: Croup and epiglottitis, Am. J. Nurs. 81(3):519–520, 1981.
This entry compares viral croup and epiglottitis in terms of age of occurrence, etiology, clinical manifestations, and diagnostic laboratory values. The therapeutic management and nursing considerations utilized throughout the clinical course of both conditions are addressed.

4. Simpkins, R.: The crisis of bronchiolitis, Am. J. Nurs. 81(3):515–516, 1981.
The author describes bronchiolitis in relation to its incidence, pathophysiology, and clinical manifestations. The rationale for using or avoiding various therapeutic methods is included in the description of treatment. Discussion of nursing care includes the criteria employed in diagnosing respiratory failure in infants and children with acute pulmonary disease.

5. Pinney, M.: Pneumonia, Am. J. Nurs. 81(3):517–518 1981.
This article describes the clinical course of bacterial, viral,

and mycoplasma pneumonia as they occur in children of various ages. A chart is included that differentiates among the various pneumonias in terms of symptoms, findings, and therapy. A general nursing care plan for the child with pneumonia is directed toward the prevention of complications.

6. Rimar, J.M.: Haemophilus influenzae Type B polysaccharide vaccine, Am. J. Maternal Child Nurs. 11(1): 57, 1986.
This MCN pharmacopoeia entry provides an overview of the infections caused by Haemophilus influenzae Type B in young children and discusses the efficacy of the HIB vaccine. Recommendations for use, dosage, and administration of the vaccine are presented with a description of its side effects and contraindications. Nursing implications associated with the vaccine's administration are described.

7. Jennings C.: Controlling the home environment of the allergic child, Am. J. Maternal Child Nurs. 7(6):376–381, 1982.
In this article, the various elements to be assessed in gathering environmental data related to children's respiratory allergy symptoms are described. Molds, dust, dust mites, animals, and aeriform substances are presented as common irritants, and suggestions for their control are provided. Assessment forms for both the general home environment and the child's bedroom are included. Mechanical devices for environmental control of allergens are discussed.

8. Kirilloff, L.H., and Tibbals, S.C.: Drugs for asthma: A complete guide, Am. J. Nurs. 83(1):55–61, 1983.
This selection emphasizes the importance of a current medication history in identifying patient teaching needs in regard to asthma medication. A series of photographs demonstrates use of the various inhalers and nebulizers. Charts provide comprehensive guidelines for the common groups of asthma medications: methyl xanthine compounds, sympathomimetic drugs, adrenal corticosteroids, cromolyn sodium, and antibiotics.

9. Simkins, R.: Asthma: reactive airways disease, Am. J. Nurs. 81(3):522–524, 1981.
This article discusses the pathophysiology, criteria for diagnosis, and treatment of asthma in children. It further describes the progression to status asthmaticus and the medications given during such an episode. Nursing responsibilities in the areas of assessment of respiratory and cardiovascular status are emphasized.

10. Larter, N.: Cystic fibrosis, Am. J. Nurs. 81(3):527–532, 1981.
This entry provides an overview of cystic fibrosis, with particular emphasis on the relationship between the pathophysiology of the various systems affected by the condition and specific clinical manifestations. A detailed nursing care plan for the child with cystic fibrosis is included. The psychosocial aspects of care are illustrated by the use of a case study.

11. Patton, A.C., Ventura, J.N., and Savedra, M.: Stress and coping responses of adolescents with cystic fibrosis, Child. Health Care 14(3):153–156, 1986.
This study examines the coping behaviors of adolescents with cystic fibrosis in response to the stresses encountered as part of the course of this chronic, potentially fatal disease. It identifies stresses in three specific areas: illness management, education, and age-specific developmental tasks. In addition, it presents coping factors identified by the subjects as either helpful or nonhelpful. The similarity between coping behaviors of adolescents with cystic fibrosis and healthy adolescents is noted.

Chapter 33

The Child with a Gastrointestinal Disorder

I. Chapter Overview

Chapter 33 introduces nursing considerations essential to the care of the child experiencing gastrointestinal dysfunction. Since disorders of the gastrointestinal tract are very common and constitute one of the largest categories of illnesses in infancy and childhood, it is important for the student to understand the care of children with such alterations in health. At the completion of this chapter, the student will be able to assess the child with alteration in gastrointestinal function and will be able to develop goals and responsibilities to help child and family cope with the physical, emotional, and psychosocial stress imposed by an alteration in gastrointestinal function.

II. Learning Objectives

Upon completion of this chapter, it is expected that the reader will be able to:

1. Develop a teaching plan for families directed at preventing the ingestion of foreign substances.

2. Plan an appropriate diet for a child with a malabsorption syndrome.

3. Outline a plan of care for a child with an obstructive disorder.

4. Describe the nursing responsibilities of caring for a child with a gastrointestinal alteration affecting motility.

5. Discuss the pathophysiology, clinical manifestations, and diagnostic evaluation of Meckel's diverticulum.

6. Compare and contrast the inflammatory diseases of the gastrointestinal tract.

7. Discuss the cause, prevention, and nursing care of hepatitis in children.

III. Review of Essential Concepts

1. List the essential functions of the gastrointestinal system.

a.

b.

c.

d.

2. The immaturity of the digestive system in the infant is demonstrated by the _____ with which swallowed food is propelled throughout the entire tract

3. _____ is more rapid in infancy than at other periods of life.

4. Digestion refers to:

5. The principal absorbing site in the gastrointestinal system is the _____.

6. Barium is the contrast medium used to provide a radiographic view of the structure of the intestinal tract. Match the following terms and definitions:

_____ Upper GI series

_____ Lower GI series

a. enables visualization of the colon

b. enables visualization of the esophagus, stomach, and the small bowel

7. The term *pica* refers to:

8. Foreign bodies that become lodged in the _____ require immediate attention.

9. _____ is a term applied to a long list of disorders associated with some degree of impaired digestion and/or absorption.

0. Absorptive defects include those conditions in which the _____ is impaired.

1. Celiac disease is characterized by an intolerance for _____.

2. In the early stages of celiac disease _____ is primarily affected, resulting in elimination of large quantities of digested fat _____ in the stool.

3. As celiac disease progresses _____ _____ are lost in the stool.

4. The clinical manifestations of celiac disease are:

. Celiac disease may be characterized by acute, severe episodes of profuse, pale, bulky, rancid, poorly formed stools and vomiting. This situation is referred to as a _____.

. The characteristic signs of acute mechanical intestinal obstruction are:

. The earliest sign of high intestinal obstruction is _____; the earliest sign of lower obstruction is _____.

. When assessing a child who has progressive abdominal distention the nurse would expect to observe:

. Intussusception can be defined as:

. The stool of the infant with intussusception is characteristically described as: _____.

. Definitive diagnosis of intussusception is based on a _____.

. Match the following terms related to constipation with their definitions by placing the appropriate letter in the blank preceding the term.

_____ constipation

_____ obstipation

_____ encopresis

a. extremely long intervals between defecation

b. constipation with fecal soiling

c. regular passage of firm or hard masses associated with symptoms

23. _____ is the most common cause of constipation in children.

24. The primary defect in congenital megacolon is the absence of _____ of the submucosal and mysenteric plexuses in one segment of the colon.

25. The functional defect in aganglionic megacolon is _____ in the affected section of the colon.

26. A _____ is performed to confirm the diagnosis of congenital megacolon.

27. The primary treatment of congenital megacolon is _____.

28. The most common symptoms of gastroesophageal reflux are:

29. The initial test to detect gastroesophageal reflux is the _____.

30. Meckel's diverticulum is defined as an _____.

31. Meckel's diverticulum results when the _____.

32. Bleeding can occur in Meckel's diverticulum because:

33. _____ is the chief presenting sign of Meckel's diverticulum.

34. Diagnosis of Meckel's diverticulum is usually based on _____.

35. Treatment of Meckel's diverticulum is _____.

36. The most significant factor associated with perforation of the appendix is _____.

37. List the clinical manifestations of appendicitis.
   a.
   b.
   c.
   d.

38. The site of most intense pain in appendicitis is _____ located at a point midway between the _____.

39. A definition of rebound tenderness is:

40. List the symptoms suggestive of peptic ulcer.
   a.
   b.

c.

d.

41. Identify at least two nursing diagnoses for the child with a peptic ulcer.

a.

b.

42. Hepatitis is caused by at least four types of viruses. List these viruses along with their abbreviations.

a.

b.

c.

d.

43. Compare the features of HAV *vs*. HBV by completing the following chart.

	TYPE A (HAV)	TYPE B (HBV)
Incub. period	a.	b.
Period of communicability	c.	d.
Mode of Transmission		
Principal route	e.	f.
	g.	h.
Less frequent route		
Onset	i.	j.
Immunity	k.	l.
Carrier state	m.	n.

44. What are the antibodies and antigens that are important in the diagnosis of HBV?

a.

b.

c.

d.

e.

f.

45. Identify which of the following statements related to hepatitis A or hepatitis B are true or false.

_____ There is no specific treatment for either hepatitis A or hepatitis B.

_____ Isolation is required to prevent transmission of the disease.

_____ If a client has had hepatitis A he has crossover immunity to hepatitis B.

_____ Immune serum globulin (ISG) is effective in preventing hepatitis A.

_____ Handwashing is the single most effective measure in prevention and control of hepatitis.

IV. Application, Analysis, and Synthesis of Essential Concepts

A. **Clinical Situation:** Edward, age 2 years, was admitted to the emergency room for treatment of ingestion of a penny.

1. What is the primary nursing intervention related to foreign body ingestion?

2. You assess that Edward has increased salivation, and is drooling, and having difficulty swallowing. These signs indicate that the foreign body is lodged in the
_____.

B. **Clinical Situation:** Patricia, age 3 years, is admitted with a diagnosis of celiac disease.

1. Patricia is going to have a peroral jejunal biopsy to definitely determine diagnosis. The nurse would intervene by preparing Patricia for this exam by:
a.
b.
c.

2. A gluten-free diet usually produces dramatic clinical improvement within 2 weeks. Your nursing goal is t teach Patricia and her parents to adhere to this diet. What foods must she avoid?

C. **Clinical Situation:** Jason, age 8 months, is admitted to the emergency room with signs of intermittent abdominal pain, vomiting, and currant-jelly stools. A diagnosis of intussusception is made.

1. As soon as the diagnosis of intussusception is made the nurse begins to prepare Jason's parents for his immediate hospitalization, the barium enema, and the possibility of surgery. What specific nursing interventions would adequately prepare the parents to deal with each of these stressors?
a. Hospitalization—

b. Barium enema—

c. Surgery—

2. What factors regarding the GI system of the infant would influence the amount and frequency of feedings?

D. **Clinical Situation:** Manuel, age 3 years, is brought to the well-child clinic with the complaint of constipation.

1. To help confirm the medical diagnosis of constipation, you would begin your nursing assessment with questions regarding which factors?
a.
b.
c.
2. Your nursing goal is to teach Manuel's father to eliminate constipating foods from his son's diet. What foods would you tell him to avoid?

E. **Clinical Situation:** Shane, age 11 months, is admitted to the pediatric unit for treatment of Hirschprung's disease.

. When doing a nursing assessment upon Shane's admission the nurse would assess certain factors related to Hirschsprung's disease. What are they?
a.
b.
. When preparing the parents for the medical treatment Shane will receive for his disease, the nurse would intervene by teaching that the repair of this defect is done in three stages. What are they?
a.
b.
c.
. List the rationale for each of the nursing interventions necessary to cleanse Shane's bowel prior to surgery.
a. Administer repeated saline enemas

b. Assist in insertion of a nasogastric tube

c. Administer an antibiotic solution through NG tube

d. Monitor irrigant and drainage

e. Insert a rectal tube

f. Take only axillary temperatures

4. The nursing interventions necessary to care for Shane's physical postoperative needs are:
a.
b.
c.
d.
e.

F. **Clinical Situation:** Stefanie, age 2 months, is admitted for treatment of gastroesophageal reflux.

1. Positioning is the recommended method of managing gastroesophageal reflux. You would intervene by teaching Stephanie's parents about positioning. What would you teach them.

2. The most important nursing intervention with Stephanie's parents is:

G. **Clinical Situation:** Gerard, age 5 years, was admitted for treatment of appendicitis.

1. Gerard tells the nurse that his abdominal pain has suddenly disappeared. The nurse continues to assess Gerard's pain because she knows that sudden relief from abdominal pain might signal _____ rather than improvement.
2. A primary nursing goal in recognizing appendicitis is to _____.
3. When assessing Gerard's pain, the nurse knows that the most reliable estimate of pain is the _____.
4. How will the nurse assess when to request discontinuance of Gerard's intermittent gastric decompression?
a.
b.

II. **Experiential Exercise:** Spend a day in an ambulatory pediatric clinic. In order to direct your nursing activities more constructively, differentiate between the two chronic intestinal disorders, ulcerative colitis and Crohn's disease, by completing the following chart.

	ULCERATIVE COLITIS	CROHN'S DISEASE
Pathologic changes	1.	2.

(continued)

	ULCERATIVE COLITIS	CROHN'S DISEASE
Clinical Manifestations		
Rectal bleeding	3.	4.
Diarrhea	5.	6.
Pain	7.	8.
Anorexia	9.	10.
Weight loss	11.	12.
Growth Retardation	13.	14.

I. **Clinical Situation:** Samuel, age 11 years, is admitted to the pediatric unit with a diagnosis of hepatitis B.

1. Nursing goals for *Samuel's* care depend on what three factors?
   a.
   b.
   c.

2. Interventions that would provide supportive care for Samuel are:
   a.

   b.

   c.

   d.

   e.

V. Suggested Readings

1. Hartwig, M.S.: Sticking to a gluten-free diet, Am. J. Nurs. **83**(9):1308–1310, 1983.

   This selection describes the usefulness of the gluten-free diet in managing both the atrophy of the jejunal mucosa and the nonabsorption of nutrients that occur in malabsorption syndromes. Foods containing gluten are listed, and substitutions are suggested. Tips on baking with gluten-free flours and some additional information sources are provided.

2. Gantt, L., and Thompson, C.: Short-gut syndrome and the infant, Am. J. Nurs. **85**(11):1263–1266, 1985.

   This article describes comprehensively the problems related to the surgical shortening of the bowel in the infant. A case study serves as the vehicle for discussing common problems related to total parenteral nutrition, bile stasis, diarrhea, stool and urine outputs, skin breakdown, infection, and oral feeding. Nursing goals are defined and specific interventions to meet these goals are discussed throughout the article.

3. Sugar, E.C.: Hirschsprung's disease, Am. J. Nurs. **81** (11):2065–2067, 1981.

   This article provides a comprehensive overview of Hirschsprung's disease in the neonate, the infant, and the older child. Discussed are the condition's etiology, pathophysiology, manifestations, diagnostic evaluation, and therapeutic management. Nursing care following the temporary colostomy and surrounding the later corrective pull-through procedure is described in detail. Psychosocial considerations related to the condition are explored.

4. Sasso, S.C.: Metoclopramide and chalasia, Am. J. Maternal Child Nurs. **8**(5):361, 1983.

   This MCN pharmacopoeia entry reviews the major features of chalasia, or gastroesophageal reflux, in the newborn. It then discusses metoclopramide and its action in treating chalasia. The drug's contraindications, adverse reactions, and administration are described, along with the nursing implications involved.

5. Lessman, M.: Painful chronicle, Am. J. Nurs. **85**(5): 551–552, 1985.

   In this entry, an adolescent graphically describes his experiences during the diagnosis, conservative treatment, and surgical management of his ulcerative colitis. His initial reactions to and problems with his ileostomy, as well as his gradual adjustment to it are discussed.

6. Gurevich, I.: Viral hepatitis: precautions, Am. J. Nurs. **83**(4):572–586, 1983.

   This comprehensive article compares and contrasts hepatitis A, hepatitis B, and non-A–non-B hepatitis in terms of modes of transmission, incubation periods, diagnosis, complications, and methods of prevention. Specific hepatitis precautions to be employed in institutions are listed. While immunization of high-risk populations with hepatitis B vaccine is recommended, this entry stresses the primary importance of preventive infection control measures.

7. Mar, D.D.: New hepatitis B vaccine: a breakthrough in hepatitis prevention, Am. J. Nurs. **82**(2):306–307, 1982.

   This article discusses the effectiveness of the hepatitis B vaccine in health-care personnel and other high-risk populations including drug addicts, sexually promiscuous persons, and homosexual males. The uses of immune serum globulin and hepatitis B immune globulin are also described, with a chart delineating specific use and dosage guidelines.

The Child with Cardiovascular Dysfunction

. Chapter Overview

Chapter 34 introduces nursing considerations essential) the care of the child experiencing cardiovascular dys-unction. This is important, because it is estimated that ongenital heart disease occurs in 8 to 10 of every thou-and live births, and the acquired conditions affect chil-ren of virtually every age group. At the completion of uis chapter, the student should have a knowledge of the ructural and physiologic changes associated with the arious cardiac disorders and will be able to develop ap-opriate nursing interventions for a child with cardiovas-ular dysfunction.

!. Learning Objectives

Upon completion of this chapter, it is expected that the udent will be able to:

◄. Identify the four components of the conduction sys-tem of the heart.

?. Design a plan for assisting a child during a cardiac diagnostic procedure.

◄. Demonstrate an understanding of the hemodynamics, clinical manifestations, and therapeutic management of congenital heart disease.

-. Describe the care of an infant or child with an acy-anotic congenital heart defect.

. Outline a plan of care for an infant or child with congestive heart failure.

. Discuss the role of the nurse in helping the child and family to cope with congenital heart disease.

. Identify the four structural defects associated with te-tralogy of Fallot.

. Describe the care of a child with rheumatic heart dis-ease.

9. Discuss the methods of assessment and management of hypertension in children and adolescents.

10. Outline a plan of care for the child with Kawasaki disease.

III. Review of Essential Concepts

1. The four components that comprise the conduction system of the heart are:

2. List the four types of information yielded by a car-diac catheterization.
   a.
   b.
   c.
   d.

3. A complication that the nurse might assess following a cardiac catheterization is _____.
   a. cardiac arrythmia
   b. rapidly rising blood pressure
   c. hypostatic pneumonia
   d. congestive heart failure

4. The two structures that influence the flow of blood in fetal circulation are the _____ and the

   _____.

5. _____ In fetal circulation, the pressure on the left side of the heart exceeds the pressure on the right side. (true or false)

6. The congenital heart defects are divided into types based on the alterations in circulation. They are _____ and _____.

7. An acyanotic heart defect is one in which there is a _____ to _____ shunting of the blood.

8. A cyanotic heart defect is one in which there is a _____ to _____ shunting of the blood.

9. Match the following physical consequences of congenital heart disease with the underlying etiologies. (Answers may be used more than once; more than one answer may apply.)

a. _____ growth retardation

b. _____ recurrent respiratory infection

c. _____ exercise intolerance

d. _____ dyspnea

e. _____ cyanosis

f. _____ tachypnea

g. _____ feeding problems

h. _____ clubbing

i. _____ tachycardia

j. _____ polycythemia

a. inadequate nutrient intake and increased caloric requirements

b. pulmonary vascular congestion

c. increased pulmonary resistance

d. compensatory mechanism to increase oxygenation

e. deoxygenation of blood

f. compensatory mechanism to increase cardiac output

g. chronic hypoxia

10. The six most common acyanotic congenital heart defects are:

11. Congestive heart failure is defined as:

12. The most common cause of congestive heart failure in children _____ secondary to structural abnormalities.

13. The two classifications of congestive heart failure are:
    a.
    b.

14. The two body systems that act to prevent cardiac decompensation are the:

15. One of the earliest signs of decompensation to assess related to impaired myocardial functioning is _____.

16. Cardiac failure may lead to pulmonary congestion, producing such signs as:
    _____.

17. Systemic congestion is a primary consequence of right-sided failure and is reflected in _____ and _____.
    _____ is the earliest sign of edema.

18. List the four goals of the therapeutic management of congestive heart failure.
    a.
    b.
    c.
    d.

19. What four interventions would the nurse utilize in helping the parents and child to adjust to the diagnosis of congenital heart disease?
    a.
    b.
    c.
    d.

20. The four structural defects of tetralogy of Fallot are:
    a.
    b.
    c.
    d.

21. The major sequela to rheumatic fever is heart damage, especially scarring of the _____.

22. Prevention or treatment of _____ infection prevents rheumatic fever.

23. Diagnosis of rheumatic fever is based on the presence of two major manifestations or one major and two minor manifestations as identified by the _____ criteria, in combinations with evidence of a recent _____ infection. The most objective evidence supporting a recent streptococcal infection is an elevated or rising _____ titer.

24. The diagnosis of hypertension in children and adolecents primarily involves the assessment of the _____ during every physical examination.

25. _____ to correct the underlying defect is the most common treatment for secondary hypertension. Essential or primary hypertension is commonly treated by _____ therapy.

26. Mucocutaneous lymph node syndrome, also known as _____, primarily affects the _____ system.

27. There is no specific diagnostic laboratory test for Kawasaki disease, so the diagnosis is based upon the presence of five or six characteristic symptoms, which must always include an elevated _____.

28. In the acute stage and the recovery period of Kawasaki disease, nursing interventions include the administration of large doses of _____.

IV. Application, Analysis, and Synthesis of Essential concepts

A. **Experiential Exercise:** Accompany a child to the cardiac catheterization laboratory.

1. List the five steps in the cardiac catheterization procedure.
    a.
    b.
    c.
    d.
    e.

2. Identify the rationale for each of the following monitoring mechanisms used during a cardiac catheterization.
a. Continuous monitoring by electrocardiogram—

b. Continuous monitoring of temperature—

B. **Clinical Situation:** Carolyn, 7 years old, is admitted to the pediatric unit for a cardiac catheterization on the following morning. She is accompanied by her parents. Both Carolyn and her parents appear anxious. A basic nursing assessment is performed.

1. In addition to the basic data, what three factors need to be assessed before giving Carolyn procedural information.
a.
b.
c.

. What are the two major nursing goals of preprocedural care?
a.
b.

. Carolyn undergoes her cardiac catheterization and returns to the pediatric unit at noon. She appears drowsy and has a pressure dressing on her right groin area. The most important nursing responsibility associated with the postprocedural care of Carolyn would be the detection of complications. Identify the rationale(s) for each of the following nursing interventions or observations.
a. Frequent vital signs—

b. Monitor blood pressure, especially for hypotension—

c. Assess pulses distal to the catheterization site—

d. Assess the temperature and color of affected extremity—

e. Observe status of dressing—

Carolyn is requesting fluids and wants to know when she can go to the playroom. What factors should be assessed in determining whether Carolyn can be given fluids?
a.
b.

5. When is the patient usually allowed to get up and walk about following a cardiac catheterization?

C. **Experiential Exercise:** Spend a day in an outpatient cardiac clinic to observe the role of the nurse in the management of children with cardiac dysfunction.

1. Place *C* before the following clinical manifestations that might indicate the presence of a congenital heart defect in an infant or young child. Mark *X* before incorrect answers.

a. _____ growth retardation   f. _____ bradypnea

b. _____ bradycardia   g. _____ decreased exercise tolerance

c. _____ difficulty with feeding

d. _____ dyspnea   h. _____ cyanosis

i. _____ dry, hot skin

e. _____ weak cry   j. _____ frequent respiratory infections

2. Identify the factors in a child's history that might be associated with an abnormally high incidence of congenital heart disease.
a. Prenatal factors—

b. Genetic factors—

3. What clinical manifestations might be seen in a child who is brought to the clinic with a diagnosed ventricular septal defect?
a

b.

4. What are five complications that could result from a ventricular septal defect?
a.
b.
c.
d.
e.

D. **Experiential Exercise**: Care for a hospitalized child with congestive heart failure.

1. Why would a child with congestive heart failure be placed on a regimen of oral digitalis and diuretics?
   a. Digitalis—

   b. Diuretics—

2. Since the margin of safety between the therapeutic and toxic dose of digitalis is narrow, the primary goal of the nurse is to prevent digitalis intoxication. What four nursing interventions would accomplish this goal?
   a.

   b.

   c.

   d.

3. What four guidelines for care would you teach the parents of a child who has vomited after receiving digitoxin?
   a.

   b.

   c.

   d.

4. What is the primary rationale for the nurse monitoring potassium levels in patients receiving potassium-losing diuretics and digoxin?

5. Diuretics are administered to the cardiac patient to promote fluid loss. What two interventions would enable the nurse to evaluate the effects of this drug therapy?
   a.
   b.

6. For each of the following nursing goals, identify at least two appropriate nursing interventions that

would be utilized when caring for a child with congestive heart failure.
   a. Assist in measures to improve cardiac functioning—

   b. Decrease cardiac demands—

   c. Reduce respiratory distress—

   d. Maintain nutritional status—

   e. Assist in measures to promote fluid loss—

   f. Provide emotional support—

E. **Clinical Situation:** Julie, an 8-year-old black child was admitted to the pediatric unit 5 days ago because of fatigue, low-grade fever, and joint pain. A heart murmur and subcutaneous nodules were discovered during her admission assessment. Laboratory tests, including an ESR, C-reactive protein, and ASO titer, helped to confirm the diagnosis of rheumatic fever.

1. The nurse is developing a home-care plan for Julie which includes the interventions listed below. Match each intervention to its appropriate rationale. (Answer may be used more than once; more than one answer may apply.)

RATIONALE	INTERVENTIONS
a. _____ prevention of permanent cardiac damage	a. Administer antibiotics as ordered.
b. _____ prevention of recurrences of the disease	b. Administer salicylates as needed.
c. _____ eradication of hemolytic streptococci	c. Enforce bed rest in the acute phase.
d. _____ palliation of symptoms	d. Initiate prophylactic measures prior to dental work
	e. Use a bed cradle.
	f. Prepare child for periodic multiple injections.

g. Position child with pillows.

e. _____ provision of emotional support

h. Explain the temporary nature of all symptoms except cardiac involvement.

i. Schedule activities to provide for adequate rest.

b. Prevent dehydration—

c. Minimize possible cardiac complications—

F. **Clinical Situation:** Johnny, age 3 years, is admitted to the pediatric unit with a diagnosis of Kawasaki disease. Upon admission, it is noted that Johnny has a fever of 102.5° F, a diffuse rash particularly evident on his trunk, and an enlargement of the cervical lymph nodes.

1. The six criteria that are used in establishing a diagnosis of Kawasaki disease are listed below. Develop a nursing diagnosis for each of these criteria.
   a. Fever for 5 or more days—

   b. Bilateral congestion of the ocular conjunctiva without exudation—

   c. Changes of the mucous membranes of the oral cavity, such as, erythema, dryness, and fissuring of the lips; oropharyngeal reddening, or "strawberry tongue"—

   d. Changes in extremities, such as peripheral edema, peripheral erythema, desquamation of palms and soles, particularly periungual peeling—

   e. Polymorphous rash, primarily of the trunk—

   f. Cervical lymphadenopathy—

2. Identify six cardiovascular changes that may occur in a child with Kawasaki disease.
   a.
   b.
   c.
   d.
   e.
   f.

3. For each of the following nursing goals, identify at least four appropriate nursing interventions to be utilized when caring for Johnny.
   a. Control of fever—

V. Suggested Readings

1. Usark, K.: A child's cardiac catheterization—avoiding potential risks, Am. J. Maternal Child Nurs. **3**(3):158–161, 1978.
   This article focuses on the role of the nurse in reducing the stressors of cardiac catheterization for the child, thus minimizing the risks of the procedure. The important elements of preparatory teaching plans for both the parents and child are described in detail.
2. Jackson, P.L.: Digoxin therapy at home: keeping the child safe, Am. J. Maternal Child Nurs. **4**(2):105–109, 1979.
   The author documents the inadequate instruction of parents who will be administering digoxin to their children at home and identifies particular areas of ignorance. A detailed guide for parent education is included.
3. Smith, K.M.: Recognizing cardiac failure in neonates, Am. J. Maternal Child Nurs. **4**(2):98–100, 1979.
   Mechanisms associated with the development of congestive heart failure in the neonate are explained in detail. A case study describes a neonate with undiagnosed congenital heart disease. Guidelines for observations that are basic to a thorough assessment and early recognition of signs of cardiac failure in the neonate are presented.
4. Gottesfeld, I.B.: The family of the child with congenital heart disease, Am. J. Maternal Child Nurs. **4**(2):101–104, 1979.
   This article discusses the implications of a child's congenital heart disease for the family prior to the actual diagnosis and after the diagnosis is made. Issues related to the prolonged stress of chronic illness are examined. The nature of continuing health team support is emphasized.
5. Botwin, E.D.: Should children be screened for hypertension? Am. J. Maternal Child Nurs. **1**(3):152–158, 1976.
   This thorough discussion of hypertension in childhood covers incidence, detection, risk factors, screening, diagnostic evaluation, and health teaching. Procedural points vital to obtaining an accurate blood pressure reading on infants and children are presented in detail.
6. L'Orange, C., and Werner-McCullough, M.: Kawasaki disease: a new threat to children, Am. J. Nurs. **83**:558–562, 1983.
   This article discusses the criteria for the diagnosis of Kawasaki disease and examines the phases of the disease in terms of their duration, clinical signs, and laboratory findings. The role of the nurse in providing emotional support, assisting with symptom relief, and preventing or detecting long-term complications is emphasized.

Chapter 35

The Child with Hematologic Dysfunction

I. Chapter Overview

Chapter 35 introduces nursing considerations essential to the care of the child experiencing a dysfunction of the blood or blood-forming organs. Since many of these conditions are inherited and chronic in nature, it is important for the student to understand the care of children with such disorders. The disorders discussed in this chapter often result in widespread systemic and structural responses within the body. A portion of the chapter deals with the hematologic system and its function, and provides an overview of the hematopoietic process and the function of the various blood cells. Upon completion of this chapter, the student will be able to formulate nursing goals and identify the responsibilities that would assist the child and his family in adjusting to a hematopoietic disorder and to prevent or cope with the resulting complications.

II. Learning Objectives

Upon completion of this chapter, it is expected that the reader will be able to:

1. Describe the major functions of the various blood elements.

2. Distinguish between the various categories of anemia.

3. Describe the pathophysiology and nursing care of children with sickle cell anemia and thalassemia major.

4. Describe the mechanisms of inheritance and nursing care of the child with hemophilia.

5. Contrast the pathophysiology and management of the deficiency disorders.

III. Review of Essential Concepts

1. What are the major functions of the hematologic system?

   a.
   b.
   c.
   d.

2. The blood is composed of two major components, a fluid portion called _____ and a cellular portion known as the _____.

3. The major blood-forming organs of the body are the _____, _____, and _____.

4. The erythrocyte is formed from the _____ in the _____.

5. What are the names applied to the various stages of erthrocytes?

   a.
   b.
   c.
   d.

6. The _____ is used as an indicator of active erythropoiesis.

7. The basic regulator of erthrocyte production is _____. The process is triggered by release of _____ by the kidneys.

8. The major function of the red blood cell is to _____.

9. _____ and _____ are the two major classifications of leukocytes.

10. There are three types of granulocytes: _____, _____, _____.

11. _____ is a term that refers to the granulocytes.

12. _____ are slightly immature forms of granulocytes.

13. Agranulocytes are comprised of two cell types, _____ and _____.

14. Match the following leukocyte cells with their specific functions by placing the correct letter in the blank. (More than one letter may apply.)

_____ neutrophils

_____ basophils

_____ eosinophils

_____ monocytes

_____ lymphocytes

a. most evident in chronic infection

b. phagocytes involved in inflammatory reactions

c. function in the immediate type of

d. most evident in acute infection

e. can destroy parasites

f. increased numbers occur during healing phase of inflammation

g. release fibrinolysin

_____ normocytic

_____ normochromic

_____ microchromic

_____ microcytic

_____ hypochromic

_____ hemolysis

_____ intracorpuscular

_____ extracorpuscular factor

_____ macrocytic

a. large size RBC

b. conditions outside RBC that cause hemolysis

c. defect within RBC

d. normal size RBC

e. pale color RBC

f. excessive destruction of RBC

g. normal color RBC

h. RBC that are pale in color

i. small size RBC

15. Platelets, also called _____, function in _____.

16. Platelets release a substance called _____ at the site of injury which causes _____ and decreases the flow of blood to the injured area.

17. List the components of the complete blood count (CBC).
a.
b.
c.
d.
e.
f.
g.
h.
i.
j.

18. In addition to the CBC, hematologic assessment includes the _____, and _____.

19. Anemia is defined as _____ volume or hemoglobin concentration to below normal levels.

20. Name the two basic categories of anemia and explain them.
a.

b.

21. List the basic causes or etiology of anemia.
a.
b.
c.

22. In order to understand the discussion of anemia, the nurse must be familiar with the terminology. Match the following terms with their definitions by placing the appropriate letter in the preceding blank.

23. There are three major reasons for a decrease in the production of red blood cells. List them.
a.
b.
c.

24. Distinguish between the various anemias by completing the following chart.

	ETIOLOGY	TREATMENT
Iron deficiency anemia	a.	b.
Pernicious anemia	c.	d.

25. In order to assess and interpret laboratory studies for integration into her client assessment, the nurse must understand the following laboratory measures. Identify what is measured by each of the following laboratory tests.
a. Mean corpuscular volume (MCV)—

b. Mean corpuscular hemoglobin (MCH)—

c. Mean corpuscular hemoglobin concentration (MCHC)—

d. Red blood cell (RBC)—
e. Hemoglobin (HGB)—
f. Hematocrit (Hct)—
g. Reticulocyte count—
h. WBC count (WBC)—

i. Differential WBC count—

j. Platelet count—

26. The basic physiologic defect caused by anemia is:

27. The clinical manifestations of anemia are directly attributable to tissue hypoxia. Identify these clinical manifestations.
    a. Four general symptoms

    b. Six central-nervous-system manifestations
        1.
        2.
        3.
        4.
        5.
        6.
    c. Circulatory system manifestations
        1.
        2.

28. The three nursing goals for the care of the child with anemia are:
    a.
    b.
    c.

29. _____ is required for the production of hemoglobin.

30. Often a baby with iron deficiency anemia is called a "milk baby." What is the meaning of this term?

31. What specific tests are used to identify the level of iron in the blood.
    a.
    b.

32. The side effects of oral iron therapy are:

33. The main nursing goal is:

34. When the proper dose of supplemental iron is reached the stools usually turn a _____.

35. List and define the 4 most common forms of sickle cell disease.

36. The basic defect in sickle cell anemia is the substitution of one amino acid, valine, for another amino acid, glutamine. Under conditions of the decreased oxygen tension and lowered pH the red blood cell changes into a _____ red cell.

37. The sickling response is reversible under conditions of adequate _____ and _____.

38. The basic pathologic changes from sickle cell anemia are primarily the result of:
    a.
    b.

39. Sickle cell crisis is usually precipitated by an _____.

40. The four types of sickle cell crisis are:
    a.
    b.
    c.
    d.

41. Since early identification of sickle cell anemia is essential, the _____ test is used for screening and case-finding.

42. The promotion of adequate _____ and _____ are necessary to prevent sickling of red blood cells.

43. Can oxygen administration reverse sickling of red blood cells? _____.

44. What is the possible negative effect of prolonged oxygen administration for the sickle cell patient?

45. Twenty to thirty percent of children with sickle cell disease under age 5 die mainly from _____ and _____.

46. Thalassemias are classified according to the _____ that is affected. Thallassemia major or _____ is a severe anemia that is _____ with life.

47. If you trace the pathologic process of thalassemia major you will see the following sequence.
    a. There is defective hemoglobin A, synthesis of which disintegrates causing damage to the _____ which causes severe _____. To compensate for the hemolytic process, the bone marrow produces large numbers of immature red blood cells which have a severely shortened _____. The increase of _____, the iron-containing pigment from the breakdown of hemoglobin, results in increased amount of iron in blood. The body stores the iron (a process called _____), resulting in cellular damage.

48. Thalassemia major causes characteristic changes in red blood cells, what are they?

49. _____, an iron-chelating agent, is given to the child with thalassemia to obviate hemosiderosis.
50. Summarize the three phases of normal coagulation.
    a. Phase I—

    b. Phase II—

    c. Phase III—

51. The definition of hemophilia is:

52. The two most common forms of hemophilia are classic hemophilia and Christmas disease.
    _____ accounts for 75% of all cases of hemophilia. What factors are defective in each form?
    a. Classic hemophilia—
    b. Christmas disease—
53. Hemophilia is transmitted as an _____.
    The most common pattern of transmission is between an unaffected male and a carrier female.
54. The most frequent site of bleeding is the
    _____; such a bleed is called a
    _____.

55. Signs and symptoms of hemarthrosis are:

56. One of the major causes of death in the hemophiliac is _____.
57. The primary therapy for the hemophiliac is preventing spontaneous bleeding by
    _____.
58. _____ is the drug of choice for the child with hemophilia A.
59. _____ and _____ are two components of adaptive immunity.
60. Humoral immunity is involved with antibody production and _____. The principal cell involved is the _____.
61. The five classes of antibodies of immunoglobins (Ig) are: _____.
62. The principal type of cell involved in cell-mediated immunity is the _____.
63. The HTLV-III is transmitted only through
    _____ with blood or blood products and
    _____ in which blood and semen mix.

64. Seventy-five percent of the cases of Acquired Immune Deficiency Syndrome (AIDS) in children are the result of _____ transmission.
65. The clinical presentation of pediatric AIDS includes:

66. Nursing considerations are primarily directed at
    _____.
67. What is the etiology, therapeutic management and prognosis of AIDS?
    a. Etiology—
    b. Therapeutic management—

    c. Prognosis—

IV. Application, Analysis, and Synthesis of Essential Concepts

A. **Clinical Situation:** Regina, age 4 years, is admitted to the pediatric unit for diagnosis and treatment of possible anemia.

1. Regina will be undergoing a battery of blood tests. The nursing goal of preparing the child for these tests can be accomplished by the following nursing interventions.
   a.
   b.
   c.

2. The nursing goal for Regina is to decrease tissue oxygen needs.
   a. What 3 assessments must the nurse make before she can intervene?

   b. What 5 interventions will accomplish this nursing goal for Regina?

3. What nursing diagnoses are appropriate for Regina?
   a.
   b.
   c.

B. **Clinical Situation:** Tonisha, age 3 years, is hospitalized with sickle cell anemia.

1. Since the major medical and nursing goals are to prevent deoxygenation and dehydration, what nursing interventions will you initiate to accomplish each of these goals?
   a. Prevent tissue deoxygenation—

   b. Prevent dehydration—

2. Tonisha has lapsed into sickle cell crisis. What nursing goals are appropriate for Tonisha?
   a.
   b.
   c.
   d.

3. Tonisha needs a blood transfusion, what are the two major nursing responsibilities?
   a.
   b.

C. **Clinical Situation:** Bradley, age 7 months, is admitted for treatment of Cooley anemia.

1. What symptoms might you expect to assess in Bradley?

2. Since there is no known cure for this disease, treatment is primarily supportive in nature. The primary objective of the supportive therapy is:

3. Bradley is going to have a blood transfusion. You would assess for signs and symptoms of a reaction. What are the signs and symptoms?

D. **Clinical Situation:** Ryan, age 3 years, is hospitalized for treatment of his hemophilia A.

1. In addition to observing for signs of hemarthrosis the nurse should intervene by teaching the family the other signs of internal hemorrhage. What are these signs and symptoms?

2. What emergency measures (interventions) could the family institute for a bleeding episode in addition to factor replacement? Include a rationale for each one.
   a.
   b.
   c.

3. One of Ryan's nursing diagnoses is "potential for hemorrhage related to injury and lack of blood coagulation." What three nursing goals are appropriate for this diagnosis?
   a.
   b.
   c.

E. **Clinical Situation:** Tony, age 4 months, is being treated for AIDS.

1. One of the nursing goals for Tony is to educate the parents, family, and the public regarding precautions to prevent transmission of the virus. List these precautions.
   a.

   b.

   c.

   d.

   e.

2. List the nursing diagnoses for Tony and his family.
   a.

   b.

   c.

   d.

V. Suggested Readings

1. McConnell, E.A.: Leukocyte studies: what the counts can tell you, Nursing 86 **16**(3):42–43, 1986.
   The article briefly reviews and explains the function of each of the five types of white cells. The white blood cell count and the differential count are explained, and their use in identifying the patient's diagnosis is explored.
2. Weeks, H.F.: Iron supplements, Am. J. Maternal Child Nurs. **5**(5):354, 1980.
   This MCN pharmacopoeia entry reviews the etiology of iron deficiency anemia in the perinatal and pediatric age groups. It presents tables that summarize the daily needs and losses of iron in menstruating women, pregnant women, infants, children, and adolescent girls and examines various factors affecting iron absorption. Nursing implications associated with administering iron supplements are described in detail.
3. Richardson, E.A.W., and Milne, L.S.: Sickle-cell disease

and the child bearing family: an update, Am. J. Maternal Child Nurs. **8**(6):417–422, 1983.

This article reviews the incidence and pathophysiology of sickle-cell disease, relating the resulting symptomatology in both infants and adults to the various body systems via an easily read chart. New developments in the treatment of the disease are outlined. Implications of the disease for the pregnant woman, fetus, and neonate are presented in detail. A sample nursing care plan for these populations is included.

4. Smith, L.G.: Reactions to blood transfusions, Am. J. Nurs. **84**(9):1096–1101, 1984.

In this entry, an extensive chart presents the types of blood transfusion reactions that occur, their signs and symptoms, the blood components involved, the pathophysiology, laboratory findings, differential diagnosis, management, and prevention. The specific reactions analyzed are hemolysis, febrile, allergic, pulmonary, circulatory overload, hypothermia, hemosiderosis, graft *vs* host disease, infection transmission, chemical toxicity, and dilutional coagulopathy.

5. McConnell, E.A.: APTT and PT: the tests of time, Nursing 86 **16** (5):47, 1986.

The activated partial thromboplastin time (APTT) and the prothrombin time (PT) tests are discussed. The article explores the coagulation process and the role of these two tests in measuring that process. Nursing considerations for patients with clotting abnormalities are identified.

6. Boland, M., and Gaskill, D.B.: Managing AIDS in children, Am. J. Maternal Child Nurs. **9**(6):384–389, 1984.

This selection examines the epidemiology of AIDS and graphically presents the nature of humoral and cell-mediated immunity. Present treatment protocols, with particular attention to avoiding the serious opportunistic infections associated with AIDS, are described. The psychological effects on the child and the family and the nurses's role in alleviating them are discussed. Specific infection-control precautions to be utilized with AIDS patients are presented.

7. Bennett, J.A.: AIDS epidemiology update, Am. J. Nurs. **85**(9):968–972, 1985.

This article presents the information that was generated at an international conference on AIDS in April, 1985. The incidence of the disease is described vis à vis sexual transmission, parenteral drug use, mother-to-child transmission, and blood and blood-product reception. Maps illustrate the geographic distribution of all AIDS cases and pediatric AIDS cases in the United States as of June, 1985. The potential risk to health-care workers and risk reduction guidelines for everyone are examined.

Chapter 36

The Child with Cancer

I. Chapter Overview

Chapter 36 discusses childhood cancers that continue to be life-threatening despite recent advances in treatment that extend the life of the afflicted child. Since many of these conditions tend to be chronic, it is important for the student to understand the necessity of providing for both the physical and emotional needs of the child and family. The chapter focuses on the etiologic factors that have been implicated in childhood cancer, and on the general properties of tumors. Various modes of therapy and the commonly encountered side effects are presented to provide the nurse with a basis for intervention. Nursing goals and responsibilities are developed that help the child and family adjust to a life-threatening disorder and cope with or prevent complications.

II. Learning Objectives

Upon completion of this chapter, it is expected that the student will be able to:

1. Identify some of the etiologic factors implicated in childhood cancer.

2. Describe the nurse's role in cancer therapy.

3. Describe the pathophysiology and clinical manifestations of leukemia.

4. Demonstrate an understanding of the rationale of therapies for neoplastic disease.

5. Outline a plan of care for the child with leukemia and his family.

6. Differentiate between Hodgkin disease and a non-Hodgkin lymphoma.

7. Describe the nursing care of a child with a brain tumor.

8. Differentiate among the various tumors found in children.

9. Differentiate between osteogenic and Ewing sarcoma.

10. Outline nursing interventions for the child with a retinoblastoma.

III. Review of Essential Concepts

1. The cause of cancer is _____.

2. List the etiologic factors implicated in childhood cancer.
   a.
   b.
   c.
   d.

3. Match the following terms regarding cancer with their definitions:
   a. invasion   b. metastasis   c. anaplasia
   a. _____ Loss of orderly differentiation and organization of cells to perform a specific function.
   b. _____ Malignant cells invade adjacent tissues and eventually the normal cells may be replaced by cancer cells that are incapable of performing the cells' original functions.
   c. _____ The phenomenon of spread of cancer to distant sites in the body and establishment of secondary colonies of malignant cells.

4. Designate the tissue or cell type from which the following neoplasms arise:
   a. Lymphoma—
   b. Leukemia—
   c. Sarcoma—
   d. Carcinoma—
   e. Adenocarcinoma—

5. Staging refers to the extent of the disease at the time of diagnosis in regard to TNM. What does TNM stand for?
   a. T—
   b. N—
   c. M—

6. The five modes of cancer therapy are:

7. Chemotherapeutic drugs are classified according to their _____ action.
8. List the classifications of the chemotherapeutic drugs.

9. The three types of bone marrow transplants are: _____, _____, and _____.

10. Serious damage often occurs to normal body tissue because chemotherapeutic agents destroy healthy as well as malignant cells. To prevent renal damage _____ is administered along with the chemotherapeutic agents.

11. The most important prognostic factors in determining long-term survival for children with ALL are:

12. The two basic pathological factors that occur in Leukemia are:
    a.

    b.

13. The three main consequences of bone marrow dysfunction are: _____, _____, and _____.

14. The clinical manifestations that result from the bone marrow dysfunction are:

15. Invasion of the meninges results in _____ _____ _____.

16. Definitive diagnosis of leukemia is based on _____ and _____.

17. List the three phases of chemotherapeutic therapy for leukemia. (a) _____, (b) _____, and (c) _____.

18. The sanctuary phase of therapy is directed toward the two anatomic areas that are protected from systemic chemotherapy. They are _____ and the _____.

19. What are the most common drugs and other therapies used in each of the three phases of chemotherapy?
    a. Induction

    b. Sanctuary

    c. Maintenance

20. Differentiate between Hodgkin disease and non-Hodgkin lymphoma.

21. Since staging is the basis for treatment protocols and expected prognoses in Hodgkin disease, define the stages.
    a. Stage I—

    b. Stage II—

    c. Stage III—

    d. Stage IV—

22. Hodgkin disease is characterized by painless _____. Systemic symptoms include:

23. _____ is essential to diagnosis and staging of Hodgkin disease, and a _____ cell is considered diagnostic of Hodgkin disease.
24. The primary modalities of therapy for Hodgkin disease are _____ and _____ used alone or in combination.
25. What are the two major forms of childhood cancer derived from neural tissue?

26. Infants with brain tumors do not display detectable symptoms; why?

27. The most diagnostic procedure for a brain tumor is the _____.

28. The treatment of choice for brain tumors is total _____.

29. After removal of a brain tumor the child is especially vulnerable to the postoperative complication of a _____.

30. When the temperature is elevated in the postoperative patient after removal of a brain tumor the nurse would suspect an _____.

31. _____ may be administered to remove excess fluid in the postoperative patient with brain tumor.

32. Headache may be severe in the postoperative patient with brain tumor. The headaches are largely due to _____.

33. Brain edema may depress the _____ necessitating _____ of oral secretions.

34. The primary site for a neuroblastoma is within the _____.

35. Because of the frequency of _____, prognosis for neuroblastoma is poor.

36. Diagnostic evaluation of neuroblastoma is aimed at locating the _____ and _____.

37. Neuroblastoma arising from the adrenal glands or from a sympathetic chain excrete catecholamines. How is the presence of catecholamines detected?

38. Identify the three methods employed to treat neuroblastoma.
    a.
    b.
    c.

39. Briefly describe the following tumors which are frequently seen in children.
    a. Neuroblastoma—

    b. Wilms tumor—

    c. Rhabdomyosarcoma—

40. In children two types of bone tumors that account for 85% of all primary malignant bone tumors are: _____ _____ and _____.

41. Compare osteogenic sarcoma and Ewing sarcoma in terms of etiology and therapeutic management.

	OSTEOGENIC SARCOMA	EWING SARCOMA
Etiology	a.	b.
Management	c.	d.

42. If an amputation is performed for osteogenic sarcoma, the child is usually fitted with a temporary _____ immediately after surgery.

43. The most frequent intra-abdominal tumor of childhood and the most common type of renal cancer is _____.

44. The most common presenting sign of Wilms tumor is a _____ in the abdomen.

45. The initial signs and symptoms of rhabdomyosarcoma are related to:

46. A frequent site for rhabdomyosarcoma is the _____.

47. Retinoblastoma is a _____ malignant tumor arising from the _____.

48. Of major concern in long-term survivors of retinoblastoma is the development of _____.

49. A characteristic clinical manifestation of retinoblastoma is:

50. Definitive diagnosis of retinoblastoma is based upon

51. Treatment of retinoblastoma depends chiefly on the stage of the tumor at diagnosis. Stages I, II, and III are treated with _____. With advanced tumor growth _____ is the treatment of choice.

IV. Application, Analysis, and Synthesis of Essential Concepts

A. **Clinical Situation:** David Greene is a 5-year-old white male admitted to the pediatric unit for treatment of acute lymphocytic leukemia.

1. Describe the nurse's role in cancer therapy of children.

2. List at least three clinical manifestations you would expect to assess in David.

3. What nursing interventions are appropriate to prevent infection in the immunosuppressed leukemia child?
   a.

   b.

   c.

   d.

   e.

   f.

   g.

   h.

   i.

4. How would you intervene to minimize the side effects of nausea and vomiting in the child receiving chemotherapy?
   a.

   b.

   c.

   d.

. David is receiving allopurinol, a xanthine-oxidase inhibitor. What is the rationale for the administration of this drug?

. David has alopecia as a result of chemotherapy and radiotherapy, what nursing interventions are appropriate?
   a.
   b.
   c.
   d.
   e.

B. **Experiential Exercise:** Spend a day in a neighborhood pediatric clinic. Answer the following questions and include specifics (examples, responses) which illustrate the concepts.

An adolescent comes to the clinic complaining of weight loss and night sweats. On the basis of this assessment data what disease would you suspect, Hodgkin disease or non-Hodgkin lymphoma?

2. Since one of the nursing goals in Hodgkin disease is "explanation of treatment side effects," what would you tell the adolescent is the most common side effect of radiation?

C. **Clinical Situation:** Amanda Brown, a 4-year-old, is hospitalized for treatment of an astrocytoma.

1. What assessment data would you gather in relation to the symptom of "vomiting" in Amanda.

2. Amanda has had surgery to remove her brain tumor. What are the seven nursing goals for postoperative care of Amanda?
   a.
   b.
   c.
   d.
   e.
   f.
   g.

3. What evaluation criteria would you expect for the achievement of the nursing goal "Prevent fluid overload or dehydration"?

4. The nurse will intervene postoperatively to observe behavior by:
   a.
   b.
   c.
   d.

5. Correct positioning after surgery is critical. What is the rationale for Amanda being positioned flat and on either side?
   a.
   b
   c.

6. Before feeding Amanda by mouth, you would assess for the presence of what reflexes?

7. List at least three nursing interventions that would prevent an increase in intracranial pressure.
   a.

   b.

   c.

D. **Clinical Situation:** Richard Patucci, age 3 years, is admitted for treatment of a Wilm's tumor.

1. Because surgery is performed within 24 to 48 hours after admission, the nurse must prepare Richard's parents for this procedure. List at least one nursing intervention that would accomplish this.
   a.

2. Because Richard is prone to intestinal obstruction, what postoperative nursing interventions are appropriate?
   a.

   b.

   c.

E. **Clinical Situation:** Thomas Block, age 17 months, is admitted for treatment of a retinoblastoma.

1. The three nursing goals for the nursing care of Thomas are:
   a.

   b.

   c.

2. List at least three nursing interventions that would accomplish these nursing goals.
   a.

   b.

   c.

V. Suggested Readings

1. Frank-Stromborg, M. et al.: Carcinogens: are some risks acceptable? Am. J. Nurs, **86**:814–817, 1986.

Most people agree on the need to regulate exposure to environmental carcinogens, but there is little agreement on how to accomplish this, nor is there agreement on what level of risk is acceptable. The government role in making laws to regulate exposure is surveyed. The authors also address the controversial questions regarding: the economics of promoting a risk-free environment; can results from animal testing be applied to humans; and are public and governmental philosophy and behavior congruent. The nurses role in this issue is explored.

2. Gaddy, D.S.: Nursing care in childhood cancer: update, Am. J. Nurs. **82**:416–421, 1982.

Although half the children diagnosed with cancer this year will survive to live productive lives, the authors feel that nurses have not integrated this hopeful attitude into their perception of patients with childhood cancer. Information may be the key to changing this perception. The balance of the article explores the clinical features, pathophysiology, diagnosis, treatment, and prognosis of leukemia, Wilms tumor, neuroblastoma, rhabdomyo sarcoma, lymphomas, and bone tumors.

3. Holmes, W.: SQ chemotherapy at home, Am. J. Nurs. **85**:168–169, 1985.

The number of hospitalizations for adults with leukemia was decreased by instituting a home program for chemotherapy using an auto-syringe. Detailed instructions regarding the use of this syringe are included.

4. Rahr, V.: Giving intrathecal drugs, Am. J. Nurs. **86**:829–831, 1986.

This article is a detailed description of the use of the Ommaya reservoir for administering chemotherapeutic drugs, antibiotics, and analgesics into the cerebrospinal fluid.

5. Hughes, C.B.: Giving cancer drugs IV: some guidelines, Am. J. Nurs. **86**:34–38, 1986.

This article is a detailed instructional unit on the nursing responsibilities for the administration of chemotherapeutic agents

6. Nuscher, R., et al.: Bone marrow transplantation, Am. J. Nurs. **84**:764–767, 1984.

The authors use the first half of the article to discuss how particular diseases respond to a bone marrow transplant. The remaining portion of the article discusses: donor and recipient matching, types of transplants, and the transplant environment.

7. Bersani, G., and Carl, W.: Oral care for cancer patients, Am. J. Nurs. **83**:533–536, 1983.

Oral problems that occur as a result of chemotherapy and radiotherapy are discussed. Detailed instructions for nursing intervention for oral problems are presented.

8. Greene, P.E., and Fergusson, J.H.: Nursing care in childhood cancer: late effects of therapy, Am. J. Nurs. **82**:443–446, 1982.

An overview of the late effects of therapy on certain key organ systems and some complications that are caused by one chemotherapeutic agent or by a combination of drugs is presented. Nursing responsibility for assessment and intervention to reduce the effects of these delayed complications during long-term follow-up are discussed.

9. Sonstegard, L., et al.: A way to minimize side effects from radiation therapy, Am. J. Maternal Child Nurs. **1**:27–31, 1976.

This study sought to find out if the physiological side effects of radiation therapy were unavoidable responses to therapy or were amenable to change with proper nursing intervention. A special care unit was created that approached the care of cancer patients with optimism and a positive attitude. Primary nursing and other interventions were instituted. Three groups of patients were compared over a period of time on their response to radiation therapy; physically, psychologically, and socially. The study found that many of the effects can be avoided with appropriate nursing intervention.

10. Cleaveland, M.J.: Nursing care in childhood cancer: brain tumor, Am. J. Nurs. **82**:422–424,1982.

The author discusses the incidence, etiology, symptoms, diagnosis and treatment of brain tumors. Specific nursing responsibilities to improve the care and relationship of the nurse with the child and his family are presented.

11. Maul S.K.: Childhood brain tumors: a special nursing challenge, Am. J. Maternal Child Nurs. **9**:123–129, 1984.

The early detection of a brain tumor is crucial to recovery. The incidence, pathology, tumor site, signs and symptoms, treatment, and prognosis of the four major brain tumors are explored. The nursing role in essential assessment, reducing postoperative complications, and enhancing recovery are discussed. Nursing responsibilities in supporting the child and family are also included.

12. Walters, J.: Coping with a leg amputation, Am. J. Nurs. **81**:1349–1352,1981.

The author discusses the phases of response—impact, retreat, acknowledgement, and reconstruction—that the patient passes through in adapting to the amputation of a leg. A variety of lower-extremity prostheses are illustrated. The nursing responsibilities in the care of the child with amputation are presented.

13. Ritchie, J.: Nursing the child undergoing limb amputation, Am. J. Maternal Child Nurs. **5**:114–120, 1980.

The article documents the patterns of behavior of five girls and two boys, aged 9 to 14 years, who underwent amputation. The preoperative reactions, anticipation and concerns, fears, postoperative reactions, and their first reactions are reviewed. The children's reaction to their stump, a phantom limb, and the artificial limb are discussed. Specific nursing approaches to deal with the child with an amputation are included.

14. Wong, D.L., and Dornan, L.R.: Nursing care in childhood cancer: retinoblastoma, Am. J. Nurs. **82**:425–435, 1982.

The incidence, etiology, tumor characteristics, diagnosis, and treatment of a retinoblastoma are presented. Special instructions regarding the home care of an eye prosthesis are included. The parent's experience with this condition is thoroughly explored, and the nurse's role of support for both the child and the parents is clearly presented.

Chapter 37

The Child with Cerebral Dysfunction

I. Chapter Overview

Chapter 37 introduces nursing considerations essential to the care of the child experiencing cerebral dysfunction. Since the brain is the center for multiple vital body functions, any disturbance in this regulating, controlling, and communicating mechanism can produce alterations in the way in which the system receives, integrates, and responds to stimuli entering the system. Since an alteration in the level of consciousness is a common finding in many cerebral disturbances, the student will be introduced to methods used to assess and diagnose neurologic function. At the completion of this chapter the student will be able to develop nursing goals and responsibilities that help the child and his family to effectively cope with the stressors imposed by an alteration in cerebral function.

II. Learning Objectives

Upon completion of this chapter, it is expected that the student will be able to:

1. Identify the three components of the nervous system.

2. Describe the clinical manifestations of increased intracranial pressure.

3. Describe the various modalities for assessment of cerebral function.

4. Differentiate between the stages of consciousness.

5. Formulate a plan of care for the unconscious child.

6. Distinguish between the types and serious complications of head injuries.

7. Outline a plan of care for the child with bacterial meningitis.

8. Differentiate among the various types of seizure disorders.

9. Demonstrate an understanding of the clinical manifestations and their management.

III. Review of Essential Concepts

1. List the three components of the nervous system.
   a.
   b.
   c.

2. The early signs and symptoms of increased intracranial pressure are subtle and assume many patterns. List these signs and symptoms for the younger and older child.
   a. Younger child—

   b. Older children—

3. As intrancranial pressure becomes progressively worse what signs would you expect to assess?

4. Since it is difficult to assess cerebral function in the infant and small child, what methods are utilized?
   a.

   b.

   c.

   d.

5. The _____ and _____ will contribute to the assessment of cerebral function.

6. Older children can be evaluated by the usual methods of neurologic examination, and in addition by _____
   _____

_____ can provide essential information about neurologic function.

7. List the abnormalities of gait that indicate cerebral dysfunction.

8. List and define the two components of consciousness?
   a.

   b.

9. Level of consciousness (LOC) is determined primarily by:

0. List the terms that describe level of consciousness.

1. The Glasgow Coma Scale (GCS) consists of what three areas of assessment?
   a.
   b.
   c.

2. The most frequently used criteria for establishing irreversible coma or a non-functioning brain are the _____.

3. List at least two of the criteria that define brain death.
   a.

   b.

4. The purpose of the neurologic examination is to:

5. What areas are assessed when performing a neurological examination?

6. The sudden appearance of a fixed and dilated pupil is a _____.

. List the diagnostic procedures, other than blood tests, that are utilized to assess cerebral function.

a.
b.
c.
d.
e.
f.

18. One of the primary concerns when caring for an unconscious patient is to maintain a _____.

19. List and define the types of head injuries.
   a.

   b.

   c.

20. List the major complications of trauma to the head.
   a.
   b.
   c.
   d.

21. Vascular rupture may occur even in minor head injuries, causing hemorrhage between the skull and cerebral surfaces. Why is the accumulation of blood between the skull and cerebral surfaces dangerous?

22. What artery is ruptured to produce epidural hemorrhage?

23. The accumulated blood is called a _____.

24. A subdural hemorrhage is bleeding _____ _____, usually as a result of rupture of the _____.

25. Compare the signs and symptoms you would assess in an epidural *vs.* a subdural hematoma.

EPIDURAL	SUBDURAL
a.	b.

26. Another major complication of head trauma is _____.

27. If cerebral edema is not detected and relieved, what is the consequence to the brain tissue?

28. The major pulmonary changes that occur in drowning are directly related to:

29. What organisms are responsible for 95% of the cases of bacterial meningitis in children older than 2 months?
    a.

    b.

    c.

30. What form of meningitis is readily transmitted to others and by what vehicle?

31. Inappropriate secretion of _____ frequently accompanies meningitis, causing _____ that intensifies the cerebral edema.

32. A definitive diagnosis of meningicoccal meningitis is made only by:

33. Identify the following statements regarding bacterial meningitis as true (T) or false (F).
    a. _____ Isolation is not needed for bacterial meningitis
    b. _____ Ampicillin is the drug of choice for treatment.
    c. _____ Seizures occur in about 30% of affected children.
    d. _____ There are no vaccines for bacterial meningitis.

34. The treatment of aseptic meningitis is primarily _____.

35. The basic mechanism of seizures is that electric discharges:
    a.

    b.

c.

36. Children seldom report an _____ or warning.

37. Muscle contraction can be one of three types; what are they?
    a.
    b.
    c.

38. What are the two major categories of seizures?

39. Psychomotor seizures are characterized by:

40. The _____ is the most useful diagnostic tool for evaluating seizure disorders.

41. What are the goals of therapeutic management?
    a.
    b.
    c.

42. What is the action of anticonvulsive drugs?

43. What precautions should be taken if the anticonvulsive drug is discontinued?

44. What is one of the major side effects of dilantin?

45. How is the dosage of anticonvulsant drugs monitored?

46. Status epilepticus is defined as:

47. Compare simple partial and complex partial seizures by completing the following chart.

	SIMPLE PARTIAL	COMPLEX PARTIAL
Duration	a.	b.
Aura	c.	d.
Impaired consciousness	e.	f.
Clonic movements	g.	h.
Postictal impairment	i.	j.
Mental	k.	l.

48. The tonic-clonic seizure is also known as
    _____.

49. The generalized seizure that is characterized by a
    brief loss of consciousness with minimal or no altera-
    tion in muscle tone and may go unrecognized is
    called _____ or _____

**IV. Application, Analysis, and Synthesis of Es-
sential Concepts**

  A. **Clinical Situation:** Beatrice McKinney, age 7
years, was admitted to the pediatric unit after sustaining
head trauma in an automobile accident. When admitted,
she was conscious and complaining that her head hurt.

1. One means of assessing neurological status is to observe Beatrice's muscular activity. What parameters of
   muscular activity would you be observing?
   a.

   b.

   c.

2. Beatrice has begun to complain of a headache and
   nausea, blurred vision, and she seems drowsy. What
   nursing diagnosis would you formulate from this assessment data?

3. Beatrice is becoming increasingly confused, dis-
   oriented, and agitated. She is suddenly fearful of the
   monitoring machines at her bedside because she thinks
   they are "wild animals." Based on this assessment
   what level of consciousness would best describe Beatrice's level of consciousness?

  B. **Clinical Situation:** Greta Kneisl, age 8 years, has
been unconscious for 3 days due to head trauma.

  List at least three nursing goals for the care of Greta.
  a.

  b.

  c.

2. What parameters are assessed to monitor Greta's neurological status?

3. What nursing interventions would achieve the nursing
   goal of "minimize intracranial pressure"?

4. What nursing interventions would achieve the nursing
   goal of "maintaining limb flexibility and function"?

5. What is the rationale for placing the child on a water-
   filled mattress?

  C. **Experiential Exercise:** Spend a day in an emergency room for pediatric clients. Answer the following
questions and include specific (examples, responses)
which illustrate these concepts.

1. Robin, age 3 years, sustained head trauma in a fall
   down some stairs. She is diagnosed as having a subdural hematoma and admitted to the pediatric unit.
   a. Three important nursing observations are frequent
      examination of:

2. Tory, age 3 years, comes to the emergency room after
   being rescued from a swimming pool.
   a. After immediate resuscitation of the child to restore
      oxygen delivery to the cells, the nurse must be
      concerned about Tory's parents. What nursing in-
      terventions would help to comfort the parents?

  D. **Clinical Situation:** Eden Capwell, age 10 months,
is admitted to the pediatric unit with a diagnosis of meningococcal meningitis.

1. What clinical manifestations would you expect to assess in Eden?

2. Identify the major nursing goals to be utilized when caring for Eden.
   a.
   b.
   c.
   d.
   e.
   f.
   g.
3. What nursing interventions are appropriate to achieve the nursing goal of "monitoring neurological status"?

E. **Clinical Situation:** Anita Sanchez, age 4 years, was admitted to the pediatric unit for diagnosis and treatment of a seizure disorder.

1. In order to assist with Anita's diagnosis the nurse should gather through a nursing history or through direct assessment what data?
   a.
   b.
   c.
   d.
   e.
   f.
   g.
2. While you are giving Anita a bath in bed she begins to have a seizure. How would you intervene to care for Anita and prevent any injury to her?
   a.
   b.
   c.
   d.
   e.
3. Anita was diagnosed as having grand mal seizures and is placed on dilantin.
   a. The nurse would formulate a teaching plan regarding drug therapy. You would intervene by teaching the following five points:

V. Suggested Readings

1. Mills, G.: Preparing children and parents for cerebral computerized tomography, Amer. J. Maternal Child Nurs. 5:403–407,1980.

In order for the nurse to prepare the child for CT scanning she must first understand the purpose of the procedure and how it is performed. This article begins with a detailed explanation of how CT scanning can help in the diagnosis of neurological problems. The cerebral CT examination technique is explained and the need for keeping the child immobile is emphasized. Guidelines for sedation of younger children are included. Suggestions for preparing both the parents and the child for this frightening procedure are discussed.

2. Scherer, P.: Assessment: the logic of coma, Amer. J. Nurs. 86:542–548,1986.

The focus of this article is accurate assessment of the patient with neurologic compromise. Definitions of arousal and awareness are presented. The steps of the coma exam and the meaning of the patient's response (or lack of response) is discussed detail for each level of the nervous system. Five levels of consciousness are defined. Principles and priorities for care of the comatose patient are outlined.

3. Surveyer, J.A.: Coma in children:how it affects parents, Amer. J. Maternal Child Nurs.1:17–21, 1976.

During the first 6 to 8 weeks following a traumatic head injury of a child with resulting coma, the parents of the child exhibit all of Lindemann's stages of grief. This article discusses how these stages manifest themselves in the parents who find themselves in a situation where the child is neither dead nor alive. The nursing role in supporting the parents through this difficult time is explored.

4. Hinkle, J.L.: Treating traumatic coma, Amer. J. Nurs. 86:551–556,1986.

The most important function of the nurse and emergency medical personnel is to prevent ischemia of the brain following a traumatic head injury. The author presents the priorities of care to accomplish this goal. The methods of monitoring and lowering intracranial pressure are outlined. The nursing role in reducing intracranial pressure and in constant assessment of the cerebral status of the child is explored.

5. Nebens, I.A. and Jackson, B.S.: A case of acute fulminating meningococcemia, Amer. J. Nurs. 82:1390–1393,198

The etiology, clinical manifestations, epidemiology, and treatment of a patient with meningococcema is discussed. A case presentation is utilized to illustrate the priorities for nursing care of a patient with this disease.

6. Wink, D.: Bacterial meningitis in children, Amer. J. Nurs 84:456–460, 1984.

The incidence, pathophysiology, clinical manifestations, diagnostic work-up, and medical management of the child with meningitis is presented. Nursing responsibilities in the care of the child with meningitis are stated along with their rationale. Need for chemoprophylaxis and long-term care are discussed.

7. Norman, S.E., and Browne, T.R.: Seizure disorders, Amer. J. Nurs. 81:984–993,1981.

The incidence and etiology of seizure disorders are outlined. The classification and the clinical manifestations of each classification of seizure disorders are introduced. The diagnosis, treatment, and terminology, associated with seizure disorders are presented. This article gives detailed explanations of status epilepticus, the EEG, and the major drugs utilized in seizure disorders. Nursing management of the child before, during, and after a seizure is thoroughly discussed.

8. Tucker, C.A.: Complex partial seizures, Amer. J. Nurs. 81:996–1000, 1981.

The etiology and clinical manifestations of the complex partial seizure are discussed in detail. Recognition of this seizure and the nursing management during the ictal and postictal phases of the complex partial seizure is presented.

9. Muehl, J.N.: Seizure disorders in children: prevention and care, Amer. J. Maternal Child Nurs. **4**:154–160,1979.

The incidence and etiology of seizure disorders are introduced. Types of seizures are listed and explained. Nursing care after a major seizure is described in detail. Medical management of seizures is discussed. The article concludes with a thorough discussion regarding phenytoin therapy and the psychological adjustment of the child and his family to a seizure disorder.

10. Coughlin, M.K.: Teaching children about their seizures and medications, Amer. J. Maternal Child Nurs. **4**:161–162, 1979.

A definition of a seizure is essential to understanding how a medication works. A list of common anticonvulsant drugs and their side effects is included in the article. The nursing responsibility of teaching the parents and the child the side effects of the drugs they are taking, and what conditions will increase the frequency of seizures is presented.

Chapter 38

The Child with Endocrine Dysfunction

I. Chapter Overview

Chapter 38 introduces nursing considerations essential to the care of the child experiencing endocrine dysfunction. Since the hormones synthesized by this system affect numerous body organs, it is important for the student to gain an understanding of the care of children with this type of alteration in health. The conditions discussed in this chapter interfere with the body's ability to produce or respond to the major hormones. The discussion of pancreatic hormone secretion is limited to diabetes mellitus, a relatively common health problem of childhood. At the completion of this chapter, the student will be able to develop nursing goals and responsibilities that will assist the child and his family to develop effective coping responses to deal with these complex disorders.

II. Learning Objectives

Upon completion of this chapter, it is expected that the student will be able to:

1. Describe the functions of the endocrine system.

2. Differentiate between the disorders caused by hypo- and hyperpituitary dysfunction.

3. Describe the manifestations and management of the child with thyroid hypo- and hyperfunction.

4. Describe the clinical manifestations and management of the child with parathyroid hypo- and hyperfunction.

5. Distinguish between the manifestations of adrenocortical hypo- and hyperfunction.

6. Describe some of the etiologic factors associated with hyperfunction of the adrenal medulla.

7. Differentiate between the categories of diabetes mellitus.

8. Describe the characteristics of the three major types of insulin.

9. Discuss the management and nursing care of the child with diabetes mellitus.

10. Distinguish between a hyper- and hypoglycemic reaction.

11. Design a teaching plan for a child with diabetes mellitus.

III. Review of Essential Concepts

1. The endocrine system consists of three components; name the components and their purpose.
   a.
   b.
   c.

2. The endocrine system controls or regulates metabolic processes governing:

3. A hormone is a _____ produced and secreted into body fluids by a cell that exerts a _____ effect on other cells.

4. Regulation of hormonal secretion is based on _____, and regulated primarily by the master gland, the _____.

5. The two regulatory systems that maintain homeostasis are:
   a.
   b.

6. The consequences of diminished or deficient secretions of the pituitary hormones depend on the degree of dysfunction and leads to:
   a.
   b.
   c.
   d.

7. _____ are the most common cause of pituitary hyposecretion.
8. The chief presenting complaint of hypopituitarism is _____.
9. Diagnosis of hypopituitarism is based on absent or subnormal reserves of _____.
10. The therapeutic management of hypopituitarism is:
    a.
    b.
11. Excess growth hormone before closure of epiphyseal shafts results in proportional _____; after closure of epiphyseal shafts results in _____, termed _____.
12. Children with a pituitary secreting tumor may also demonstrate signs of _____.
13. The primary nursing responsibility regarding hypopituitarism and hyperpituitarism is:

14. The principal disorder of the posterior pituitary hypofunction is _____ which causes hyposecretion of antidiuretic hormone (ADH), producing a state of uncontrolled _____.
15. The cardinal signs of diabetes insipidus are: _____ and _____.
16. The usual treatment of diabetes insipidus is hormone relacement with _____.
17. SIADH = _____ _____which results in _____ and _____.
18. The _____ gland is the only endocrine gland capable of storing excess amounts of hormones for release as needed.
19. The main physiologic action of thyroid hormone is:

    and thereby controls multiple processes of growth and tissue differentiation.
20. A *goiter* is:

    The synthesis of thyroid hormone depends upon the availability of _____ and _____.
21. Graves disease is usually associated with an enlarged _____ and _____.
22. List the symptoms that may occur if the patient with thyroid hyperfunction develops thyrotoxicosis.

23. A possible complication of thyroidectomy is _____ due to mistaken removal of the _____ glands.
24. The objective of therapeutic management of hypopara-

thyroidism is to maintain normal serum _____ and _____ levels with minimal complications.
25. _____ can be secondary to chronic renal disease and congenital anomalies of the urinary tract.
26. Identify whether the following hormones are secreted by the adrenal medulla or the adrenal cortex by matching the following:

a. _____ Glucocorticoids (cortisol)   a. Adrenal cortex

b. _____ Catecholamine (epinephrine)   b. Adrenal medulla

c. _____ Catecholamine (norepinephrine)

d. _____ Mineralocorticoid (aldosterone)

e. _____ Sex steroids

27. Identify whether the following clinical manifestations are indicative of (a) adrenocortical insufficiency or (b) hyperfunction of the adrenal gland.
    a. _____ Increased irritability, headache, diffuse abdominal pain, weakness, nausea and vomiting, diarrhea, fever and CNS symptoms
    b. _____ Moon face, hyperglycemia, decreased protein stores, increased mobilization and utilization of fatty acids for energy, increased storage of adipose tissue, decreased inflammatory and allergic actions, regulation of fluid and electrolytes by promoting sodium retention and potassium excretion, increased gastric acid and pepsin, and suppression of lymphocytes, eosinophils, and basophils but increased neutrophils, erythrocytes, and thrombocytes.
28. The administration of excessive amounts of exogenous corticosteroids can result in

29. A procedure which can be utilized to establish a more definitive diagnosis of Cushing syndrome is the _____ test.
30. Insufficient amounts of _____ and _____ are produced by the child with salt-losing congenital adrenogenital hyperplasia.
31. Untreated congenital adrenogenital hyperplasia results in early _____ maturation.
32. A sex is assigned to the child with adrenogenital hyperplasia that is consistent with the _____.
33. Urinary levels of 17-ketosteroids are abnormal in _____.
34. Compare the actions of epinephrine and norepinephrine.

	EPINEPHRINE	NOREPINEPH-RINE
Cardiac activity	a.	b.
Constriction of blood vessels	c.	d.
Blood pressure	e.	f.
Cardiac output	g.	h.
Metabolic rate	i.	j.

35. Pheochromocytomas arise from chromaffin cells of the adrenal medulla and there is a _____ transmission as an autosomal _____ trait.

36. The clinical manifestations of pheochromocytoma are caused by: _____.

37. The islets of Langerhans of the pancreas have three major functioning cells. List the hormones produced by each of these cells and its function.
a.

b.

c.

38. There are three types of diabetes mellitus, they are: _____, _____, and _____.

39. Compare the characteristics of Type I and Type II of diabetes mellitus by completing the following chart.

CHARACTERIS-TIC	TYPE I (IDDM)	TYPE II (NIDDM)
Age of onset	a.	b.
% of population	c.	d.
Family history	e.	f.

Presenting symptoms	g.	h.
Nutritional status	i.	j.
Insulin (natural) Pancreatic content Serum insulin Primary resistence	k.	l.
Therapy Insulin Oral agents Diet only	m.	n.
Ketoacidosis	o.	p.

40. Trace the pathophysiology of diabetes mellitus by describing the etiology underlying each of the following physical consequences of the absence of insulin.
a. Insulin is absent—

b. Hyperglycemia—

c. Glycosuria—

d. Polyuria—

e. Polydipsia—

f. Metabolizes proteins and fats—

g. Glucogenesis—

h. Ketonuria and acetone breath—

i. Metabolic acidosis—

j. Polyphagia—

41. What are the three "polys" of diabetes mellitus?

42. Differentiate between the three types of insulin by completing the following chart:

TYPE	ONSET	PEAK	DURATION
Short-acting: regular insulin	a.	b.	c.
Semilente	d.	e.	f.
Intermediate-acting: NPH	g.	h.	i.
Lente	j.	k.	l.
Long-acting: Ultralente	m.	n.	o.
Protamine zinc	p.	q.	r.

3. Exercise is beneficial to the diabetic child because it _____ blood sugar levels.

4. Differentiate between ketoacidosis and a hypoglycemic reaction by completing the following chart.

	HYPOGLY-CEMIA (insulin reaction)	HYPERGLY-CEMIA (ketoacidosis)
Onset	a.	b.
Cause	c.	d.
Manifestations	e.	f.
Ominous features	g.	h.
Urinary findings	i.	j.
Blood glucose	k.	l.

Define the Somogyi effect.

46. The therapeutic management of ketoacidosis consists of:
a.
b.
c.
d.

47. After hydrating the child, a normal serum _____ level must be re-established.

48. What type of insulin is utilized in treating ketoacidosis? _____.

49. What are the long-term complications of diabetes mellitus?
a.
b.
c.
d.

IV. Application, Analysis, and Synthesis of Essential Concepts

A. **Experiential Exercise:** Spend a day in a pediatric endocrine clinic. Answer the following questions and include specific (examples, responses) which illustrate these concepts.

1. List the clinical manifestations you would expect to assess in a child with hypopituitarism.
a.
b.
c.
d.
e.

2. List the clinical manifestations you would expect to assess in a child with hyperpituitarism before epiphyseal closure.
a.
b.
c.

3. List the clinical manifestations you would expect to assess in an infant with diabetes insipidus.
a.
b.
c.
d.

4. What piece of assessment data would alert you to the possibility of an infant having hypothyroidism?

5. The primary nursing goal in relation to hypothyroidism is:

6. Nursing interventions that would achieve the nursing goal of "maintaining the safety of the patient" in a patient experiencing a deficiency in parathyroid would be:
   a.
   b.
   c.
   d.

7. What is the rationale for the nursing intervention "institute safety precautions" with the child who has secondary hyperparathyroidism.

B. **Experiential Exercise:** Care for a child with adrenocortical insufficiency. Answer the following questions and include specifics (examples, responses) which illustrate these concepts.

1. You would take the child's vital signs every 15 minutes. What is the rationale for this intervention?

2. When administering cortisol to the child the nurse carefully checks the dosage and the rate of administration. What is the rationale for these actions?

3. As treatment progesses, you continually assess the child for signs of hypokalemia. What are these signs?

C. **Experiential Exercise:** Care for a child with the Salt-losing form of congenital adrenogenital hyperplasia.

1. A primary nursing goal in relation to the child with adrenogenital hyperplasia is:

2. The rationale for administering cortisone to the child with adrenogenital syndrome is:

3. The nurse would intervene by teaching the parents how to administer cortisol to their child daily. The parents should be taught that in times of stress the cortisol dosage must be _____.

D. **Clinical Situation:** Bobby Lee Jones, an 8-year-old, is on the pediatric unit for diagnosis and treatment of diabetes mellitus.

1. When Bobby arrived on the unit he was displaying symptoms of ketoacidosis.
   a. What are four nursing goals for the care of Bobby?

   b. What evaluation data would you expect for the nursing goal of "Ensure adequate hydration"?

2. Bobby is placed on NPH insulin twice a day. The nurse must intervene by monitoring whether the insulin dose is appropriate. What is the best method to this?

3. Bobby will be maintained on a balanced diet utilizing the exchange system of the American Diabetic Association. The nursing goal regarding this diet is to:

4. Bobby is experiencing a hypoglycemic reaction.
   a. What symptoms would you expect to assess in Bobby?

   b. How would you intervene to treat the hypoglycemia?

E. **Experiential Exercise:** Design a teaching plan f the child with diabetes mellitus.

1. What nursing goals are appropriate to include in thi teaching plan?
   a.
   b.
   c.
   d.
   e.
   f.
   g.
   h.
   i.

V. Suggested Readings

1. McElroy, D., and Davis, G.: SIADH and the acutely ill child, Amer. J. Maternal Child Nurs. **11**:193–196, 1986.
   This thorough discussion of SIADH covers the pathophysiology, detection, and treatment of this complex disease.
2. Burnett, J.: Congenital adrenocortical hyperplasia, Amer Nurs. **80**:1304–1308, 1980.
   The first portion of this article is an anecdotal description a boy with congenital adrenocortical hyperplasia and how the illness affected his family and his growth and development. second part of the article describes the etiology and therapeut management of CAH.
3. Camunas, C.: Pheochromocytoma, Amer. J. Nurs. **83**:88 891,1983.
   This article describes the incidence and etiology of the ph chromocytoma. Diagnostic tests for pheochromocytoma are d

ussed, and drug and surgical therapy are described. Management of the child before and after surgery is explored. Discharge planning is an essential postoperative action that would include the nurse and the parent.

4. Miller B.K., and White, E.: Diabetes assessment guide, Am. J. Nurs. **80**:1314–1316,1980.

This article explains how a questionnaire developed by these authors can be utilized to assess the knowledge as well as the skills regarding diabetes that a child and his family have acquired. The questionnaire addresses six areas of knowledge: history of diabetes, insulin, oral hypoglycemics, diet, diagnostic tests, and general information. Both the patient and the nurse can readily identify those areas of knowledge and skill that are well understood and those areas that need reinforcement through further teaching.

5. Dexter, D.: The new insulins, Am. J. Nurs. **81**:146–148,1981.

This article compares all of the insulin products produced by Lilly and Squibb companies. The insulin products are identical to those produced in the past, except for the purity factor. The importance of this factor is explained in detail. The implications for modification of the normal dosage of insulin due to increased purity is essential knowledge for the nurse and her patient.

6. Fredholm, N.: The insulin pump: new method of insulin delivery, Am. J. Nurs. **81**:2024–2026,1981.

This article explains the two models of insulin pumps being used at the Joslin Clinic, the Mill Hill Infusion Insulin Pump and the Auto Syringe AS6C. Detailed instructions for use of these pumps, and the advantages and disadvantages of their use are discussed. It is hoped that this method of insulin administration will prevent diabetic complications such as neuropathy, retinopathy, and nephropathy.

7. Stevens, A.D.: Monitoring blood glucose at home, who should do it? Am. J. Nurs. **81**:2026–2027, 1981.

This article advocates the use of home blood glucose monitoring (HBGM) as a more accurate and reliable method of monitoring blood glucose than urine testing. The two brands of testing strips, Dextrostix and Chemstrip bG, are discussed and compared on the basis of ease of use and cost.

8. Plasse, N.: Monitoring blood glucose at home, a comparison of three products, Am. J. Nurs. **81**:2028–2029,1981.

This article summarizes the results of a study done at El Camino Hospital to compare three glucose testing devices: Chemstrip bG, Ames Dextrostix, and the Ames Dextrometer. The study compared the performance of 16 nurses and 12 patients on the ease and accuracy of use of the three products. The accuracy of use was checked against laboratory readings on blood glucose. The findings of the study are presented along with recommendations for use for patients whose visual acuity, dexterity or color perception are compromised.

9. Thatcher, G.: Insulin injections, the case against random rotation, Am. J. Nurs. **85**:690–693,1985.

Based on cited research findings the author recommends a non-random rotation method of insulin injection. The disadvantages of the random method are discussed, and a detailed description of the new method of administration is presented.

10. Kiser, D.: The Somogyi effect, Am. J. Nurs. **80**:236–238, 1980.

The clinical clues indicative of the Somogyi effect are presented. The article gives a clear, detailed description of how to teach patients to recognize and deal with the rapid hyperglycemia and hypoglycemia due to the Somogyi effect.

11. Miller, V.G.: Diabetes, let's stop testing urine, Am. J. Nurs. **86**:54,1986.

This article quotes research findings from 1939 through 1986 that discourages the use of urine testing as the means of determining needed insulin dosage. The research documents that there is no correlation between blood glucose and urine glucose readings. The author concludes by recommending urine testing only for ketones.

12. Fendya D.G., and Flynn K.: Nursing care for children with hypoglycemia due to hyperinsulinism, Am. J. Maternal Child Nurs. **6**:100–105, 1981.

The article begins by describing the action of insulin and the diagnosis of hypoglycemia due to hyperinsulinism. Four children of various ages are discussed to illustrate the following concepts of hyperinsulinism-induced hypoglycemia: initial treatment; immediate postoperative care; maintaining glucose levels; psychosocial considerations; and discharge teaching.

Chapter 39

The Child with Neuromuscular, Musculoskeletal, or Articular Dysfunction

I. Chapter Overview

Chapter 39 introduces nursing considerations essential to the care of the child with a disorder of neuromuscular, musculoskeletal, or articular function. Since childhood is the age of onset for a variety of physically disabling conditions, it is important for the student to gain an understanding of the care of children with this type of alteration in health. The conditions discussed in this chapter may result from defects in the muscle itself, defective transmission of nerve impulses to muscles, dysfunction of peripheral motor or sensory nerves, damage to the central nervous system, or damage to the skeletal system. At the completion of this chapter, the student will be able to formulate nursing measures directed toward helping the child and his family develop effective coping responses to deal with alterations in neuromuscular function.

II. Learning Objectives

Upon completion of this chapter, it is expected that the student will be able to:

1. Discuss the role of the nurse in helping parents deal effectively with a child with cerebral palsy.

2. Outline a plan of care for the child with Guillain-Barré syndrome.

3. Discuss the prevention and treatment of tetanus.

4. Differentiate among the various types of muscular dystrophy.

5. Describe the therapeutic management and nursing care of the child with scoliosis.

6. Outline a plan of care for the child with osteomyelitis.

7. Describe the nursing care of a child with juvenile rheumatoid arthritis.

8. Demonstrate an understanding of the management of systemic lupus erythematosus.

III. Review of Essential Concepts

1. Cerebral palsy is:

2. Is there a characteristic pathologic picture of cerebr palsy? _____.

3. The clinical manifestations of cerebral palsy fall int five major areas, what are they?
   a.
   b.
   c.
   d.
   e.

4. What is the relationship between cerebral palsy and mental retardation?

5. List and define the classifications of cerebral palsy.
   a.

   b.

c.

d.

e.

6. The broad aims of therapy for the child with cerebral palsy are:
   a.

   b.

   c.

   d.

7. The most frequently employed conservative treatment modality is _____.

8. Guillain-Barré syndrome is an

9. Identify the clinical manifestations of Guillain-Barré syndrome.

10. Treatment of Guillain-Barré syndrome is symptomatic but _____ may be needed to preserve life.

11. Tetanus is:

12. The characteristic symptom of tetanus that gives the disease its common name is:

13. The specific prophylactic therapy for tetanus after trauma is: _____. The unimmunized child who sustains a "tetanus-prone" wound should receive _____.

14. Proper surgical cleansing of contaminated wounds will reduce _____.

15. What specific nursing interventions are utilized to prevent seizures in the child with tetanus?
    a.

    b.

All of the muscular dystrophies have a genetic origin

in which there is a gradual degeneration of _____ and all are characterized by:

_____

_____.

17. In all forms of muscular dystrophy there is insidious loss of strength, the various forms differ in regard to:

18. The most severe and most common muscular dystrophy of childhood is:

19. The cause of death in Duchenne's muscular dystrophy is:

20. _____ of the hips, knees, and ankles occur early in the disease and compromise mobility.

21. The primary goal of therapy is:

22. What are the two classifications of scoliosis?

23. Scoliosis is currently managed by straightening and realignment of the vertebrae by either:

24. _____ is the primary mode of therapy for minor curvatures.

25. _____ is often used before spinal fusion to provide partial correction and more flexibility.

26. Following Harrington instrumentation the child is immobilized on a _____. Children with Dwyer instrumentation are cared for in _____.

27. What is the primary advantage and disadvantage of the Lugue segmental instrumentation?

28. Osteomyelitis is an _____ which can be acquired from _____ or _____ sources.

29. When the infective agent of osteomyelitis is identified, vigorous _____ is initiated with an appropriate _____. Therapy is continued for at least _____ weeks.

30. In addition to antibiotic therapy the child with osteomyelitis is placed on _____ and the affected extremity is _____.

31. The latex fixation test is diagnostic for rheumatoid arthritis in the adult. In children the latex fixation test is _____.

32. What are the clinical manifestations of juvenile rheumatoid arthritis?

33. Growth disturbances are often present in the child with JRA. What are the reasons?

a.

b.

34. What is the prognosis for children with JRA?

35. What are the major goals of therapy for the child with JRA?
a.

b.

c.

36. Iridocyclitis is an _____.

37. The primary group of drugs prescribed for JRA are: _____. What are the desired effects of these drugs?

38. The levels of these drugs are monitored regularly because:

39. The second group of drugs used to treat JRA are:

40. Why are corticosteroids not a drug of choice for JRA?

41. Systemic lupus erythematosus (SLE) is:

42. SLE can affect almost any tissue, so the clinical manifestations vary according to the tissue affected. However, a characteristic cutaneous response of SLE is:

43. Identify the gravest prognostic sign in SLE.

44. Identify the objectives of therapeutic management of SLE.
a.

b.

45. Identify the principal drugs utilized to control the inflammation of SLE.

46. Identify the principal nursing goal for the child with SLE.

47. Identify the relationship of rest to the status of SLE.

IV. Application, Analysis, and Synthesis of Essential Concepts

A. **Experiential Exercise:** Spend a day in a clinic that treats children with cerebral palsy.

1. What specific nursing interventions would help parents to cope with a child with cerebral palsy?
a.
b.
c.
d.
e.
f.
g.

2. List at least two nursing diagnoses for a child with cerebral palsy.
a.

b.

B. **Clinical Situation:** Victor Morris, age 13 years, has been admitted to the Pediatric Unit with a diagnosis of Guillain-Barré syndrome.

1. The primary nursing goal is:

2. List at least two nursing interventions to achieve the above nursing goal.
a.
b.

C. **Experiential Exercise:** Spend a day in a clinic serving children with muscular dystrophy.

1. Because parents of children with muscular dystrophy tend to overprotect their child, how would you intervene to assist both child and family?

2. Because of the genetic etiology of this disease you would intervene by:

D. **Clinical Situation:** Jane Roberts, age 14 years, is admitted to the adolescent unit for the Harrington rod procedure.

1. What is an important nursing diagnosis that may be evident when the nurse considers the interaction of Jane's physical defect and psychological growth and developmental processes of the adolescent.

   a.

   or:

   b.

2. What nursing interventions are appropriate to promote the nursing goal of "Help the child develop a positive self-image"?

   a.
   b.
   c.
   d.
   e.

E. **Clinical Situation:** Emmanuel Rogerio, age 10 years, is admitted for treatment of osteomyelitis.

. What clinical manifestations would you expect to assess in Emmanuel if the diagnosis is correct?

. What nursing interventions are appropriate for the nursing goal of "Maintain intravenous infusion"?

   a.
   b.
   c.
   d.
   e.
   f.

F. **Clinical Situation:** Robin Monteira, age 11 years, admitted to the pediatric unit for treatment of JRA.

Identify evaluation date that would evidence accomplishment of the nursing goal of "Preserve joint function".

   a.
   b.

Identify an appropriate nursing diagnosis related to nutrition in Robin.

Since Robin is on high doses of aspirin, you would assess for aspirin toxicity. Identify the signs of aspirin toxicity and their underlying etiology.

   a.

   b.

c.

d.

V. Suggested Readings

1. Hussey, C.G.: Surviving a handicap in everyday life: how to help, Am. J. Maternal Guild Nurs. **4**:46–50, 1979.

   Although this article describes the case history of a child with Legg-Calvé-Perthes disease, the concepts presented can be applied to the nursing care of any child with a handicapping condition. The article describes how a mother, who was also a nurse, planned and implemented a plan of care for this child that addressed the growth and development needs of the child in the physical, psychological, emotional, and social realms. The role of the nurse in helping the parents and child to cope with a handicapping condition is outlined.

2. Brady, M.H.: Lifelong care of the child with Duchenne muscular dystrophy, Am. J. Maternal Child Nurs. **4**:227–230, 1979.

   After a discussion of the etiologic and genetic considerations for the child with Duchenne muscular dystrophy, this article explores the nurse's role in helping the parents to provide life-long nursing care for this child. Special emphasis is given to the parental problems of adjustment and to the prevention of complications in the child.

3. Lenox, A.C.: When motor nerves die, Am. J. Nurs. **83**:540–546, 1983.

   This article begins by describing five diseases that involve motor cell degeneration. The focus of the remaining portion of the article is on assisting the client to adjust and cope with his handicap. The role of the nurse in helping this client achieve the maximal level of function possible is described. Boxed material on support devices, head and neck exercises, and equipment resources would be helpful to the nurse planning care for a client with this handicap. The role of the nurse in augmenting physical therapy and dealing with complications is discussed.

4. Allar, J.L., and Dibble, S.L.: Scoliosis surgery: a look at Luque rods, Am. J. Nurs. **84**:609–611, 1984.

   Through the case of a 13-year-old girl with scoliosis, the authors illustrate the advantages, disadvantages, and nursing care of the child undergoing the placement of Luque rods for correction of scoliosis.

5. Davis, S.E., and Lewis, S.A.: Managing scoliosis: fashions for the body and mind, Am. J. Maternal Child Nurs. **9**:186–187.

   Through the presentation of a case of an adolescent female with scoliosis the authors illustrate the necessity for nursing care focused on preserving the adolescent's physical and emotional wellbeing, while insuring compliance with medical treatment of the scoliosis.

6. Gorman, T.K., and March, M.E.: Arthritis at an early age, Am. J. Nurs. **84**:1472–1477, 1984.

   The three major types of juvenile rheumatoid arthritis (JRA) are listed and explained. Detailed discussion of current drug therapy for JRA is included. Boxed material on the drugs is very helpful. The nurse's role in prevention of deformity and the enhancement of the psychosocial growth of the child is addressed.

Chapter 40

The Immobilized or Traumatically Injured Child

I. Chapter Overview

Chapter 40 introduces nursing considerations essential to the care of the child immobilized with a traumatic injury. Since childhood is the time for the occurrence of a variety of physical conditions caused by trauma, it is important for the student to understand the care of children with these types of alterations in health. The conditions discussed in this chapter may be either temporary or permanent, however, they all affect the child's locomotive ability to a greater or lesser extent. Nursing goals and responsibilities are developed to assist the child and family to effectively cope with the physical, emotional, and psychosocial stressors imposed by a traumatic injury.

II. Learning Objectives

Upon completion of this chapter, it is expected that the student will be able to:

1. Identify the major complications of immobilization.

2. Identify the major etiologic factors that contribute to the incidence of trauma in childhood.

3. Identify the rationale for the immediate assessment of traumatic injuries.

4. Describe the types of fractures that are most frequently seen in children.

5. Develop a teaching plan for the parents of a child in a cast.

6. Explain the functions of the various types of traction.

7. Devise a nursing care plan for a child in traction.

8. Describe the staging of spinal cord injuries according to physiologic responses.

III. Review of Essential Concepts

1. List the consequences of immobilization of the child.

   a.

   b.

   c.

2. Shallow respirations and obstruction of the airway with mucus contributes to the development of secondary complications such as:_____, _____, and _____.

3. The psychological and emotional consequences of immobilization to the child can severely affect normal growth and development. One of the most useful interventions to help children cope with immobility to encourage the child to _____.

4. _____ is the leading cause of death in children.

5. List the three major causes of trauma in children.

   a.
   b.
   c.

6. Many serious accidents are caused by:

7. It is important to immediately assess the child who has sustained a traumatic injury in order to:

8. Spinal cord injury is suspected if there is:

9. The first priority upon admission to an emergency facility is assessment of the ABC status. What does ABC refer to?

   a.

   b.

   c.

10. Identify the features of children's fractures that are not observed in the adult.

a.

b.

c.

d.

e.

f.

1. List and describe the most frequently seen fractures in children.
   a.

   b.

   c.

   d.

2. The three goals of therapeutic management are:
   a.
   b.
   c.

3. In children, the bone fragments are usually realigned and immobilized by _____ or by _____ and _____ until adequate callus is formed.

4. During the first few hours after a cast is applied the nurse must observe the cast and the involved extremity for signs of neurovascular integrity. What signs would indicate compromise in the extremity?

5. What signs would you assess in the casted extremity to indicate the possibility of a developing infection?

6. What are the three primary purposes for use of traction?
   a.

   b.

   c.

17. What are the three methods of applying pull to the distal bone fragment for traction?
    a.
    b.
    c.

18. Compare the functions of the various types of traction for the lower extremity by matching the following:
    a. Balance suspension
    b. 90-degree-90-degree traction
    c. Buck's extension
    d. Russell traction
    e. Bryant's traction

    a. _____ A form of running traction utilized for children less than 2 years of age
    b. _____ A form of running traction in which hips are not flexed
    c. _____ A form of skin traction that has two lines of pull, one along the longitudinal line of the lower leg and one perpendicular to the leg
    d. _____ Lower leg is put in a boot cast and a skeletal Steinmann pin is placed in the distal fragment of the femur.
    e. _____ Suspends the leg in a desired flexed position to relax the hip and hamstring muscles and does not exert any traction directly on a body part

19. Identify the major complication that can occur in a child with multiple fractures: _____

20. Two terms that describe neurologic deficits in spinal cord injury are paraplegia and quadriplegia. Define these terms.
    a. Paraplegia:—

    b. Quadriplegia:—

21. The extent of paralysis is determined by both _____ and _____ assessment.

22. Describe the stages of physiologic response to spinal cord injury by completing the following chart.

STAGE	RESPONSES
First (spinal shock)	a.
Second	b.

STAGE	RESPONSES
Third	c.

c.

d.

e.

23. The three goals of rehabilitation of a child with acquired spinal injury are:
   a.

   b.

   c.

B. **Clinical Situation:** You arrive at the scene of an automobile accident before the rescue squad. An 8-year-old child has been injured in the crash and is seated in the front seat of the automobile with his seat belt still fastened.

1. What would you assess before intervening to move the child out of the car?
   a.

   b.

   If you decide to move the child, how should it be done?
   c.

IV. Application, Analysis, and Synthesis of Essential Concepts

A. **Experiential Exercise:** Spend a day on the neurological unit observing the care of immobilized children.

The nurse must plan the care of the immobilized child with the knowledge that immobilization causes functional and metabolic responses in most of the body systems.

1. Identify nursing interventions that would help the child to minimize the effects of venous stasis.
   a.
   b.
   c.
   d.
   e.
   f.
   g.
   h.

2. What is the rationale for monitoring vital signs every 4 hours in the immobilized child?

3. What manifestations of tissue ischemia of the skin would you assess to detect and prevent skin breakdown?
   a.

   b.

2. It is important to assess the injured child for bleeding. You discover that there is a bleeding wound on his left leg. What is the most appropriate way to stop the bleeding?

3. You decide to assess the left leg for possible function. What factors would you assess?
   a.
   b.
   c.
   d.
   e.

4. Upon further assessment there appears to be a fracture of the left leg. How would you intervene to treat this fracture?

C. **Experiential Exercise:** Spend a day on a pediatric orthopedic unit.

1. A 5-year-old child with a fractured right leg has just had a cast applied. The nurse must intervene by teaching the parents how to care for the cast. What elements would you include in your teaching plan regarding methods to decrease the swelling under the cast.
   a.

b.

c.

d.

2. What elements would you include in a teaching plan regarding maintaining the integrity of the cast?
   a.
   b.
   c.

D. **Clinical Situation:** Roger Trudeau, age 13 years, is in 90-degree-90-degree traction for treatment of a fracture of the right femur.

1. Identify the nursing interventions that will achieve the nursing goal of "maintaining the traction."
   a.
   b.
   c.
   d.
   e.
   f.
   g.
2. Identify a nursing diagnosis in which the primary nursing goal is "prevent complications."

3. You would assess the Steinmann pin for signs of bleeding or for inflammation to detect problems.

E. **Clinical Situation:** Anthony Romero, age 15 years, is hospitalized in a rehabilitation center for treatment of paraplegia secondary to a spinal cord injury.

1. The primary nursing goals for care of Anthony in the acute period are:
   a.
   b.
2. What nursing interventions would accomplish the nursing goal of "prevention of skin breakdown?"
   a.
   b.

c.
d.
3. What is the rationale for administering ascorbic acid daily to Anthony?

V. Suggested Readings

1. Drehoble, P.: Quadriceps contracture, Am. J. Nurs. **80**:1650–1654, 1980.
   A case study is presented to illustrate how quadriceps contractures can occur; and how a combination of surgery and physical therapy is utilized to decrease the contractures and increase function. Nursing interventions to prevent these contractures from occurring are outlined.
2. Farrell, J.: Orthopedic pain, what does it mean? Am. J. Nurs. **84**:466–469, 1984.
   How to differentiate between pain from an injury or from a complication is the focus of this article. How to assess and intervene effectively in the manangement of pain is discussed for four common orthopedic conditions: total knee replacement, total hip replacement, fractured femur, and fractured tibia. A comparison is made between expected pain and signs of complications for each of these conditions.
3. Wise, L.B.: A comparison of orthopedic casts: breaking the mold, Am. J. Maternal Child Nurs. **11**:174–176, 1986.
   The author compares the plaster-of-Paris cast and the synthetic casts on five parameters. General nursing goals and nursing care considerations for care of the child in a cast are introduced.
4. Howard, M., and Corbo-Pelaia, S.A.: Psychological after effects of halo traction, Am. J. Nurs. **82**:1839–1843, 1982.
   The purpose and nursing considerations for halo traction in spinal cord injury are presented. When halo traction is removed the patient experiences an entity called post-halo-traction depression. Nursing interventions to deal with this depressive state are discussed.
5. Birdsall, C.: How do you teach female self-catheterization? Am. J. Nurs. **85**:1226–1227, 1985.
   The variables that the nurse must consider when teaching self-catheterization are outlined. A step-by-step procedure for performing the self-catheterization is included.

Answer Key

Chapter 1

QUESTION		ANSWER

Section III

1.   b
2.   accidents
3.   developmental stage
4.   b
5.   a
6.   a.   family advocacy
      b.   illness prevention and health promotion
      c.   health teaching
      d.   support and counseling
      e.   therapeutic role
      f.   coordination and collaboration
      g.   research
      h.   health care planning
7.   a.   assessment
      b.   nursing diagnosis
      c.   plan formulation
      d.   implementation
      e.   evaluation
8.   primary nursing

Section IV A

1.   a.   the number of individuals who have died over a specific period of time
      b.   the prevalence of a specific illness in the population at a particular time.
2.   Knowledge of these two concepts can help to identify high-risk age groups for certain disorders or hazards, identify advances in prevention and treatment, direct energies into specific areas of health counseling, and guide more effective planning and delivery of care.
3.   The most effective approach to reducing morbidity and mortality is through the nurse's role in educating parents and promoting optimal health practices.

Section IV B

1.   a.   Ensure families' awareness of various health services; inform families of treatments and procedures; involve families in child's care; change or support existing health-care practices.
      b.   Practice within the overall framework for preventive health; utilize an approach of education and anticipatory guidance.
      c.   Provide health education and evaluate the status of and need for health knowledge.
      d.   Provide support through listening, touching, and physical presence; utilize counseling as the basis for mutual problem solving.
      e.   Continual assessment and evaluation of the health status of the client; implementation of care-giving activities to facilitate optimal level of wellness.
      f.   Work with professionals in other disciplines to formulate and implement a plan of care that meets the child's needs.
      g.   Become involved in policy and decision-making on the community and national levels to enhance health care delivery.
2.   a.   to identify any problems the client may be experiencing and thus develop a comprehensive means of achieving an optimal outcome

    b.   to provide continuity of nursing care

3.   a.   the collection, classification, and analysis of data from a variety of sources

    b.   identification of problem areas that may include unmet needs, unrealized expectations, interrupted processes, or community crises

    c.   decision-making phase of the process in which a plan of action is developed to a specific goal

    d.   selecting and performing interventions that are most likely to achieve a desired outcome

    e.   analysis of data to determine whether the goal has been met, the plan requires modification, or another alternative should be considered

4.   Primary nursing involves 24-hour responsibility and accountability for the care of a small group of patients. In this capacity, nurses are responsible for their actions, in both the legal and ethical sense. If the nurse's responsibilities are shared with other staff, it is usually with an associate primary nurse who maintains continuity of care and assumes only temporary accountability.

Chapter 2

QUESTION		ANSWER

Section III

1.   culture

2.   a.   b

    b.   d

    c.   c

    d.   a

3.   T

4.   a.   ethnicity

    b.   social class

    c.   occupational role

5.   a.   teaches the child how to deal with dominance and hostility

    b.   teaches children to relate with persons in positions of leadership and authority

    c.   relieves the child's boredom

    d.   provides recognition that individual members do not receive from teachers and other authority figures

6.   a.   anger

    b.   low self-esteem

7.   susceptible; resistant

8.   a.   proximity to disease

    b.   environmental factors

    c.   general physical status

9.   a.   cultural standards and values

    b.   families' past experiences with health care

    c.   family structure and function

10.   F

Section IV A

1.   The culture in which children are reared determines the types of food they will eat, the language they will speak, the ideals of behavior, and the way in which social roles should be conducted. It also outlines the roles of their parents, structures their relationships with other people, and determines much of the behavior they acquire.

2.   a.   ethnicity

    b.   social class

    c.   economic status

    d.   occupation

    e.   religion

    f.   education

    g.   peer influences

3.   a.   emphasizes a group-oriented and other-directed philosophy

    b.   results in a future orientation with the possibility of upward social mobility

    c.   results in less reliance on tradition

    d.   results in the child's exposure to a number of adults who differ from one another but who all provide input as role models and teachers

    e.   strongly influences adult relationships with children and produces changing philosophies of child-rearing

    f.   exert a major force in providing continuity between generations; prepare children to carry out traditional social roles expected of adults in society

    g.   produces vulnerability to hostility, derogation, and discrimination from children and adults of the social majority

Section IV B

1.   a.   hereditary factors—may be the result of an inherent lack of resistance to a disease organism, a trait that is an advantage in one environment but places the possessor at a disadvantage in another, or the consequence of intermarriage in a relatively narrow range of geographic, ethnic, or religious restrictions.

    b.   socioeconomic factors—such aspects of lower-class living conditions as crowding, poor sanitation, access to lead-containing substances, inadequate access to health services.

2.   a.   result in a diet lacking in essential nutrients, especially proteins, vitamins, and iron, leading to nutritional deficiencies and growth retardation

    b.   leads to erratic food intake and a disproportionately large consumption of non-nourishing snacks

    c.   leads to dental problems and lack of standard immunization.

    d.   contribute to a higher incidence and perpetuation of illness

3.   a.   beliefs about birth and death

    b.   beliefs about diet and food practices

4.   Nurses are products of their own cultural backgrounds and educations, which influence their values, thoughts, and actions. When they are aware of their own culturally founded behavior, they are likely to be more sensitive to cultural behavior in others. They identify behaviors as characteristic of a culture rather than as ''abnormal'' and thus can relate more effectively with the families.

5.   a.   establishing a resource file of pertinent information about the cultural and subcultural characteristics of the community

    b.   establishing a close relationship with families and other influential persons in the community

    c.   assessing his or her own attitudes and behaviors and those of other health workers toward people of varying cultures

Chapter 3

QUESTION		ANSWER

Section III

1.   a.   developmental theory
    b.   structural-functional theory
    c.   interactional theory

2.   a.   c
    b.   f
    c.   e
    d.   a
    e.   b
    f.   d

3.   a.   caregiving
    b.   nurturing
    c.   training

4.   c

5.   a.   c
    b.   e
    c.   b
    d.   f
    e.   a
    f.   d

6.   F

7.   socialization

8.   d

9.   a.   family size
    b.   spacing of children
    c.   ordinal position
    d.   multiple births

10.   T

11.	a.	promotion of physical survival and health of the children; ensuring that they will live long enough to reproduce
	b.	fostering of skills and behavioral capacities needed for economic self-maintenance as an adult
	c.	fostering of behavioral capabilities for the maximization of cultural values and beliefs
12.	a.	anticipation
	b.	honeymoon
	c.	plateau
	d.	disengagement
13.	a.	parental age
	b.	previous experience
	c.	marital relationship
	d.	father involvement
	e.	effects of stress
	f.	infant characteristics
	g.	support systems
14.	a.	Parents try to control their children's behavior and attitudes through unquestioned mandates.
	b.	Parents exert little or no control over their children's actions.
	c.	Parents combine some practices from both the authoritarian and permissive styles, directing children's behavior and attitudes by emphasizing the reason for rules and negatively reinforcing deviations.
15.		T
16.	a.	b
	b.	c
	c.	a
	d.	e
	e.	d
17.		reciprocal role relationship
18.		T
19.		T
20.		F
21.		adolescence
22.	a.	age and sex of children
	b.	the outcome of the divorce
	c.	the quality of parental care following the divorce
	d.	the love and understanding that continue after the parents' separation
	e.	the genuine concern and affection that exist for the child
23.	a.	efforts on the part of one parent to subvert the child's loyalty to the other
	b.	abandonment to other caregivers
	c.	need for adjustment to a step-parent
24.	a.	Task 1—acknowledge the marital disruption
	b.	Task 2—regain a sense of direction and freedom to pursue customary activities
	c.	Task 3—deal with the loss and feelings of rejection
	d.	Task 4—forgive the parents
	e.	Task 5—accept the permanence of the divorce and relinquish longings for the restoration of the predivorced family
	f.	Task 6—resolve issues of relationship
25.	a.	Parent—assumed in matters of discipline, planning family experiences, and setting limits on behavior
	b.	Step-parent—assumed when plans and activities must be shared with the absent natural parent
	c.	Non-parent—assumed when the step-parent steps aside to allow the spouse to manage things that the step-parent is not or does not wish to be a part of
26.		52%
27.		F

Section IV A

1.	a.	caregiving
	b.	nurturing
	c.	training
2.		individuals with socially recognized statuses and positions who interact with one another on a regular, recurring basis in socially sanctioned ways
3.		events such as marriage, divorce, birth, death, abandonment, and incarceration
4.		Roles must be redefined or redistributed
5.	a.	This predominant American family structure is highly adaptable, having the ability to adjust and reshape its structure when needed. It is free to move where there is opportunity and is not dependent on the cooperative effort of other

members. When there is wide geographic separation from the extended family, parents are faced with having no relatives readily available for advice, assistance, and child care.

b.   More liberal attitudes have made it possible to rear children without both parents being present in the home. Frequently children in these families are absorbed into the extended family.

c.   More functional in areas where land is the basis of wealth and sustenance. Here the family serves as the basic social, educational and productive unit, providing services and sharing resources. The needs of the individual are sublimated for the welfare of the family. Children learn early in life to respect their elders. Child rearing is a shared responsibility.

6.   In the upper classes, the nuclear family is firmly embedded and primarily patrifocal. In the middle classes, the family ties are more loosely attached, allowing for social, economic, and geographic mobility. The tendency in lower classes is toward matrifocal family units with multiple generations living in an extended structure to share the economic burden and child care.

7.   a.   In a small family, more emphasis is placed on the individual development of the child, parenting is intensive, and there is constant pressure to measure up to family expectations. In a large family, more emphasis is placed on the group and less on the individual. The number of children reduces one-to-one contact between parent and individual children.

b.   Older siblings tend to dominate so that the younger children develop better interpersonal skills, the ability to negotiate, and the ability to accept unfavorable outcomes. Later-born children seem to be more outgoing and make friends more easily, while firstborn children are more achievement-oriented and exhibit strong drive and ambition.

c.   The narrower the spacing between siblings, the more the children influence each other. When there is wider spacing between children, the parent has the greater influence.

Section IV B

1.   Parents apply direct or indirect pressures in an attempt to either induce or force children into desired patterns of behavior. They might also direct their efforts toward modification of the role responses of the child on a mutually accepted basis.

2.   a.   by rewards such as love, affection, friendship, and honors
     b.   by ridicule, withdrawal of love, expressions of disapproval, and banishment

3.   a.   These strictly defined roles apply to general traits such as sex, age, kinship, social class and ethnic origins.
     b.   These are acquired through effort and include education, occupation, religion, and recreation.
     c.   These may be transient or become fixed into character roles and apply to unique behaviors displayed in a given situation such as leader, follower, prankster, or show-off.
     d.   These are related to fantasy and are roles of persons whom children observe within their environment.

4.   The times at which adult behaviors are learned vary greatly. Roles may be discontinuous; that is, children are taught roles in direct opposition to those they are expected to assume as adults. In other cultures, roles are continuous, with the same behaviors encouraged in children and adults. Attitudes toward sexuality vary across cultures.

Section IV C

1.   a.   simple assumption that all normal people get married and have children
     b.   proof of biological adequacy and demonstration of adulthood
     c.   fulfills a parent's wish for grandchildren and to perpetuate the family name and fortune
     d.   an attempt to save a tenuous marriage

2.   a.   survival goal
     b.   economic goal
     c.   self-actualization goal

3.   a.   young couple thinks about and discusses becoming parents and how they will rear their children
     b.   early adjustment to the infant in which an attachment is formed and new role learning takes place; transition from non-parent to parent is made
     c.   period of parental development that parallels the child's development
     d.   phase ending the active parental role, usually at the time of the child's marriage

4.   a.   parental age
     b.   previous experience
     c.   marital relationship
     d.   father involvement
     e.   effects of stress
     f.   infant's characteristics

5.   Factors include cultural influences, social class, and economic resources.

6.   They are most effective when they are appropriate to the age of the child and to the magnitude of the transgression. They are also effective when administered early rather than late. Disciplinary action should be consistent and tempered with affection.

Section IV D

1.   altered self-image; need for realignment of role; feelings of anger, remorse, guilt, retaliation, and sorrow for oneself
2.   Parents tend to devote extra attention to the child because of feelings of guilt and lowered self-esteem. As a result, children often feel that the burden of the parent's happiness is on their shoulders.
3.   overload, time demands, and scheduling
4.   a.   age of the child
     b.   attitude of the father toward the wife's employment
     c.   regularity with which the mother is away from home
     d.   availability and quality of substitute child care

Chapter 4

QUESTION		ANSWER

Section III

1.   a.   f
     b.   c
     c.   a
     d.   e
     e.   b
     f.   d
2.   a.   conception to birth
     b.   birth to 28 days
     c.   1 month to 12 months
     d.   1 to 6 years
     e.   1 to 3 years
     f.   3 to 6 years
     g.   6 to 11 years
     h.   10 to 13 years
     i.   13 to 18 years
3.   a.   cephalocaudal, or head-to-tail
     b.   proximodistal, or near-to-far
     c.   mass to specific, or differentiation
4.   sensitive periods
5.   a.   b
     b.   a
     c.   d
     d.   c
6.   physical growth
7.   a.   the creation of new cells and tissues (growth)
     b.   the consolidation of tissues into a permanent form (maturation)
8.   F
9.   a.   growth
     b.   calcification
     c.   eruption
     d.   attrition
10.   Catch-up growth
11.   110; 120; 40; 50
12. a.   reflexive or rudimentary movement
     b.   general fundamental skills
     c.   specific skills
     d.   specialized skills
13. a.   the difficult child
     b.   the slow-to-warm-up child
     c.   the easy child
14. a.   oral stage—birth to 1 year
     b.   anal stage—1 to 3 years
     c.   phallic stage—3 to 6 years
     d.   latency period—6 to 12 years

	e.	genital stage—12 years and over
15.	a.	trust vs mistrust
	b.	autonomy vs shame and doubt
	c.	initiative vs guilt
	d.	industry vs inferiority
	e.	identity vs role confusion
	f.	intimacy vs isolation
	g.	generativity vs stagnation
	h.	ego integrity vs despair
16.	a.	c, e
	b.	a, h
	c.	d, g
	d.	b, f
17.	a.	Preconventional morality
	b.	Postconventional level
	c.	Conventional level
18.	a.	an intact and discriminating auditory apparatus
	b.	intelligence
	c.	a need to communicate
	d.	stimulation
19.		F
20.		T
21.	a.	a dietary intake that is quantitatively and/or qualitatively inadequate
	b.	disease that interferes with appetite, digestion, or absorption while increasing nutritional requirements
	c.	excessive physical activity or inadequate rest
	d.	disturbed interpersonal relationships and other environmental or psychologic factors
22.		developmental retardation
23.	a.	b
	b.	e
	c.	a
	d.	d
	e.	c
24.	a.	sensorimotor development
	b.	intellectual development
	c.	socialization
	d.	creativity
	e.	self-awareness
	f.	therapeutic value
	g.	moral value
25.	a.	physical and biologic needs
	b.	love and affection
	c.	security
	d.	discipline and authority
	e.	dependence and independence
	f.	self-esteem

Section IV A

1. Although children vary in both their rate of growth and their acquisition of developmental skills, certain predictable patterns are universal and basic to all human beings. These predetermined trends in direction, sequence, and pace help to predict the child's physical development and maturation of neuromuscular function.

2.	a.	d, f
	b.	a, b, e, f
	c.	b, c, e
	d.	b, e
	e.	d, g
3.	a.	trust vs mistrust (consistently meet the child's basic needs, provide loving care)
	b.	autonomy vs shame and doubt (allow the child the opportunity to make choice, avoid criticizing and demeaning the child)
	c.	initiative vs guilt (encourage exploration of the environment; set realistic limits in a nonjudgmental manner)
	d.	industry vs inferiority (encourage competition and cooperation; assist in setting achievable goals)

e.   identity vs role confusion (provide positive feedback regarding appearance and activities; encourage exploration of future goals and career opportunities)

4.   a.   no concept of right or wrong evident
      b.   imitation of religious gestures and behaviors of others without comprehension of meaning
      c.   imitation of religious behavior and following of parental religious beliefs as part of daily lives without real understanding of basic concepts
      d.   strong interest in religion with acceptance of a deity; petitions to this deity made and expected to be answered
      e.   realization that prayers are not always answered; initiation of modification or abandonment of religious practices; question the religious standards of their parents

5.   a.   the toys should suit the skills, abilities, and interests of the child
      b.   toys should be safe for the child's specific developmental age

Section IV B

1.   Infants with difficult or slow-to-warm-up patterns of behavior are more vulnerable to the development of behavior problems in early and middle childhood. However, any child can develop behavior problems if there is dissonance between his or her temperament and the environment. When parents are unable to accept and deal with the child's behavior, there is a greater likelihood of subsequent behavioral problems.

2.   a.   even-tempered, regular and predictable habits, positive approach to new stimuli, adaptable to change
      b.   highly active; irritable; irregular in habits; has negative withdrawal responses; slow to adapt to new routines, people, or situations
      c.   inactive, moody, moderately irregular in functions, passive resistance to novelty or changes in routine, reacts negatively with mild intensity to new stimuli but adapts slowly with repeated contact

Section IV C

1.   a.   providing adequate nutrition, maintaining or restoring hydration, promoting adequate ventilation, regulating temperature status, promoting normal elimination, providing for adequate rest and activity, promoting physical safety
      b.   communicating unconditional acceptance of the child, promoting parent-child attachment, supporting and reassuring the parents
      c.   providing a consistent caregiver, meeting physical needs, allowing for expression of feelings, setting limits, identifying realistic expectations for behavior and achievement, assessing threats to sense of security
      d.   setting reasonable rules, demanding acceptable behavior, providing consistent and unconditional discipline, supporting and guiding parents in planning and carrying out effective discipline
      e.   conveying acceptance of regression and dependence, providing opportunities for autonomy, adjusting expectations to meet changing needs, supporting efforts to achieve self-control
      f.   communicating pride in achievements and understanding of limitations, counseling parents in regard to realistic expectations, seeking a balance between adequate protection and allowing for independent exploration, providing encouragement for efforts

2.   Children do not have the resources for coping with the changes caused by illness and hospitalization. Their universal needs are magnified, and special needs are generated by these changes. Meeting their needs provides a sense of security that enables them to withstand the crises superimposed by illness on the anticipated course of development.

Chapter 5

QUESTION	ANSWER

Section III

1.   a.   c
      b.   e
      c.   a
      d.   f
      e.   h
      f.   g
      g.   d
      h.   i
      i.   b
2.   F
3.   T
4.   F
5.   b

6.   basic mendelian principles

7.   T

8.   a.   X-D
      b.   A-D, X-D
      c.   A-D, A-R
      d.   X-R
      e.   A-R
      f.   A-D, X-D
      g.   A-R
      h.   X-R
      i.   A-R, X-R
      j.   A-D

9.   Monozygotic

10.   a

11.   T

12.   a.   d
      b.   e
      c.   a
      d.   h
      e.   b
      f.   g
      g.   c
      h.   f

13.   Eugenics; euthenics

14.   d

15.   a.   hyperplasia
      b.   hypertrophy
      c.   differentiation
      d.   organogenesis

16.   F

17.   Teratogenesis

18.   tissue differentiation

19.   a.   to detect the presence of disease, incipient or overt
      b.   to provide reproductive information
      c.   to gain information about the incidence of a disorder in the population

20.   genetic counseling

21.   F

22.   c

Section IV A

1.   a.   disorder present at birth that may be brought about by genetic causes, nongenetic causes, or a combination of these
      b.   disorder that may or may not be apparent at birth that is caused by a single harmful gene, several genes, or a deviation in chromosomal number or structure

2.   a.   G
      b.   C
      c.   G
      d.   M
      e.   M
      f.   G
      g.   G
      h.   M
      i.   C
      j.   M

3.   This requires a strong genetic predisposition that places susceptible individuals at a point of risk where environmental influences determine whether or to what extent they will be affected.

4.   a.   congenital heart disease, pyloric stenosis, facial and limb deformities, retinoblastoma
      b.   phenylketonuria, galactosemia, maple-syrup-urine disease, hereditary lactase deficiency
      c.   hypothyroidism, hemophilia, pituitary dwarfism, adrenogenital syndrome, diabetes mellitus
      d.   hemochromatosis, Wilson disease
      e.   hereditary polycystic kidneys, hepatic atresia, cardiac myopathy, thalassemia
      f.   beta thalassemia, sickle cell anemia

Section IV B

1.   Hemophilia is caused by a recessive gene on the X chromosome.
2.   a.   unaffected
      b.   carrier of the disorder
      c.   unaffected and cannot transmit the disorder
      d.   either unaffected or carrier of the disorder
3.   a.   unaffected and cannot transmit the disorder
      b.   carriers
4.   a.   Screening can determine whether Billy's sister is a carrier. This will either assure her that she does not carry the defective gene or provide her with the information necessary for family planning decisions if she is found to be a carrier.
      b.   In future pregnancies, the prenatal screening of fetal sex would allow the parents to determine whether the child is male. Since there is a 50% chance that a male offspring will be affected, the parents may choose whether to terminate or continue the pregnancy.

Section IV C

1.   a.   comprehension of the medical facts, including the diagnosis, probable course, and available management of the disorder
      b.   appreciation of the way heredity contributes to the disorder, and the risk of recurrence in specified relatives
      c.   understanding of the options for dealing with the risk of recurrence
      d.   choice of the course of action that seems correct for them in view of their risk and their family goals, and action in accordance with that decision
      e.   making the best possible adjustment to the disorder in an affected family member or to the risk of recurrence of the disorder
2.   a.   to advise families with genetic disorders
      b.   to identify special risk situations
      c.   to reduce numbers of affected children
3.   a.   an accurate diagnosis
      b.   a thorough family history
      c.   an extensive knowledge of genetics
4.   a.   identification of potential hereditary problems
      b.   assistance in obtaining diagnosis and treatment
      c.   provision of counseling by genetics nurse specialists
      d.   provision of follow-up care
5.   Time and understanding are essential in dealing with the anxiety these disorders generate. Knowledge of and the ability to deal with the range of psychologic responses and their ramifications are necessary. The timing of counseling needs careful evaluation. The extent and type of information needed and desired by the clients must be assessed. Guilt and self-blame must be dealt with. Sympathetic and supportive listening is vital.
6.   a.   religious attitudes toward conception, sterilization, and abortion
      b.   the right of the fetus to come to full term and the right of parents to conceive
      c.   differences in the ability to comprehend what is said
      d.   biases and judgmental attitudes of the counselor

Chapter 6

QUESTION   **ANSWER**

Section III

.   a.   the appropriateness of the nurse's introduction to the child and family
      b.   the nurse's explanation of her role in the health care setting and the purpose of the interview
      c.   the inclusion of preliminary acquaintance conversation
      d.   the nurse's assurance of privacy and confidentiality of the interview material
.   a.   allows the nurse to obtain information concerning the health and developmental status of the child, factors that may influence the child's life, and cues to aspects in the child's health and development that may be a source of concern to the parents
      b.   permits the nurse to allow for maximum freedom of expression while not allowing the interview to go off on tangents
      c.   allows the nurse to make objective judgments concerning the perception of the parents, is useful in preventing the nurse's views from being interjected into the interview process, and aids in detecting cues from the parents that may aid in identifying problem areas
      d.   allows the interviewee to sort out thoughts and feelings
      e.   allows the nurse to see the problem from the parents' perspective
      f.   informs the parents that their feelings and concerns are shared by other parents

g.   facilitates the formulation of solutions, because, in order for a problem to be solved, the nurse and parent must agree that one exists

h.   includes the parents in the problem-solving process and allows solutions to be proposed that will be adhered to by parents

i.   provides preventive methods so problems will not occur

j.   prevents the quality of the helping relationship from being altered

3.   F

4.   d

5.   b
    a
    c
    d

6.   d

7.   writing; drawing; playing

8.   T

9. a.   identifying information
    b.   chief complaint
    c.   present illness
    d.   past history
    e.   review of systems
    f.   family history
    g.   personal and social history
    h.   patient profile
    i.   nutritional assessment

10.   F

11.   dietary history; clinical examination; biochemical analysis

12.   c

Section IV A

1.   An appropriate introduction is crucial to establish a setting that is conducive to the interview process. The first component to this process is an introduction of the interviewer to the parents.

2.   Some of the more common blocks to communication include giving unrestricted advice, offering premature reassurance, using stereotypic comments, using close-ended questions, interrupting the client, talking more than the interviewee, and deliberately changing the focus.

3.   A number of techniques are effective. These include; third-person technique; story telling; neurolinguistic programming; using books, fantasy, dreams, three wishes, word association games, drawing, and playing.

4.   It is important to include the parent in the problem-solving process, because a parent who is included will be more likely to follow through on a course of action. In addition, a parent may have already tried a particular solution. Encouraging participation may prevent the nurse from suggesting a solution that the patient has already tried.

Section IV B

1. a.   role clarification and explanation of the interview to the interpreter
    b.   introduction and preliminary acquaintance
    c.   communicate directly with the parent
    d.   respect cultural differences
    e.   communicate directly with the interpreter
    f.   continuity

2.   The nurse can redirect the focus of the interview by saying that they can talk about the other children later in the interview.

3.   Since Susan has been in this country only 6 months, she may have not received her immunization. It is extremely important for the nurse to obtain an accurate record of immunizations from Mrs. Fernandez.

4.   The nurse should obtain information concerning the state of health, age, and presence of illness of first-degree relatives. This section may also include a general overview of family interaction.

Section IV C

1.   A dietary history should include information regarding the family mealtime, preparation of food, pattern of eating and of meals, likes and dislikes of the child, appetite, allergies, feeding problems, family history of illnesses, pattern of weight gain, the child's pattern of exercise, and the amount of money spent on food.

2.   The three methods include 24-hour recall, food diary, and food frequency record

3. Anthropometry is the measurement of height, weight, head circumference, proportions, skin-fold thickness and arm circumference. Skin-fold thickness is a measurement of the body's fat content and would be useful in determining whether Gwen is obese.

4. Gwen should be told what is being done and why. She should be told that various measurements such as height, weight, and skin-fold thickness will be taken to determine how big and tall she has become. If blood is to be drawn she should be told why.

5. a. nutrition, alteration in: more than body requirement related to eating practices
    b. Nutrition, alteration in: related to knowledge deficit of parents

Chapter 7

QUESTION   **ANSWERS**

Section III

1. a. families of diverse socioeconomic backgrounds
    b. one-parent families
    c. children who have chronic illnesses or disabilities
2. a. minimizing the stress and anxiety associated with body part assessment
    b. fostering a trusting nurse-child-parent relationship
    c. allowing for maximum preparation of the child
    d. preserving the essential security of the parent-child relationship
    e. maximizing the accuracy and reliability of the assessment findings
3. a. talk to parent first, ignoring the child, then gradually focus on the child
    b. make a complimentary remark about the child's dress or appearance
    c. tell a funny story
    d. utilize a puppet
    e. allow for choices
    f. begin the exam with activities that can be viewed as games
4.   F
5.   T
6. a. growth measurements
    b. physiologic measurements
    c. general appearance
    d. skin
    e. lymph nodes
    f. head
    g. neck
    h. eyes
    i. ears
    j. nose
    k. mouth and throat
    l. chest
    m. lungs
    n. heart
    o. abdomen
    p. genitalia
    q. anus
    r. back and extremities
    s. neurologic assessment
7.   respiration, pulse, then temperature
8.   d
9.   for a full minute
).   b
    .   b
        c
        d
        a
2.   d
3.   F
    .   F

15.   When assessing the head of an 8-month-old, the nurse should record the general shape, symmetry, head control and/or posture, range of motion, presence of patent sutures, fontanels, fractures and swellings, and the condition of the scalp.
16.   primitive
17.   F
18.   birth through 6 years
19.   T
20.   a

Chapter 7

QUESTION	ANSWER

Section IV A

1. Tia should be brought to the clinic more frequently because she is from a different cultural background and is from a family that at this time has only one parent.
2. Since this is Tia's first visit to the clinic an initial health history should be obtained. She should have her height and weight taken. These should be plotted on growth charts, and her weight should be charted against height. Tia should have her blood pressure taken. She should also have her sight, hearing, speech, and development assessed. An initial dental examination should be recommended at this visit.
3. You should observe Tia for signs of readiness such as her willingness to talk to you, make eye contact, accept the offered equipment, allow physical contact, smile or choose to sit on the examining table. Several methods might be used to facilitate the exam process. You could tell a story or utilize a puppet. Since Tia needs to have a developmental assessment, you might want to begin with this aspect of the exam since it might be perceived by Tia as a game.
4. Methods that you could utilize to relax Tia include positioning her in a semireclining position on her mother's lap, telling her a story, teaching her to deep breathe, or using the nonpalpating hand to comfort the child.
5. Additional assessment information might include: Tia's parents' patterns of growth, whether her growth pattern has been steady, and her nutritional intake. In addition, you might want to utilize growth charts standardized for Asian populations to see if her height and weight are normal for this group.
6. Tia is 3 years of age, so she can have her height taken standing. She should be encouraged to stand as tall and straight as possible.
7. Tia may not understand that she should not bite down on the thermometer or that she has to keep the thermometer under her tongue.
8. Tia should have a complete vision assessment that includes binocularity and acuity. To test for binocularity, you might use the corneal light reflex test. Visual acuity can be assessed using Allen Picture Cards.

Section IV B

1. After the general appearance section the skin is assessed.
2. The infant's height is obtained in the recumbent position by fully extending the child's body. The school-age child's height is obtained by having the child stand straight. Height should be recorded to the nearest 1/8 in. or 1 mm.
3. Radial pulses can be obtained if the child is over 2 years of age. The infant's pulse should be taken apically, and the school-age child's can be taken radially.
4. Information in this area includes the child's personality, level of activity, reaction to stress, interaction with others, degree of alertness, and response to stimuli.
5. To complete an assessment of the ears, you must screen for hearing ability. Audiometry can be utilized for the school-age child. The infant's hearing can be assessed by making a loud noise and noting the child's reaction to it.
6. quality, intensity, rate, and rhythm
7. Instruct the child to hold his breath, this causes the heart rate to remain steady.
8. Deep tendon reflexes are recorded as: 4+, extremely brisk; 3+, brisker than normal; 2+, average normal; 1+, diminished; 0+, absent.

Section IV C

1. The parent is told that the purpose of the test is to help the nurse observe what the child can do at this age and that the results of the performance will be explained after all items have been completed. It should be emphasized that this is not an intelligence test.
2. The parent is asked whether the child's performance is typical of his behavior at other times.
3. The method that is utilized is a failure to perform an item that is passed by 90% of children the child's age or any item that falls completely to the left of the age line.
4. Items are scored as follows: P, passing; F, failing; N.O., the child has no opportunity to perform an item; and R, the child refuses.

5.   All children with questionable or abnormal results should be rescreened before a referral for further diagnostic testing is done.

Chapter 8

QUESTION		ANSWER

Section III

1.   the entrance of air into the upper airway replacing the lung fluid, initiation of breathing, and a lowering of the surface tension in the alveoli

2.   F

3.   a

4.   a.   large surface area
     b.   greater metabolic rate
     c.   thin layer of subcutaneous fat
     d.   inability to shiver

5.   d

6.   T

7.   heart rate, respiratory effort, muscle tone, color and reflex irritability

8.   10

9.   6 to 8

10.   an alert and active infant, active gag reflex, increased heart and respiratory rate, increased gastric and respiratory secretions, and passage of meconium

11.   The six external signs include skin, lanugo, plantar creases, breast, ear, and genitalia.

12.   F

13.   T

14.   b

15.   posture, behavior, skin, head, fontanels, eyes, ears, nose, mouth, chest, lungs, heart, abdomen, genitalia, back and rectum, and extremities.

16.   two arteries

17.   F

18.   a.   maintenance of patent airway
     b.   maintenance of stable body temperature
     c.   protection from injury and infection
     d.   provision of optimal nutrition

19.   the acid mantle of the skin

20.   F

21.   b

22.   T

23.   the expectations the parents have for this child, the parents' relationships with their own parents, whether the pregnancy was planned, the presence of a support system, views on child affecting the parents' lifestyle, and views regarding child rearing

24.   postpartum hospitalizations are shorter, and more deliveries are being performed at home

25.   maternal fatigue and depression, attachment, neonatal jaundice, breast feeding, and excessive infant crying

Section IV A

.   heart, respiratory effort, muscle tone, reflex irritability, and color

.   below 100 beats/min

.   7 to 10

.   The behaviors that are observed include an initial period of alertness, vigorous suck, initially elevated heart and respiratory rates, active bowel sounds, and falling temperature

.   c

Section IV B

.   perinatal mortality and morbidity are related to gestational age and weight

.   30 and 42 hours of age

.   resting posture, square window, arm recoil, popliteal angle, scarf sign, and heel-to-ear maneuver

.   T

.   c

.   his weight falls between the 10th and 90th percentile

Section IV C

1.   30.5 and 33 cm (12 and 13 inches); microcephaly or craniostenosis should be suspected.
2.   Information that should be gathered is the presentation of the infant during delivery. The observations listed are commonly seen with frank breech deliveries.
3.   reversible blood flow
4.   The areas to assess include: observing the lids for edema, upward slope of the eyes, symmetry of the eyes, presence of tears, presence of discharge, cornea, pupillary reflex, nystagmus, strabismus, and color of the iris.
5.   The infant is able to respond to his environment by moving his head and/or limbs and staring at objects in the environment such as a mobile or a face.

Section IV D

1.   a.   Injury, potential for, related to immature temperature control, deficient immunologic defenses, immature regulatory mechanisms, and environmental factors
     b.   Nutrition, alteration in, potential for less than body requirements related to immaturity
     c.   Ineffective airway clearance, related to excess mucus or improper positioning
2.   a.   maintain stable body temperature
     b.   ensure infant's identity
     c.   protect from infection and trauma
3.   b
4.   a.   position on right side or abdomen after feeding
     b.   keep diapers, clothing, and blankets loose
     c.   clean nares of crusted material
     d.   check for patency of nares
5.   The reason that clothes are kept loose is that infants are abdominal breathers; this intervention allows for maximal expansion of the lungs.
6.   The infant is in the first stage of reactivity. During this time he is alert and awake and can establish eye-to-eye contact with the parents, facilitating the development of attachment.
7.   Criteria include: breathing that is regular and unlabored, normal respiratory rate, and gastric aspirates of 20 ml or less.
8.   The parents should be instructed in routine baby care such as feeding, bathing, and umbilical and circumcision care. They should also be encouraged to participate in parenting classes. The use of care restraints should be discussed as well.

Section IV E

1.   Specific behaviors that might be assessed include: the parent reaching out for the baby when she is brought into the room, referring to the infant by name, talking about who the child looks like, speaking about the uniqueness of the infant, the type of body contact used, types of stimulation, and whether or not the parents avoid eye contact.
2.   This is important, because the ability to parent is largely dependent on the type of parenting the parents received as children, as this may influence the attachment process.
3.   parenting; alteration in: related to knowledge deficit of lack of available role models.
4.   a.   Allow parents to see and hold the infant as soon as possible.
     b.   Perform eye care after the parents have met the infant.
     c.   Identify the infant's unique behaviors.
     d.   Observe and assess the reciprocity of cues between infant and parent.
     e.   Assess variables affecting the attachment process.
     f.   Observe for behaviors indicating attachment.

Chapter 9

QUESTION	ANSWER

Section III

1.   presenting part; maternal pelvis
2.   a
3.   clavicle
4.   facial nerve paralysis
5.   proper positioning
6.   a.   C
     b.   I
     c.   I

d.	C
e.	C
f.	I
g.	I

7. hyperbilirubinemia
8. 20 mg/dl
9. jaundice
0. This occurs because of the immaturity of hepatic function combined with increased hemolysis of excess red blood cells.
1. phototherapy
2. calcium gluconate
3. a. Administer slowly over a period of 5 to 10 min to prevent nausea, vomiting, bradycardia, and circulatory collapse.
   b. Ensure placement of the needle within the vein before administering calcium gluconate, because extravasation into the surrounding tissue will cause local calcification and sloughing.
4. T
5. caloric expenditure; adequate caloric intake
6. T
7. phenylalanine hydroxylase
8 screening
9. F

ection IV A

1. a. a vaguely outlined area of edematous tissue situated over the portion of the scalp that presents in a vertex delivery. The swelling consists of serum, blood, or both, accumulated in the tissues above the bone, and it may extend beyond the bone margins. It is present at or shortly after birth.
   b. formed when blood vessels rupture during labor or delivery to produce bleeding into the area between the bone and its periosteum. The boundaries are sharply demarcated and do not extend beyond the limits of the bone. Swelling is usually minimal at birth and increases on the second or third day.
2. a. detection of complications, such as subdural hematoma
   b. parental support

ection IV B

. a. children with anomalies such as cleft lip or palate
   b. children who have received prolonged antibiotic therapy
   c. children with immunologic deficiencies
   d. newborns of diabetic mothers
. a. infection, related to presence of *Candida albicans*
   b. alteration in comfort, pain, related to oral lesions
   c. alteration in nutrition, less than body requirements, related to pain in the mouth
   d. knowledge deficit, related to hygiene practices
   e. alterations in oral mucous membranes, related to candidiasis
   f. potential impairment of skin integrity, related to spread of infection

ction IV C

. a. the administration of systemic and local antibiotics
   b. isolation of the infant and initiation of meticulous handwashing techniques
. a. Systemic and local antibiotics should be used according to instructions.
   b. The hands should be washed meticulously after caring for the infant, and the infant's clothing should be laundered separately.
   c. The infant's arms may need to be restrained with elbow restraints or by pulling the undershirt sleeves over the hands and securing the openings with tape.
   d. The infant should be freed from restraints periodically to allow for movement with close supervision; when restrained, the infant should be held and cuddled as much as possible.

ction IV D

. a. immaturity of hepatic functions
   b. increased bilirubin load from increased hemolysis of red blood cells
. a. after 24 hours
   b. by the second to third day
   c. from the fifth to the tenth day
. a. after 48 hours

    b.   by the fifth day
    c.   from 6 days to 1 month
4. a.   Shield the infant's eyes with an opaque mask.
    b.   Place infant nude under the fluorescent light.
    c.   Monitor body temperature.
    d.   Place a protective Plexiglass shield between the fluorescent light and the infant.
    e.   Maintain accurate charting during therapy.
5. a.   to protect the eyes of the infant from possible damage
    b.   to allow maximum contact of the light with skin surfaces
    c.   to ensure that the infant's temperature remains normothermic
    d.   to minimize the amount of undesirable ultraviolet light reaching the infant's skin and to protect the infant from acciden-
          tal bulb breakage
    e.   to provide documentation of correct use of equipment and monitoring of the treatment

Section IV E

1.   The Guthrie blood test is performed on a fresh heel blood specimen obtained after the infant has ingested cow's or
          human milk for 24 to 48 hours.
2. a.   infants tested in the first 24 hours of life
    b.   infants whose levels were greater than 20 mg/dl
    c.   infants with phenylketonuric siblings
3. a.   False-positive results can occur if large amounts of ketones are present or certain brands of disposable diapers are used.
    b.   By the time the serum phenylalanine level is high enough to produce phenylpyruvic acid in the urine, brain damage
          may have occurred.
4. a.   It must meet the child's nutritional need for optimal growth.
    b.   It must maintain phenylalanine levels within a safe range.
5.   These measures evaluate the effectiveness of the child's dietary treatment.
6. a.   Investigate the possibility of total or partial breast feeding with close monitoring of phenylalanine levels.
    b.   Recommend the use of a blender or mixer for the preparation of the formula.
    c.   Powdered Tang, fruit punch, or Quik may be added. The flavored mixture may then be heated or frozen into popsicles.
    d.   Stress the need for continuing contact with the PKU clinic or a health team that includes a nutritionist.
    e.   Stress the importance of genetic counseling.

CHAPTER 10

QUESTION   **ANSWER**

Section III

1.   Preconceptional factors include: hereditary diseases, socioeconomic factors, high altitude, maternal size, grand multi-
          parity, history of obstetric complications, and uterine abnormalities.
2.   F
3.   size, gestational age, and mortality
4.   F
5.   100 and 180
6.   Observations include: feeding behavior, abdominal distention, behavior, skin manifestations, character and location of
          heart sounds, and respiratory data.
7.   determining the presence of abdominal distention, determining any signs of regurgitation, describing any emesis, de-
          scribing the stools, and describing bowel sounds
8.   d
9.   higher
10.   acid mantle of the skin
11.   c
12.   (1) gestational age at birth; (2) head circumference, weight, and length at birth; (3) length of growth delay; (4) days
          necessary to regain birth weight; (5) measurements at term dates; and (6) head circumference, weight, and length at
          discharge
13.   F
14.   a
          c
          b
15.   c
16.   b

7.   T
8.   meningitis, pyarthrosis, and shock
9.   abdominal distention, blood in the stools, bile-stained vomitus, gastric retention, and absence of bowel sounds
0.   this may prevent the occurrence of necrotizing enterocolitis
1   T
2.   b
3.   withdrawal of blood for specimens
4.   bulging fontanel, seizures, apnea, twitching and lethargy
5.   the metabolic control of the mother
6.   d
7.   the gastrointestinal symptoms
8.   T

ection IV A

1.   The most meaningful method of classification is one that encompasses all three methods, i.e., size, gestational age, and fetal outcome.
2.   High-risk infants have deficient immunologic defenses and are also exposed to many sources of nosocomial infections.
3. a. placing infant in a humidified Isolette or radiant warmer
    b. monitoring temperature hourly, if unstable
    c. changing temperature in relation to temperature of heating unit
    d. avoiding situations that predispose to chilling
        A shift in the point of maximum intensity indicates a mediastinal shift and is often used to diagnose pneumothorax.
        nutrition, alteration in: less than body requirements related to inability to ingest nutrients
        The infant would be weighed daily and should exhibit a steady weight gain.
        Assessment of the skin reveals that the skin remains clean and intact with no evidence of breakdown.
    a. placing colorful mobiles and toys within the visual field
    b. holding face within 9 to 12 inches of infant's face and stimulating the infant to follow head movements
    a. keep parents informed of infant's progress
    b. facilitate sibling-infant attachment
    c. prepare for discharge
        Since the infant is in an ICU, the parents may not have had time to become acquainted with and attached to their infant. Encouraging visitation counteracts interruptions of the bonding process.

ection IV B

.   Physical findings include: the absence of lanugo; little if any vernix caseosa; abundant scalp hair; long fingernails; whiter, cracked parchmentlike skin; depletion of subcutaneous fat, and vernix that is stained yellow or green.
.   the presence of meconium in the airways which results in obstruction and inhibition of normal air flow
.   a. the shape of the chest
    b. use of accessory muscles
    c. respiratory rate and regularity
    d. breath sounds
    e. whether suctioning is needed
    f. description of the cry
    g. the presence of ambient oxygen and method of delivery
        Tommy is probably npo and also is receiving oxygen, which has a drying effect on the mucus membranes.
.   a. position for optimum air exchange
    b. observe for signs of respiratory distress
    c. suction as necessary
    d. perform percussion, vibration, and postural drainage
    e. maintain ambient oxygen levels
    f. carry out respiratory regimen as prescribed
        The nurse would assess Tommy's color and obtain an oxygen level utilizing a transcutaneous monitor, an arterial sample, or a capillary sample.
.   Tommy has been stressed in utero, may be hypothermic, and because of his respiratory distress, has an imbalance between oxygen supply and demand.

ction IV C

        cross-contamination. The sources of this could include: humidifying apparatus, suction machines, indwelling catheters, poor hand washing and inadequate housecleaning.

2.   Some of the signs of sepsis include poor temperature control, pallor, hypotension, edema, respiratory distress, diminished or increased activity, full fontanel, poor feeding, vomiting, diarrhea, jaundice, and an infant not doing well.

3.   recognition of the existing problem, sepsis

4.   a.   prevent or control infection
    b.   maintain a neutral thermal environment
    c.   maintain hydration
    d.   support respiratory efforts

5.   These may include suctioning, head positioning, and not maintaining good body alignment.

Section IV D

1.   Michael experienced severe asphyxia at birth.

2.   early recognition

3.   monitoring the abdomen for distention, measuring residual gastric aspirates, and presence of bowel sounds

4.   a.   assisting with the diagnostic procedures
    b.   monitoring vital signs
    c.   avoiding rectal temperatures
    d.   avoiding pressure on abdomen
    e.   administering antibiotics
    f.   providing hydration and nutrition
    g.   control of infection

5.   The infant would not exhibit signs of dehydration such as weight loss, poor skin turgor, increased urine output, and an elevated specific gravity.

6.   Anemia is a common problem caused by hemorrhage during delivery, a drop in the production of fetal hemoglobin, diminished erythropoietin activity, and loss of blood as a result of too many specimens.

7.   careful monitoring of all blood drawn for tests

8.   a.   observing for feeding difficulties
    b.   monitoring respiratory status
    c.   monitoring activity level
    d.   weighing
    e.   assessing color

Section IV E

1.   It occurs as a result of the hyperplasia and hypertrophy of the islet cells in utero. The islet cells continue to excrete large amounts of insulin after birth, resulting in decreased blood glucose levels.

2.   Feeding is begun early to prevent hypoglycemia.

3.   hypoglycemia, respiratory distress, and hyperbilirubinemia

4.   a.   assessing readiness of family to care for infant
    b.   teach necessary techniques
    c.   arrange for public health referral
    d.   reinforce follow-up care
    e.   encourage involvement with parent groups

5.   The family would demonstrate the ability to care for the infant, avail themselves of services, and keep follow-up appointments.

CHAPTER 11

QUESTION	ANSWER

Section III

1.   death of a child

2.   d

3.   b

4.   Hydrocephalus

5.   a.   impaired absorption of CSF fluid within the subarachnoid space
    b.   obstruction to the flow of CSF within the ventricles

6.   a.   bulging fontanels
    b.   positive MacEwen sign
    c.   setting-sun sign
    d.   sluggish pupils with unequal response to light
    e.   irritability, lethargy, and changes in level of consciousness

f. persistence of early infantile reflex acts

. T

. T

. a. acetabular dysplasia or preluxation

b. subluxation

c. dislocation

. Ortolani; Barlow

. a. d

b. a

c. b

d. c

. a. correction of the deformity

b. maintenance of the correction

c. follow-up observation to avert possible recurrence

. defective speech

. feeding

. a. excessive salivation

b. drooling that is frequently accompanied by choking, coughing, and sneezing

. a. coughing

b. choking

c. cyanosis

. Biliary atresia

. a. c

b. a

c. e

d. b

e. f

f. d

. Hypospadias

a. history

b. physical examination

c. buccal smear

d. chromosomal analysis

e. endoscopy and x-ray contrast studies

f. biochemical tests

g. laparotomy or gonad biopsy

a. toxoplasmosis

b. other (hepatitis, varicella zoster, measles, mumps)

c. rubella

d. cytomegalovirus infection

e. herpes simplex

F

prevention

ction IV

a. prevention of infection

b. determination of neurologic status and identification of associated anomalies

c. dealing with the impact of the anomaly on the parents

a. the neurologic deficit present at birth, including motor ability and bladder innervation

b. the presence of associated cerebral anomalies

neurogenic bladder dysfunction; renal disease

a. maintaining temperature through use of an Isolette or warmer

b. applying a sterile, moist, nonadherent dressing to the sac

c. inspecting the sac for leaks, abrasions, irritations, or signs of infection

d. placing child in prone position to minimize tension and trauma to the sac

e. keeping the diaper area dry and free of irritation; diapering is contraindicated

f. providing appropriate means of stimulation

a. difficulty in sucking and feeding

b. a shrill, brief, high-pitched cry

c. emesis

d. somnolence

e. seizures

f.   cardiopulmonary embarrassment

6.   a

7.   Alteration in family process, actual, related to the birth of a defective child.

8.   a.   encourage parents to express feelings; refer to genetic counseling service

b.   assess family's ability to care for child; teach essential aspects of infant's physical care

c.   discuss developmental expectations; teach family to observe for signs of complications

d.   assist parents in planning activities appropriate to the child's developmental level; assist with educational placement

e.   arrange for ongoing contact with family; refer parents to appropriate groups and organizations

f.   plan for home visits as needed; maintain contact with family; make referrals to special agencies

Section IV B

1.   a.   leg shortening

b.   asymmetry of the thigh and gluteal folds

c.   limited abduction

2.   a.   correcting abnormal hip position

b.   preventing complications

3.   teaching the parents to apply and maintain the reduction device

4.   a.   observe for tightness or irritation that indicates a need for adjustment of the device

b.   apply a protective covering to the device during feeding, toileting, and bathing

c.   carry out appropriate skin care; avoid use of powders and lotions

d.   modify clothing and methods of transportation to accommodate the appliance

e.   provide appropriate stimulation and activities for age and limitations

Section IV C

1.   a.   feeding difficulties

b.   dealing with the parents' reaction to the defect

2.   The feeding process is often time-consuming and very difficult. Clefts of the lip or palate reduce the infant's ability to suck, which interferes with compression of the areola and usually renders both breast-and bottle feeding difficult.

3.   The infant should be held in an upright position, and special nipples or feeding devices should be used.

4.   protecting the operative site

5.   a.   prevents aspiration of secretions

b.   prevents trauma to the suture line

c.   prevents infection

d.   prevents inflammation and tissue breakdown

e.   provides adequate nutrition and prevents trauma to suture line

f.   provides for comfort and normal development

Section IV D

1.   A catheter is gently passed into the esophagus. It will meet with resistance if the lumen is blocked but will pass unobstructed if the lumen is patent. The exact type of anomaly is determined by roentgenographic studies.

2.   a.   prevention of pneumonia

b.   repair of the anomaly

3.   a.   aspirate secretions from oropharynx; position for optimal lung expansion; observe for signs of respiratory distress

b.   administer nothing by mouth; position in supine position with head elevated 30 degrees; aspirate secretions

4.   a.   a, c, h

b.   e

c.   a, c

d.   d, f

e.   b, g

Section IV E

1.   a.   to enable the child to void in a standing position by voluntarily directing the stream in the usual manner

b.   to improve the physical appearance of the genitalia for psychologic reasons

c.   to produce a sexually adequate organ

2.   The prepuce provides valuable skin for reconstructive surgery.

3.   Six to 18 months—before the child has developed body image and castration anxiety

4.   a.   the type of procedure to be done

b.   the expected cosmetic result

5.   a.   alteration in urinary elimination patterns, actual, related to structural defect and surgery

b.   impairment of skin integrity, actual, related to surgical incision

c.   alteration in comfort. pain, actual, related to surgical procedure

d.   alteration in family process, actual, related to physical defect and hospitalization

HAPTER 12

JESTION	ANSWER

ction III

doubled

12 months

d

a.   greater proportion of extracellular fluid

b.   immaturity of the kidney

b

a

F

c

(1) the ability to discriminate the mother from other individuals and (2) object permanence

F

the infant's displaying displeasure when the mother leaves the room

a

a.   plays games such as peekaboo

b.   extends arms to signal desire to be picked up

c.   shows displeasure when toy is removed

mirrors, bright toys to hold, rattles or bells, soft squeeze toys, and swings

Parents should be aware that this child will have to be watched more closely, and that extra precautions regarding safety will need to be taken. This child benefits from increased opportunity for gross motor activities.

F

age of child − 6 = number of teeth

protection

fluoride; 25 mg

F

a.   the digestive tract is not able to digest them

b.   food allergies may develop

c.   the extrusion reflex is still strong

d.   inability to push food away

cereal; iron

T

b

F

c

local tenderness, erythema, and swelling at the injection site and a low-grade fever

c

asphyxiation by foreign material

d

T

ction IV A

Yes. Jerry should have at least doubled his birth weight by at least 6 months. The average infant gains at least 2 lb a month till 6 months and about 1 lb a month from 6 months to 1 year.

Jerry's developmental milestones are assessed as follows: when supine lifts head off table, sits erect momentarily, bears full weight on feet, transfers objects from hand to hand, rakes at a small object, bangs cube on table, produces vowel sounds and chained syllables, vocalizes four distinct vowel sounds, plays peekaboo, fears strangers when mother disappears, and imitates simple acts.

You should stress to Mrs. Backer that this behavior is normal and indicates good parental attachment. Mrs. Backer should be encouraged to allow clingy behavior and to find a suitable baby sitter who can visit often.

a.   a cold metal spoon or frozen teething ring to chew on

b.   topical analgesics such as Anbesol

5.   Jerry's lack of interest in breast feeding may indicate his desire to be weaned. You should suggest that Jerry might be weaned to a cup, that it should be done gradually by replacing one feeding at time, with the night-time feeding the last to be replaced, and not allowing the child to take a bottle to bed.

6.   a.   give fluoride supplements of 0.25 mg a day
      b.   clean teeth with a damp cloth
      c.   do not include concentrated sugars in the diet
      d.   do not coat pacifiers with honey
      e.   never allow a bottle to be taken to bed or during a nap

7.   The major nursing goals are to prepare the parents for stranger-anxiety and accident prevention.

Section IV B

1.   Behaviors include searching for objects that have fallen, imitating sounds, showing great interest in mirror image.

2.   a.   administer the Infant Temperament Questionnaire
      b.   discuss results with mother
      c.   suggest that she adhere to structured care giving and scheduled feedings

3.   a.   the reason for the concern
      b.   the frequency and duration of waking
      c.   the usual bedtime routine
      d.   the number of night-time feedings
      e.   the interventions Rachel's mother attempted

4.   a.   Rachel should be started on cereal first
      b.   cereal should be mixed with formula
      c.   spoon feeding should be first introduced after the infant has had some formula
      d.   the infant will at first push spoon away but to be persistent
      e.   new foods are fed in small amounts (about 1 tsp) and for a period of 4 to 7 days
      f.   as the amount of solids increases, she should decrease the amount of formula

5.   a.   supporting Rachel's social responses
      b.   developing a reciprocal relationship with Rachel
      c.   investigating the infant's habits
      d.   begin discussing new foods and potential sources of injury

Section IV C

1.   Live virus vaccines should not be given to infants with a febrile illness, acquired passive immunity, a known allergic response to a previously administered vaccine or substance in the vaccine, or who have immunodeficiency diseases or who have received immunosuppressive therapy or who have a sibling at home receiving such therapy.

2.   a.   proper storage such as refrigeration and exposure to light
      b.   DPT vaccines should always be administered intramuscularly with a needle of adequate length to deposit the antigen deep in the muscle mass. Care should be taken to prevent tracking of fluid into the skin.

3.   The safest site for the administration of immunizations is the vastus lateralis muscles.

4.   a.   inquire about reactions to previously administered DTP vaccines
      b.   advise parents of side effects such as fever, soreness, redness and swelling at site, malaise
      c.   recommend the use of antipyretics if fever occurs
      d.   advise parents to notify the physician if any unusual symptoms such as loss of consciousness, convulsions, high fever or systemic allergic reaction occur

Section IV D

1.   Such developmental landmarks include: crawling, standing, cruising, walking, pulling on objects, throwing objects, picking up small objects, exploring by mouthing, exploring away from parent, helplessness in water

2.   a.   place guard around heating appliances, fireplace, or furnace
      b.   keep electrical wires hidden
      c.   keep hanging tablecloth out of reach
      d.   apply a sunscreen when infant is exposed to sunlight

3.   The infant is now mobile and could drown in a tub if allowed to get in the bathroom. He is also helpless in water.

4.   a.   do not allow the infant to use a fork for self feeding
      b.   use plastic cups or dishes
      c.   check the safety of toys and toy box
      d.   protect from young children and animals

5.   Infants at this age still explore objects by mouthing them and might choke on a small object.

6.   The child may think the medication is candy and eat some and might accidentally be poisoned.

7.   You might visit the family again and see whether the parents have accident-proofed their home.
8.   You should suggest that the grandparents' homes be accident-proofed as well.

Chapter 13

QUESTION   **ANSWER**

Section III

1.   a.   economic factors, such as poverty
     b.   sociocultural factors, limitation of food due to preference
     c.   social factors, such as a detached parenting style
     d.   geographic location—hunger is very prevalent in underdeveloped countries
     e.   education—lack of parental knowledge concerning nutrition predisposes infants to nutritional disturbances
2.   T
3.   injudicious use of vitamin supplements
4.   b
5.   F
6.   loss of appetite, diminished taste sensation, delayed healing, skin lesions, growth failure, and retarded sexual maturity
7.   liver, red meat, shellfish, egg yolks, leafy vegetables, dried fruits, nuts, enriched cereals and breads, and whole grains
8.   d
9.   from the findings of the history
10.   c
           c
           d
           a
           b
     a.   investigation of cause, such as cow's milk allergy
     b.   obtaining a diet history that includes the time of day of occurrence, presence of specific family members, activity of
           parents during crying, and mother's diet if breast feeding
     c.   encouraging the mother to feed the infant in a quiet environment
     d.   encouraging the mother to place child over a hot-water bottle or heating pad, administer glycerin suppository, or give 1
           to 2 oz of diluted tea
     e.   assessment of the feeding process
     f.   administration of Bentyl
           T
           to terminate the ruminating behavior and restore normal feeding patterns
           d
           F
           socially isolated, have inadequate support systems, have difficulty assessing the needs of their infants, and have little
           knowledge regarding normal development
           is the provision of adequate nutrition
     a.   provide a quiet, unstimulating environment
     b.   maintain a calm, even temperament
     c.   talk to child by giving directions about eating
     d.   follow child's rhythm of feeding
     e.   develop a structured routine
     f.   be persistent
     g.   maintain a face-to-face posture with the child
           b
           a
           c
           removal of specific allergens
     a.   removal of allergen
     b.   place on hypoallergenic diet
     c.   reduce skin irritation
     d.   control itching
     e.   prevent of skin drying and irritation
     f.   reduce inflammation
           those who have ceased breathing and been saved, siblings of SIDS infant, and infants with infantile apnea

24. the usual sequence of events that occur after the infant is found
25. to avoid any suggestions of responsibility on the part of the parents
26. a
27. F
28   cardiopneumogram
29. home monitoring
30. (1) removal of leads from infant when not attached to monitor; (2) unplugging the power cord from electrical outlet when not plugged into monitor; (3) using safety covers on electrical outlets
31. a. onset before age 30 months
     b. serious lack of social response
     c. language deficit
     d. speech peculiar, if present
     e. no delusions or hallucinations
32. b

Section IV A

1. The nurse should have assessed the cultural food preferences of the Bacons. Seventh Day Adventists are often vegeta(ri)ans. They may also have a lack of knowledge of how to meet their child's nutritional needs on this type of diet.
2. exactly what the diet includes and excludes
3. a. teaching the Bacons to include grains, legumes, milk products (if allowed) and seeds to meet protein and niacin requ(ire)ments
    b. teaching the Bacons to include iron-fortified cereals
    c. teaching the Bacons to include juices containing vitamin C
    d. suggesting that they utilize soy-based formulas
    e. suggesting that they utilize a variety of foods in the diet
    f. teaching them about the safety and digestibility of solid foods
4. If the interventions were successful, the infant would begin to gain weight; the infant would not exhibit signs of niac(in) deficiency such as the stomatitis, scaly dermatitis, diarrhea, or lethargy; and the parents would be able to verbalize a(nd) provide a nutritionally adequate diet for the child.

Section IV B

1. the identification of potential milk sensitivity and appropriate counseling
2. a. advising parents to buy small quantities of substitute formulas
    b. advising parents that the child will receive adequate nutrition from the new formula
    c. advising the parents to carefully read all food labels
    d. advising the parents to check with the pharmacist regarding the presence of potential allergic proteins in medications (and) ointments
3. a. skin integrity: impairment related to immunologic deficit
    b. diversional activity, deficit related to restrictive movement and restraining devices
    c. sleep pattern disturbance related to discomfort and restlessness
    d. sensory perceptual alteration: tactile, related to skin lesions, dressings, and/or restraining devices
    e. self-care deficit: feeding, bathing, related to developmental level and special needs
    f. family process, alteration in, related to situational crisis
4. prevent or minimize scratching
5. The nurse would assess whether the child engages in activities appropriate for his age, such as tracking tubes, mirror(s), rattles, a crib exerciser, soft mobiles, and music boxes.
6. a. bathe with tepid water, little or no soap
    b. dress in loose-fitting, one-piece, long-sleeve and long-pant clothing
    c. eliminate any woolen or rough garments
    d. launder all clothes in mild detergent and rinse well

Section IV C

1. a. identify mothers and fathers at risk
    b. recognize characteristics of parents
    c. identify children who fail to thrive
2. Some of the characteristics would include; (1) growth failure; (2) developmental retardation; (3) apathy; (4) poor hygiene; (5) withdrawal behavior; (6) feeding or eating disorders, such as rumination; (7) avoidance of eye-to-eye conta(ct); (8) no fear of strangers; and (9) minimal smiling.
3. the child gains a minimum of 1 to 2 oz a day and whether the infant responds positively to feeding practices
4. a. assess the child's developmental age

   b.   apply primary care

   c.   provide gentle, sure, and loving handling

   d.   perform physical care with as much holding and rocking as child will allow

   e.   employ consistent schedule

   f.   provide sensory stimulation appropriate to child's developmental level

5.   Parenting, alteration in: actual, related to poverty, neglect, or lack of knowledge.

6.   a.   providing stimulation to the child after feedings

   b.   introducing new foods of various textures, consistencies, and flavors gradually

   c.   giving the child a small quantity of milk immediately followed by teaspoon of solid, if solid acceptance is a problem

ection IV D

1.   The nurse assessed Sean's skin and noted the presence of a rash on the convex surfaces of the diaper area but not in the folds.

2.   the wetness, pH, and fecal irritants

3.   a.   do change diapers as soon as they become wet

   b.   do expose the area to light and air

   c.   do not use rubber pants

   d.   do clean the area well after each soiling

   e.   do use an occlusive ointment

4.   to take a thorough, detailed history of the usual day's events

5.   She should be encouraged to follow a milk-free diet for 5 days, and if that is successful, she may need calcium supplements.

ection IV E

.   a.   inform the parents that the child probably died from SIDS

   b.   ask as few questions as possible

   c.   avoid giving any indication of guilt

2.   to allow them an opportunity for a last visit with the child

3.   a.   make home visits as soon as possible

   b.   provide literature about SIDS

   c.   refer parents to local foundation

.   There might be changes in the parent-child relationship such as anger, altered sleep patterns, or changes in social behavior.

ection IV F

.   Characteristics include: development at about the 1-month level; lack of anticipatory movements; being unyielding to cuddling; the presence of a blank, detached look; absence of stranger-anxiety; and poor or absent language development.

.   are retarded

.   increasing social awareness, teaching verbal skills, and decreasing unacceptable behavior.

ection IV G

.   educating the parents regarding the equipment, observing the infant's status, and immediately intervening during apneic periods

.   Monitors can cause electrical burns and electrocution.

.   The utility company is informed because, if there is a power outage, some provision of emergency power may be provided. The rescue squad is notified because in the event that the infant stops breathing, they will be aware of the problem, and help may arrive more quickly.

.   encouraging other family members to become familiar with the equipment, read and interpret signals, administer CPR, and stay with infant

.   Vomiting usually refers to the forcible ejection of stomach contents. Spitting up refers to the dribbling of unswallowed formula from the infant's mouth immediately after feedings.

hapter 14

JESTION	ANSWER

ction III

.   12 months; 2 years of age

.   2

3.   T

4.   Because the abdominal musculature is not yet well developed and because the legs, though elongating, are still short in relation to the rest of the body.

5.   20/20; 20/40

6.   elimination

7.   locomotion

8.   a.   differentiation of self from others, particularly the mother
       b.   toleration of separation from the parent
       c.   ability to withstand delayed gratification
       d.   control over bodily functions
       e.   acquisition of socially acceptable behavior
       f.   verbal means of communication
       g.   ability to interact with others in a less egocentric manner

9.   autonomy; doubt; shame

10   a.   negativism
       b.   ritualism

11.   b

12.   e

13.   preconceptual phase

14.   a.   consists of repeating words and sounds for the pleasure of hearing oneself and is not intended to communicate
       b.   used to communicate about themselves to others

15.   a

16.   a.   b
       b.   d
       c.   a
       d.   f
       e.   e
       f.   c

17.   reward; punishment

18.   T

19.   a.   the child's emergence from a symbiotic fusion with the mother
       b.   those achievements that mark children's assumption of their own individual characteristics in the environment

20.   F

21.   300; 66

22.   independence

23.   d

24.   parallel

25.   15 months

26.   latter half of the second year

27.   T

28.   firstborn; 2

29.   F

30.   a.   establishing the rules or guidelines for behavior
       b.   the action taken to enforce rules following noncompliance

31.   a.   helps the child test limits of control
       b.   helps the child to achieve in areas appropriate for mastery
       c.   serves to channel undesirable feelings into constructive activity
       d.   protects the child from danger
       e.   teaches socially acceptable behavior

32.   a

33.   physiologic anorexia

34.   1 Tbsp

35.   2

36.   brushing; flossing

37.   fluoride

38.   F

39.   d

40.   Injuries

41.   There is a need to emphasize safety awareness in parents.

42.   The rule of fours is a guide to determining when a child has outgrown a special car restraint system. According to the rule, a child should use this restraint until he weighs about 40 pounds, is 40 inches tall, or is 4 years old.

43.   Scald burns
44.   improper storage

Section IV A

1.   a.   slightly below the 75th percentile
      b.   falls at the 75th percentile
2.   Growth slows considerably during the toddler years. A toddler gains approximately 4 to 6 pounds and grows 3 inches per year. Growth occurs in spurts and plateaus during toddlerhood.
3.   a.   goes up and down stairs alone, using both feet on each step; picks up objects without falling; and can kick a ball forward without overbalancing
      b.   can build a tower of 6 to 7 cubes; turns the pages of a book one at time; and can imitate vertical and circular strokes when drawing.
      c.   uses two- to three-word phrases; uses the pronouns *I*, *me*, and *you*; and talks incessantly
4.   This is characteristic of parallel play, which is typical during the toddler years.
5.   a.   toys should be purchased using safety and developmental level as guidelines
      b.   child should be allowed to choose the toys he wishes to play with a a given time
      c.   child should be allowed unrestricted motor activity within safe limits
6.   b
7.   a.   if drinking water is not fluoridated, provide fluoride supplements
      b.   arrange a visit to the dentist so the child may become familiar with the equipment
      c.   introduce the use of a soft toothbrush as part of the child's bedtime regime
      d.   encourage the consumption of a low-cariogenic diet

Section IV B

1.   By their persistent *no* response to every request.
2.   negative response
3.   As an assertion of self-control and an attempt to control the environment, it increases independence.
4.   Toddlers assert their independence by violently objecting in this manner to restrictions on their behavior.
5.   a.   frequency of occurrence
      b.   precipitating factors
      c.   typical parental responses
6.   a.   extinguishing the behavior
      b.   preventing physical injury
7.   establish realistic and concrete rules
8.   a
9.   a.   no physical punishment is involved
      b.   no reasoning or scolding is given
      c.   separation from the child facilitates the parents' ability to consistently apply this punishment
      d.   provides both the parent and the child with a ''cooling off'' period
10.   Because the growth rate slows, there is a decrease in nutritional needs.
11.   a.   food fads or jags
      b.   rituals involving mealtime and utensils
      c.   inability to sit through family mealtimes
      d.   unpredictable table manners
12.   Because the eating habits established in the first 2 or 3 years of life tend to have lasting effects.

Section IV C

1.   a.   child protection
      b.   parent education
2.   The toddler is unrestricted because of increased locomotion and is unaware of danger in the environment.
3.   a.   motor vehicle injuries
      b.   drowning
      c.   burns
      d.   poisoning
      e.   falls
      f.   aspiration and suffocation
4.   a.   matches and cigarette lighters
      b.   sources of water—tubs, swimming pools
      c.   medications, toxic agents, plants

    d.   unguarded stairways

    e.   tools, garden equipment, and firearms

5. a.   d, g

    b.   a, f

    c.   c, h

    d.   b, e

Chapter 15

QUESTION   **ANSWER**

Section III

1.   3; fifth

2.   slow; stabilize

3. a.   how to interact and relate to other children and adults

    b.   appropriate sex role functions and socially acceptable behavior

    c.   right and wrong and the types of reward or punishment associated with each

4.   initiative

5.   superego; conscience

6.   c

7. a.   the preconceptual phase (ages 2 to 4)

    b.   the phase of intuitive thought (ages 4 to 7)

8.   There is a shift from totally egocentric thought to social awareness and ability to consider other viewpoints.

9.   centration

10.   F

11.   magical

12.   In this stage, the child's actions are directed toward satisfying his needs and, less frequently, the needs of others.

13.   T

14. a.   They can relate to unfamiliar people easily

    b.   They tolerate brief separations from parents with little or no protest.

15.   T

16.   Telegraphic

17.   2100

18. a.   The preschooler is able to verbalize his request for independence

    b.   The preschooler can perform many tasks independently

19.   associative

20.   T

21.   2; 3

22. a.   they become friends for the child in times of loneliness

    b.   they accomplish what the child is still attempting

    c.   they experience what the child wants to forget or remember

23.   a

24. a.   learning group cooperation

    b.   adjusting to various sociocultural differences

    c.   coping with frustration, dissatisfaction, and anger

25. a.   whether the facility is licensed

    b.   qualifications of the staff

    c.   the center's daily program

    d.   student-to-staff ratio

    e.   environmental safety precautions

    f.   provision of meals

    g.   sanitary conditions

    h.   adequate indoor and outdoor space per child

    i.   fee schedule

26.   personal observation

27. a.   determine what the child thinks

    b.   be honest with responses

28.   Masturbation

29.   130

30. a.   frustration

	b.	modeling
	c.	reinforcement
31.		2; 4
32.		**The child is using his rapidly growing vocabulary to interact with the environment. However, the rate of vocabulary acquisition does not parallel the child's advancing mental ability of degree of comprehension.**
33.		prevention; early detection
34.	a.	structuring the child's schedule to allow for adequate rest
	b.	preparing the child for changes
35.	a.	fear of the dark
	b.	fear of being left alone
	c.	fear of animals
	d.	fear of ghosts
	e.	fear of sexual matters
	f.	fear of objects or persons associated with pain
36.		Actively involve them in finding practical methods to deal with frightening experiences.
37.		toddlers; Four; 5
38.		The quality of the food consumed is more important than the quantity.
39.	a.	they have difficulty going to sleep after daytime activity and stimulation
	b.	they develop bedtime fears
	c.	they awaken during the night
	d.	they have nightmares
	e.	they prolong going to sleep through elaborate rituals
40.	a.	to preserve the deciduous teeth
	b.	to teach good dental habits
41.		T

Section IV A

1.	a.	slightly above the 25th percentile
	b.	falls at the 25th percentile
2.		Physical growth slows and stabilizes during this time. The average weight gain is about 5 lb (2.3 kg) per year and height increases by about 2 to 3 in (6.75 to 7.5 cm) per year.
3.	a.	skips and hops on alternate feet; throws and catches ball well; and walks backward with heel to toe
	b.	ties shoelaces; uses scissors well; and prints a few letters, numbers, or words
	c.	has a vocabulary of 2100 words; uses 6- to 8-word sentences; and names four or more colors
4.		The functions served by these playmates are accomplished as the child gets older. Most children give up these friends when the group process becomes more important, usually when they enter school.
5.	a.	balls, shovels, ladders, swings, slides, sleds, wagons, blocks
	b.	blocks, cars, sandboxes, old adult clothes
	c.	paper, crayons, finger paints, chalk, paste, musical toys
	d.	books, puzzles, records, table games
6.		Because of improved gross motor skills and increasing independence, the preschooler is susceptible to injuries from such activities as playing in the street, riding tricycles, chasing after balls, or forgetting safety regulations when crossing streets.

Section IV B

1.		The social climate, type of guidance, and attitude toward the children that is fostered by the teacher or leader rather than whether or not structured learning is imposed.
2.	a.	licensing of the facility
	b.	the center's daily program
	c.	teacher qualifications
	d.	child-to-staff ratio
	e.	environmental safety
	f.	sanitary conditions
	g.	provision of meals
	h.	indoor and outdoor space per child
	i.	fee schedule
3.	a.	meet the director
	b.	meet some of the caregivers or teachers
	c.	systematically evaluate the facility in comparison with others
	d.	oberve the program in action

4.   a.   present the idea of school as exciting and pleasurable
      b.   talk to the child about the activities that he will participate in at school
      c.   provide the school with detailed information about the child's home environment, such as familiar routines, food prefer-
            ences, etc.
      d.   introduce the child to the teacher and familiarize him with the school
5.   a.   behave confidently with no hesitancy or self-doubt about the decision to send the child to school
      b.   spend some part of the first day with the child until he is at ease with the school situation

Section IV C

1.   At about age 3, children are aware of anatomic differences between the sexes and are concerned with how the anatomy
            of the opposite sex works. They are really concerned about eliminative functions. This leads to physical exploration and
            questioning to obtain more information.
2.   a.   giving no answers
      b.   giving too much information
3.   a.   this allows parents to identify the child's beliefs, and enables them to reinforce or correct the information
      b.   this avoids the establishment of a double standard in which the child receives conflicting information
4.   Inability to fall asleep, bedtime fears, waking during the night, nightmares, prolonging bedtime through rituals.
5.   a.   ignore attention-seeking behavior
      b.   establish and consistently apply a reasonable bedtime ritual
      c.   alleviate sources of fear by keeping a light on, providing a favorite toy, etc.
      d.   decrease levels of stimuli prior to bedtime
      e.   comfort child if nightmares occur, but leave him in his own bed
6.   The decreased quantity of food that the preschooler consumes.
7.   Advise parents to keep a weekly record of the child's diet in order to accurately estimate the intake of food at each
            meal. This should be evaluated at the end of a week's time. In most instances, the child has consumed more than the
            parent realizes.

Chapter 16

QUESTION	ANSWER

Section III

1.   a.   f
      b.   e
      c.   a
      d.   g
      e.   b
      f.   h
      g.   d
      h.   c
2.   a.   identification of the communicable disease
      b.   provision of comfort
      c.   prevention of spread to others
      d.   prevention of complications
3.   to help parents provide care for the child at home
4.   a.   recent exposure to a known case
      b.   history of prodromal symptoms or evidence of constitutional symptoms
      c.   history of previous immunizations
      d.   previous history of having the disease
5.   immunization
6.   a.   instructing parents regarding isolation techniques
      b.   instituting early appropriate treatment
7.   a.   those undergoing steroid or other immunosuppressive therapy
      b.   those who have a generalized malignancy
      c.   those who have an immunologic disorder
8.   Inflammation of the conjunctiva.
9.   a.   obstruction of the nasolacrimal duct
      b.   bacterial infection
10.   purulent drainage
11.   T

12.		F
13.		b
14.	a.	keeping the eye clean
	b.	properly administering ophthalmic medication
15.		prevention of infection in other family members
16.		Intestinal parasitic diseases
17.	a.	their hand-to-mouth activity
	b.	their uncontrolled evacuation habits
18.	a.	life cycle of the infecting parasite
	b.	mode of transmission
	c.	site in the body where it becomes established
	d.	symptomatology displayed by the host
	e.	habits of the host
19.		ingestion
20.	a.	identification of the parasite
	b.	treatment of the infection
	c.	prevention of initial infection or reinfection
21.		preventive education of children and families regarding good hygiene and health habits
22.		Giardiasis
23.		Enterobiasis; pinworm
24.		T
25.	a.	general irritability
	b.	restlessness
	c.	poor sleep
	d.	bedwetting
	e.	distractibility
	f.	short attention span
26.		tape test
27.		mebendazole
28.		It provides that certain potentially hazardous drugs and household products be sold in child-resistant containers.
29.	a.	infants and toddlers explore their environment through oral experimentation
	b.	the sense of taste is less discriminating in small children, and many unpalatable substances are ingested
	c.	toddlers and preschoolers are developing autonomy and initiative which increases their curiosity and exploration
	d.	imitation is a powerful motivator, especially when combined with a lack of awareness of danger
30.	a.	assessment
	b.	gastric decontamination
	c.	family support
	d.	prevention of recurrence
31.		ipecac syrup
32.	a.	used in young infants in whom ipecac is contraindicated
	b.	used if the patient is comatose or convulsing or requires a protected airway
	c.	used if the ingested poison is rapidly absorbed
33.		F
34.		aspiration
35.		T
36.	a.	the use of child-resistant closures
	b.	the limitation of the quantity of drug per container
	c.	the association of Reye's syndrome with aspirin use
37.	a.	adult-strength aspirin
	b.	time-released aspirin
38.		hyperventilation
39.		F
40.		Acetaminophen; hepatic
41.		emesis; lavage; N-acetylcysteine (Mucomyst)
42.	a.	providing supportive care during the critical stages of intoxication
	b.	providing family counseling to prevent recurrence
43.	a.	environment characteristics
	b.	characteristics of the child
	c.	parental characteristics
44.		twice
45.	a.	the blood lead concentration
	b.	the erythrocyte protoporphyrin level

46. a.   urgent risk requiring immediate medical evaluation
     b.   high risk, need further diagnostic tests but are not in immediate danger
     c.   moderate risk, need further diagnostic tests but are not in immediate danger
     d.   low risk, not usually given further tests
47.   T
48. a.   calcium disodium edetate (EDTA)
     b.   dimercaprol (BAL)
     c.   D-penicillamine
49.   Child maltreatment
50.   T
51. a.   parental characteristics
     b.   characteristics of the child
     c.   environmental characteristics
52.   c
53.   d
54. a.   preventing maltreatment from occurring
     b.   identifying the occurrence of maltreatment
     c.   protecting from further maltreatment
55. a.   incest
     b.   molestation
     c.   exhibitionism
     d.   child pornography
     e.   child prostitution
56.   F

Section IV A

1.   Through a tape test or inspection of the anal area while the child sleeps
2.   a.   teach parent to inspect perianal area while child is sleeping; provide instructions for the tape test; and provide for examination of specimen
     b.   administer drug of choice to infected child and all household members; provide complete instructions regarding administration and side effects of medications; repeat administration of drug in 2 weeks
     c.   instruct parents to wash bedding and underwear in hot water; instruct parents to clean washable bedroom and bathroom surfaces with a disinfectant; instruct family members to wear clean, snug underclothing to sleep; cut child's fingernails; encourage hand washing before eating and after toileting

Section IV B

1.   To treat the child first, not the poison.
2.   Respiratory assistance, circulatory support, control of seizures.
3.   a.   obtain history regarding ingestion and identify poison; obtain vital signs and initiate any needed support; institute measures to reduce effects of shock; anticipate and prepare for potential problems
     b.   induce vomiting if indicated; administer antidotes; assist with gastric lavage; be aware of indications and contraindications for the various decontamination procedures
     c.   unaccusingly explore the circumstances of the accident; avoid premature attempts at education regarding prevention of recurrence; remain calm and support child and parent; avoid admonishing for negligence
     d.   discuss difficulties of constantly safeguarding young children; make a follow-up home visit for assessment of potential hazards; ask specific questions to isolate risk factors; emphasize proper storage
4.   a.   S
     b.   A
     c.   S
     d.   S
     e.   A
5.   b
6.   a.   "If you suspected that your child ingested a poison, what would you do first?"
     b.   "Do you have ipecac syrup in your home?"
     c.   "Should you always make the child vomit following the ingestion of poison?"
     d.   "If you suspected that your child had taken a poison, but there were no signs of illness and the child denied doing so, what would you do?"

Section IV C

1.   a.   dilapidated housing
     b.   presence of a lead smelter nearby

    c.   proximity to heavily trafficked roadways

    d.   presence of lead plumbing and piping

    e.   use of unglazed pottery

    f.   use of folk remedies

2.   a.   high level of oral activity; presence of pica; dietary deficiencies of iron and calcium; young developmental age

    b.   poor hygiene practices; inadequate health seeking behavior; poor knowledge of nutrition; few resources to stimulate child; immature attitude toward maintaining discipline

3.   a.   behavioral changes such as aggression, hyperactivity, lethargy, or loss of interest in play

    b.   developmental delays or recent loss of acquired skills

    c.   clumsiness and loss of newly acquired motor skills

    d.   constitutional symptoms such as headache, abdominal pain, vomiting, constipation, and anorexia

4.   To refer the child immediately for examination and lead screening.

5.   By the Centers for Disease Control's classification of risk.

6.   a.   inpatient chelation therapy would be initiated

    b.   either inpatient or outpatient chelation therapy may be initiated

    c.   chelation therapy is not required; however, removal of lead sources and careful follow-up is necessary

    d.   require periodic rescreening until their sixth birthday

7.   a.   c

    b.   e

    c.   a

    d.   d

    e.   e

    f.   d

    g.   c

    h.   b

    i.   a

    j.   b

Section IV D

1.   a.   type of parenting received; negative relationship with own parents; low self-esteem; inadequate knowledge of normal development; concept of role reversal; lack of knowledge of parenting skills; social isolation

    b.   temperament; position in the family; additional physical and/or emotional needs; activity level; illegitimacy; reminds parents of someone they dislike; prematurity; product of difficult delivery

    c.   chronic stress from divorce, financial deficits, unemployment; lack of support systems; absence of a parent; alcoholism; drug addiction

2.   a.   a thorough physical examination

    b.   detailed history

3.   a.   conflicting stories about the accident or injury

    b.   an injury inconsistent with the history

    c.   history inconsistent with the child's developmental level

    d.   inappropriate parental concern for the degree of injury

    e.   a complaint other than the obvious injury; excessive delay in seeking treatment

    f.   refusal of the parents to sign for additional tests

    g.   inappropriate response of child

    h.   previous reports of abuse in family

    i.   repeated visits to emergency facilities with injuries

4.   a.   potential for injury related to presence of risk factors

    b.   alteration in parenting: actual, related to abuse and/or risk factors

    c.   potential for violence: directed at others, related to presence of risk factors

    d.   ineffective family coping: compromised, related to abusive behaviors and/or risk factors

5.   The record of the hospital admission or home visit may be the most supportive evidence of abuse that can be obtained.

6.   a.   victim and family are referred for appropriate intervention; victim is removed from environment

    b.   families avoid precipitating situations; families exhibit positive interaction with child

    c.   child exhibits evidence of decreased distress; child engages in positive relationships with caregivers

    d.   parents demonstrate an attitude of concern for child; parents demonstrate appropriate parenting activities

    e.   parents demonstrate an understanding of normal expectations for their child; parents demonstrate the ability to care for the child

    f.   parents seek group and individual support; parents receive assistance with problems

7.   a.   self-help groups, such as Parents Anonymous

    b.   psychiatric or mental health intervention

    c.   group therapy sessions

Chapter 17

QUESTION		ANSWER

Section III

1.		d
2.		first deciduous tooth; permanent teeth
3.		F
4.	a.	a decrease in head circumference in relation to standing height
	b.	a decrease in waist circumference in relation to height
	c.	an increase in leg length related to height
5.		10; 13
6.		12; 14
7.		d
8.		inferiority
9.		T
10.		c
11.		T
12.	a.	identity
	b.	reversibility
	c.	reciprocity
13.		The ability to group objects according to the attributes that they share
14.		T
15.		d
16.		b
17.		peers
18.		F
19.	a.	to appreciate the numerous and varied points of view that are represented in the peer group
	b.	to become increasingly sensitive to the social norms and pressures of the peer group
	c.	to form intimate friendships between same-sex peers
20.		formalized groups; gangs
21.		team games; sports
22.	a.	subordination of personal goals to group goals
	b.	the division of labor as an effective strategy for the attainment of a goal
	c.	the nature of competition and the importance of winning
23.		family
24.	a.	to help the child interrupt or inhibit a forbidden action
	b.	to point out a more acceptable form of behavior so that the child knows what is right in a future situation
	c.	to provide some reason, understandable to the child, that explains why one action is inappropriate and another action is more desirable
	d.	to stimulate the child's ability to empathize with the victim of the misdeeds
25.		T
26.	a.	inner feelings
	b.	behavior of others
	c.	objective situations
27.	a.	doing nothing
	b.	acting impulsively without thought
	c.	problem-solving
28.	a.	an assessment of growth progress
	b.	vision screening
	c.	evaluation of hearing
	d.	evaluation of posture
	e.	assessment of general health status
29.		Health education
30.	a.	learn about his body
	b.	recognize how his behavior affects his health
	c.	recognize that adaptation may be needed to protect health
31.		obesity
32.		sleepwalking (somnambulism); sleeptalking
33.		T
34.	a.	human sexuality
	b.	her own attitudes and feelings toward sexuality

35. a. health appraisal
     b. emergency care and safety
     c. communicable disease control
     d. counseling and guidance
     e. adjustment to individual student needs
36.   T
37. a. a
     b. c
     c. b
     d. b

Section IV A

1. a. falls at the 50th percentile
    b. falls at the 50th percentile
2.   While 20/20 vision is usually established by 9 to 11 years of age, controversy exists as to the exact age at which it occurs. Mrs. Douglas should be reassured that 20/30 vision is not abnormal for Jimmy, but she should be encouraged to have his vision tested again within a year.
3.   At Jimmy's stage of development, he needs and wants real achievement. When he has access to tasks that need to be done, and is suitably rewarded, he will be able to achieve a sense of industry and accomplishment.
4. a. able to bathe and dress himself
    b. can keep room and personal belongings reasonably neat
    c. often gets up early to have time to himself before school
5.   Lying, cheating, and stealing are frequent occurrences in the young school-age child. Children of this age do not understand why dishonesty is wrong. This behavior usually disappears as they mature.
6. a. provide the child with support as unobtrusively as possible without feeling rejected, hurt, or angry
    b. respect the child's need for privacy and independence while maintaining limit-setting and discipline
    c. prepare the child for the body changes of pubescence.
    d. make certain that the child's sex education is adequate and accurate
    e. allow for some regressive behavior
    f. reinforce earlier safety teaching

Section IV B

1.   The child needs to fit into a peer group and gain a sense of industry through individual, cooperative performance. It is necessary to move away from the familiar relationships of the family group in order to increase the scope of interpersonal interactions and explore the environment.
2.   This is the first time that children are able to join in group activities with unrestrained enthusiasm and steady participation. Formerly, interactions were limited to short periods under considerable adult supervision.
3.   It provides children with comfortable places in a society.
4. a. gangs are small, loosely organized groups with changing membership and little formal structure. There may be a mixture of both sexes.
    b. rigid rules are imposed on the members. There is exclusiveness in the selection of members and acceptance may be based on social or behavioral criteria. Conformity is the core of the gang structure.
    c. formal structure and prolonged cohesiveness. They demonstrate elements of give and take, cooperation, and order and are composed predominantly of children of the same sex.
5.   the need for conformity
6.   Peer pressures may force children into taking risks, even against their better judgment. Minor infractions are often a normal part of gang activity.
7. a. they must relinquish their hold on the child
    b. they find it difficult to face rejection
    c. they resent the child's preference for peer activities
    d. they become the target of the child's intolerance and criticism
    e. their knowledge and authority are questioned

Section IV C

1. a. health supervision
    b. health counseling
    c. health education
2. a. health appraisal
    b. emergency care and safety
    c. communicable disease control

      d.   counseling and guidance

      e.   adjustment to individual student needs

3.   a.   level of understanding and cognitive development

      b.   health beliefs and behaviors

      c.   actual health practices

4.   a.   teach child about the basic food groups; encourage child to participate in food preparation at home; promote nutritious snacks as substitutes for junk food

      b.   assess child's age, activity level, etc., to determine amount of sleep required; allow a later bedtime in deference to the child's age as a measure to resolve bedtime resistance

      c.   encourage child to participate in activities that he is capable of performing; substitute physical activities for television watching; rest adequately following strenuous exercise

      d.   teach correct brushing and flossing techniques; emphasize measures to decrease the development of dental caries; encourage routine dental examinations

5.   a.   assessment of the group's level of understanding regarding sexuality

      b.   conveyance of a nonjudgmental and accepting attitude toward the students

      c.   discussion of normal human anatomy and physiology

      d.   explanation of the maturational changes expected, allowing for normal variations

      e.   exploration of sexuality in a social context

      f.   provision for the expression of student concerns

Chapter 18

QUESTION   **ANSWER**

Section III

1.   a.   dental caries

      b.   malocclusion

      c.   periodontal disease

      d.   trauma

2.   F

3.   a.   the host

      b.   microorganisms

      c.   substrate

      d.   time

4.   a.   frequent, regular observation by a dentist beginning when all primary teeth have erupted, but at least by 3 years of age

      b.   halting the progression of a carious lesion by surgical removal of all affected portions of involved teeth as soon as detected

      c.   oral hygiene that emphasizes thorough mechanical removal of plaque and other material from tooth surfaces

      d.   elimination of concentrated sugars between meals and reducing the mealtime ingestion of sweets to a minimum

      e.   sound nutritional practices

      f.   systemic administration and topical application of fluoride to the teeth

5.   Inflammatory and degenerative conditions involving the gums and tissues supporting the teeth.

6.   gingivitis; periodontitis

7.   Refers to teeth that are uneven, crowded, or overlapping or that interfere with the ability to meet their opponents in the opposite jaw in the appropriate relationships.

8.   a.   elimination of habits that aggravate the deformity

      b.   corrective therapy at the optimal time

9.   a.   Rinse tooth while holding the crown and then gently place in socket.

      b.   Place tooth in cold milk for transport to the dentist.

      c.   Place under child's tongue, or parent's tongue, if child is too young or anxious and transport to the dentist.

10.   T

11.   a.   protection

      b.   impermeability

      c.   heat regulation

      d.   sensation

12.   a.   c, d

      b.   a, e, g

      c.   b, f

13.   a.   contact with injurious agents such as infectious organisms, toxic chemicals, and physical trauma

      b.   hereditary factors

c.   external factor that produces a reaction in the skin
d.   a systemic disease of which the lesions are a cutaneous manifestation

14. a. d
b. b
c. a
d. e
e. c

15. glucocorticoids
16. c
17. F
18. a. to prevent the spread of infection
b. to prevent complications
19. a. administering parenteral antibiotics
b. applying warm compresses
c. maintaining the intravenous infusion
20. a. with inflammation and vesiculation
b. by proliferating to form growths, such as warts
21. b
22. health; hygiene
23. griseofulvin
24. An inflammatory reaction of the skin to chemical substances, natural or synthetic, that evoke a hypersensitivity response or to those agents that cause direct irritation.
25. to prevent further exposure of the skin to the offending substance
26. ammonia, putrefactive enzymes acting on urinary amino acids, laundry products
27. F
28. d
29. Further doses of the medication should be withheld and the rash reported to the attending physician.
30. a. to stop the burning process
b. to decrease the inflammatory response
c. to rehydrate the skin
31. a. cuts on the face
b. a gaping cut longer than ¼ in.
c. cuts that bleed persistently
32. a. when they cause symptoms that interfere with the child's normal activities
b. when they signify the presence of a contagious skin disease
c. if the parasite is able to transmit other diseases
d. when the venom causes a life-threatening immune response
33. scabies; pediculosis capitis
34. a. Interdigital surfaces
b. axillary-cubital area
c. popliteal folds
d. inguinal region
35. lindane (Kwell)
36. b
37. Term applied to various behavior problems that in some way impair the child's capacity to profit from new experiences, occurring with or without hyperactivity.
38. a. family education and counseling
b. medication
c. remedial education
d. environmental manipulation
e. psychotherapy
39. Repeated involuntary urination, usually nocturnal, beyond the age when voluntary bladder control should normally have been acquired.
40. a. c
b. a
c. b
d. e
e. d
41. Repeated voluntary or involuntary passage of feces of normal or near-normal consistency into places not appropriate for that purpose in the individual's own sociocultural setting and not the result of any physical disorder.
42. constipation; environmental change

43.   To return the child to school.
44.   a.   the home situation
      b.   peer relationships
      c.   the school situation
      d.   antecedent events
45.   Providing support and reassurance to the family.

Section IV A

1.   Because all of the permanent teeth (except the wisdom teeth) erupt during this period.
2.   a.   hereditary factors
      b.   abnormal growth
      c.   habits such as thumb-sucking and tongue thrusting
3.   Because the last primary teeth have been shed, yet growth has not ceased.
4.   a.   injury is usually secondary to falls or child abuse
      b.   injury is most often subsequent to bicycle and playground accidents
      c.   injury is usually secondary to fights, athletic injury, and automobile accidents
5.   a.   refer children for dental services; encourage good oral hygiene by teaching correct tooth cleaning to children and parents. (Also, emphasize the importance of regular administration of fluoride; provide nutritional guidance regarding the restriction of cariogenic foods.)
      b.   provide education regarding good dental hygiene; encourage regular inspection of the gingival tissue for signs of early inflammation.
      c.   encourage children with evidence of malocclusion to be examined by a dentist for possible orthodontia; suggest ways to eliminate habits such as thumb- or finger-sucking.
      d.   instruct parents regarding correct methods of replanting evulsed teeth; encourage immediate dental follow-up.

Section IV B

1.   a.   the active ingredient of choice must be safe and suited to the specific disorder
      b.   the proper vehicle for applying the active ingredient to the area must reach and maintain sufficient contact with the affected area and be nonirritating to both affected and healthy skin
      c.   the cosmetic effect of the preparation should not be more unsightly than the lesion
      d.   the cost must be maintained within the means of the family
      e.   instructions for use of the preparation must be clear
2.   a.   injury: potential for infection, related to presence of pathogens
      b.   impairment of skin integrity: actual, related to intrinsic or extrinsic factors
      c.   alteration in comfort: pain or itching, related to skin lesions
      d.   disturbance in self-concept: body image, related to perception of appearance of lesions
      e.   alteration in family process, related to child's skin disorder
3.   a.   provides a soothing film that reduces external stimuli
      b.   provides a palliative anti-inflammatory effect
      c.   prevents autoinoculation and secondary infection
      d.   helps to cool the skin by evaporation, relieve itching and inflammation, and cleanse the area by loosening and removing crusts and debris
      e.   increases the penetration of the medication by promoting moisture retention, nonevaporation of the vehicle, and maceration of the epidermis.
      f.   prevents skin breakdown by absorbing moisture and reducing friction
      g.   provides information and motivation for parents to complete the course of therapy at home
4.   The development of a positive self-concept

Section IV C

1.   Because of their social nature and proximity to other children
2.   The crawling insect and the insect's saliva on the skin
3.   Kwell
4.   a.   educational
      b.   reinfestation-prevention
5.   The pediculocide is not effective against nits. Therefore, it is necessary to retreat in order to eliminate newly hatched lice.
6.   a.   Kwell should be applied to wet hair, lathered generously, and left on for 4 to 5 minutes before rinsing.
      b.   Remove remaining nits and dead lice with a fine-tooth comb.
      c.   Launder clothing and bed linens that have come in contact with the child in hot water and dry in a hot dryer.

d.   Soak all combs and brushes in pediculocide for 1 hour or in very hot water for 5 to 10 min.

e.   Vacuum all mattresses and upholstered furniture thoroughly to remove any living lice or nits.

Section IV D

1.   a.   the child's developmental level

b.   the manner in which training is carried out

c.   the personality makeup of the child

d.   the emotional climate of the home environment

2.   a.   there has never been a long dry or symptom-free period

b.   occurs after a dry period of at least a year

3.   Urgency that is immediate and accompanied by acute discomfort, restlessness, and sometimes, urinary frequency

4.   Structural disorders of the urinary tract, urinary tract infections, major neurologic deficits, nocturnal epilepsy, disorders such as diabetes mellitus and diabetes insipidus.

5.   a.   education

b.   support

c.   communication with the child

6.   a.   help child and parents to understand the problem

b.   explain the advantages and disadvantages of the various treatment modalities

c.   help the child deal with feelings of shame, guilt, and parental disapproval

Chapter 19

QUESTION		ANSWER

Section III

1.   secondary sex characteristics; somatic growth

2.   a.   the maturational, hormonal, and growth processes that occur when the reproductive organs begin to function and secondary sex characteristics develop

b.   means "to grow into maturity" and is generally regarded as the psychologic, social, and maturational process initiated by the pubertal changes

3.   hormonal activity

4.   a.   increased physical growth

b.   appearance and development of secondary sex characteristics

5.   a.   the external and internal organs that carry on the reproductive functions

b.   the characteristics that distinguish the sexes from each other but play no direct part in reproduction

6.   Estrogen; androgens

7.   growth spurt

8.   8; 14

9.   9½; 16

10.   10; 15; 12

11.   nocturnal emissions

12.   height; arms and legs; shoulder; hip development

13.   T

14.   Sebaceous; acne

15.   T

16.   b

17.   group; personal

18.   acceptance; roles

19.   When the individual is unable to formulate a satisfactory identity from the multiplicity of aspirations, roles, and identifications.

20.   peers; adults

21.   c

22.   formal operations

23.   a.   can think beyond the present

b.   is capable of scientific reasoning and formal logic

c.   is capable of mentally manipulating more than two categories of variables at the same time

d.   is to differentiate the thoughts of others from his own and are able to interpret the thoughts of others more accurately

e.   can imagine the possible, a sequence of events that might occur

24.   F

25.   Serious questioning of existing moral values and their relevance to society and the individual
26.   By a period of rejection of the parents.
27.   a.   provides a sense of belonging and a feeling of strength and power
       b.   forms a transition between dependence and autonomy
       c.   is a support for conformity and for questioning adult values
28.   As a means of enhancing their own sex role identity.
29.   a.   an increase in moods and sentiments
       b.   periodic regression to childlike behavior
       c.   mild antisocial behavior
30.   a.   verbalize conceptually
       b.   establish independence
       c.   become comfortable with his body
       d.   build new and meaningful relationships
       e.   seek economic and social stability
       f.   develop a workable value system
31.   a.   body image
       b.   sexuality conflicts
       c.   scholastic pressures
       d.   competitive pressures
       e.   relationships with family and peers
32.   a.   sexual experimentation
       b.   use of hard drugs, alcohol, and cigarettes
       c.   potentially dangerous physical activities
33.   a.   withholding privileges
       b.   contracting
       c.   negotiation
34.   T
35.   a.   calcium
       b.   iron
       c.   zinc
36.   Through the high incidence of anemia.
37.   a.   growth and development
       b.   education process
       c.   better health
38.   Visual refractive difficulties.
39.   a.   biologic
       b.   social
       c.   health
       d.   personal adjustments and attitudes
       e.   interpersonal associations
       f.   establishment of values
40.   physical injury
41.   motor vehicles
42.   a.   inexperience
       b.   lack of defensive driving skills
       c.   inexperience with drinking
43.   a.   understanding of the changes taking place
       b.   understanding and acceptance of detachment behaviors
       c.   preparation for ''letting the child go''
       d.   awareness of the change from dependency to mutuality

Section IV A

1.   a.   between the 50th and 75th percentile
      b.   at the 95th percentile
2.   Nonlean body mass, primarily fat, increases in adolescence.
            Fatty tissue deposition is more pronounced in girls, particularly in the regions over the thighs, hips, buttocks, and
            breast tissue. While the 95th percentile is the top of the normal range, nutritional counseling to prevent additional
            weight gain and/or eating disorders should be instituted.
3.   a.   recommend participation in sports and other physical activities; encourage to practice correct posture in front of a mirror

b.   encourage good hygiene practices; explain the need for deodorant; avoid oily applications to the skin; assist in a well-balanced diet

c.   prepare the adolescent girl for the onset of menarche; encourage good hygiene practices; assess knowledge and answer questions

Section IV B

1.   A sense of group identity is essential to the later development of personal identity. Younger adolescents must resolve questions concerning relationships with a peer group before they are able to resolve questions about who they are in relation to the family and society.

2.   a.   wearing clothes, make-up, and hairstyles according to group criteria
b.   enjoying music and dancing that is exclusive to the age group
c.   using the same language
d.   conforming to the peer group rather than to the adult world

3.   They serve as a strong support to the adolescent, individually and collectively, providing a sense of belonging and a feeling of strength and power. They form a transitional world between dependence and autonomy.

4.   Most of this behavior is related to the struggle for independence and the external restrictions that are placed on this maturation process. On the one hand, adolescents are allowed privileges and increasing responsibilities. On the other, they must conform to regulations set by adults. In their attempt to escape from parental controls, adolescents are critical, argumentative, and remote with both parents.

5.   a.   support and reassure
b.   be available when needed
c.   expect turbulent, unpredictable behavior
d.   accept rejecting behavior as evidence of struggle for independence
e.   allow increasing independence while maintaining suitable limit setting

Section IV C

1.   a.   necessary to support accelerated skeletal growth
b.   necessary for meeting the needs of increased muscle and soft-tissue growth and the demands of the expanding red cell mass
c.   essential for growth and sexual maturation

2.   A distorted body image, inappropriate nutritional information and/or consumption, and the popularity of "fad" diets combine to precipitate these problems.

3.   Rapid physical growth, increased activity, and a propensity for staying up late tend to contribute to this.

4.   This is a period when orthodontic appliances are usually worn, so it is important to provide instructions regarding use and care of the appliances and emphasize attention to tooth brushing.

5.   a.   motor vehicle accidents
b.   drowning
c.   burns
d.   poisoning
e.   falls
f.   bodily damage

6.   The need for independence, coupled with the propensity for risk taking and feelings of indestructibility, makes the adolescent vulnerable. The need for peer approval often causes the adolescent to attempt hazardous feats.

7.   a.   simple, correct explanations of sexual functions
b.   accurate information about pregnancy, including contraception
c.   the transmission, symptoms, and treatment of sexually transmitted diseases
d.   information about sexuality in the opposite sex
e.   reassurance regarding thoughts, fantasies, and masturbation

8.   a.   involve adolescent in diet planning; discuss four basic food groups and their importance in daily diet; associate proper diet with improved physical appearance
b.   educate to the need for sleep in proportion to physical activity; stress importance of a regular sleep pattern
c.   encourage participation in sports; educate to the release of tension through physical activity
d.   explain physical changes occurring in adolescence that require increased bathing and shampooing; assess knowledge of menstrual hygiene
e.   stress necessity of using car restraint systems; reinforce the dangers of drugs; discourage smoking; advise regarding excessive exposure to sunlight; encourage use of protective equipment; encourage practice of safety principles and prevention

Chapter 20

<u>**QUESTION**</u>   <u>**ANSWER**</u>

Section III

1.   acne vulgaris
2.   a.   hereditary factors
   - b.   androgens
   - c.   emotional stress
   - d.   winter weather
   - e.   stimulant drugs
   - f.   the premenstrual period
3.   b
4.   a.   improving the adolescent's general health
   - b.   removing the comedones
   - c.   preventing the formation of comedones
   - d.   controlling excessive sebaceous gland activity
   - e.   controlling infection
   - f.   preventing scar formation
5.   benzoyl peroxide; tretinion
6.   a.   reducing the risk of future inflammatory lesions and scarring
   - b.   producing a prompt improvement in the adolescent's appearance
7.   a.   imitation of smoking behavior of parents, peer pressure, association with maturity
   - b.   low socioeconomic status, low academic goals and performance, failure to participate in school activities
   - c.   emulation of traits popularly attributed to smokers, desire for inclusion in peer groups
   - d.   the initial harshness and irritation may represent a challenge to overcome, nicotine produces dependence
8.   a.   preparation
   - b.   initiation
   - c.   experimentation
   - d.   regular smoking
9.   F
10. a.   peer-led programming
    - b.   use of media, such as video tapes and films
11.   Epstein-Barr virus
12. a.   fatigue
    - b.   lack of energy
    - c.   sore throat
13.   Monospot
14.   prevention, treatment; rehabilitation; prevention
15.   F
16. a.   c
    - b.   a
    - c.   e
    - d.   b
    - e.   d
17. a.   rest
    - b.   ice
    - c.   compression
    - d.   elevation
    - e.   support
18. a.   rest or alteration of activities
    - b.   physical therapies
    - c.   medication
19. a.   in sports with a high inherent risk for sport-related sudden death
    - b.   in children with recognized or unknown underlying medical problems
    - c.   in the sport environment, which may be a contributing or causal factor
20.   T
21. a.   family history
    - b.   child's history
    - c.   previous growth pattern
    - d.   physical examination

	e.	bone age
	f.	endocrine studies
22.		familial short stature; constitutional delay
23.		10; 8
24.	a.	short stature
	b.	sexual infantilism
	c.	amenorrhea
25.	a.	tall, eunuchoid figure with disproportionately long legs
	b.	sparse facial and pubic hair, often with female distribution pattern
	c.	gynecomastia of some degree
	d.	small, firm, and insensitive testes; small penis in childhood
	e.	aspermia or oligospermia
26.		T
27.		Testicular
28.		pituitary
29.		Primary dysmenorrhea
30.		prostaglandins
31.		gonococcal; chlamydial
32.		14; Papanicolaou smear
33.		T
34.		preeclampsia
35.		smaller stature; incomplete growth process
36.		prematurity; low birth weight
37.		T
38.	a.	lack of information
	b.	anxiety regarding contraception
	c.	conflict about sexual activity
	d.	desire for pregnancy
39.		T
40.	a.	all right
	b.	not being blamed for the situation
41.	a.	the acute phase of disorganization of life style
	b.	the long-term process of reorganization
42.		Gonorrhea
43.	a.	d, k
	b.	a, h
	c.	b, i
	d.	e, k
	e.	f, j
	f.	c, g

Section IV A

On the basis of clinical manifestations, an absolute increase in atypical lymphocytes, a positive heterophil agglutination test, and a positive Monospot test.

	a.	disappear within 7 to 10 days
	b.	subsides within 2 to 4 weeks
	c.	usually 2 to 3 months

A short course of oral penicillin, gargles, hot drinks, analgesic troches, and mild analgesics.

	a.	to relieve the symptoms
	b.	to establish appropriate activities
	a.	assist in determining activities according to condition and interests
	b.	promote comfort measures
	c.	provide diet counseling
	d.	prevent secondary infection by limiting exposure
	e.	allow to express feelings, concerns, and anger
	f.	reassure that limitations are only temporary

Section IV B

	a.	acute overload, which includes dislocations, sprains, and muscle pulls
	b.	chronic overload (overuse syndrome), which includes stress fractures, tendonitis, bursitis, and fasciculitis

2. a.   training errors
    b.   muscle-tendon imbalance
    c.   anatomic malalignment
    d.   incorrect footwear or playing surface
    e.   an associated disease state
    f.   growth
3.   c
4.   To alleviate the repetitive stress that initiated the symptoms.
5.   As reduced activity and use of alternative exercise to keep the athlete mobile and maintain conditioning.
6.   Whether running provides both pleasure and physical benefits for him at the present time and into adulthood.
7. a.   collaborate with coaches to ensure safety measures
    b.   assess for environmental safety risks
    c.   counsel child and parents regarding the choice of appropriate sports activities
    d.   recommend alternative activities when appropriate

Section IV C

1. a.   infections, especially sexually transmitted diseases
    b.   problems related to menstruation: delay, discomfort, or irregularities
2. a.   the girl and her parents can be assured that her body is normal, contributing to a positive body image
    b.   it provides an opportunity for health teaching in the areas of hygiene, body functions, and sexuality
    c.   it provides an opportunity for the girl to ask questions about her changing body and the implications of those changes
    d.   if any reproductive system problems arise during adolescence, experience makes the exam less stressful
3. a.   the delay of menarche beyond the age of 17
    b.   absence of menstruation for 12 months or more between periods in the first 2 years following menarche or when more than three periods have been missed following the establishment of menses
4. a.   endometriosis
    b.   pelvic inflammatory disease
5. a.   reassurance about the normalcy of menstrual function
    b.   education about menstrual physiology and hygiene
    c.   education about importance of diet, exercise, and general health maintenanace for menstrual normalcy
    d.   assessment for problems that indicate referral
    e.   education about nonprescription drugs for dysmenorrhea
6.   Because they often delay seeking medical attention. Both gonorrhea and chlamydial infections can result in pelvic inflammatory disease and possible occlusion of the fallopian tubes or abscesses if the infection is untreated or repeated.
7. a.   finding and treating affected persons
    b.   locating and examining contacts of affected persons
    c.   educating adolescents regarding the diseases and their transmission
    d.   encouraging the use of barriers in sexually active adolescents
8. a.   health maintenance deficit, related to knowledge deficit regarding the reproductive system
    b.   rape trauma syndrome, related to sexual abuse
    c.   sexual dysfunction, related to misinformation or disorder of the reproductive system
    d.   injury: potential for tissue damage, related to infection of the reproductive system

Section IV D

1.   The pregnant adolescent must still cope with the developmental tasks of adolescence. When the tasks of motherhood are superimposed on adolescent needs, the girl is ill-prepared to deal appropriately with either.
2. a.   motivation reflects a complex relationship with her own mother and a testing of new and mysterious body functions. Tends to disavow responsibility for and often denies her pregnancy.
    b.   motivation may reflect resurgence of oedipal feelings and expression of independence from parents. Disavows responsibility for but is very conscious of her pregnant state and may view it romantically.
    c.   motivation may reflect an attempt to force a reluctant boyfriend into a permanent commitment or a genuine wish to love and care for a child. Takes responsibility for and views pregnancy as a happy event.
3. a.   forced early marriage that is unstable and at risk
    b.   increased dependency demands on parents for physical, emotional, and financial support
    c.   school dropout with resulting knowledge and skill deficits
    d.   isolation from peers and the adolescent social system
4. a.   provide supportive, nonjudgmental abortion counseling
    b.   provide guidance to an agency and emotional support
    c.   provide assistance and support in caring for herself and baby
5. a.   obtaining medical care for the girl

 b.   establishing a trusting relationship
 c.   establishing good communication with girl and family
 d.   providing information and support
. a.   daily physical care
 b.   protection from injury
 c.   how to care for a child who is ill
 d.   child development
 e.   nutrition
 f.   stress management

Chapter 21

1. a.   age
 b.   sex
 c.   genetically controlled body build
 d.   culturally determined diet and caloric intake
 e.   amount of exercise
 f.   emotions
2.   Obesity
3.   Overweight
4.   A caloric intake that consistently exceeds caloric requirements and expenditure.
5. a.   defective body image
 b.   low self-esteem
 c.   social isolation
 d.   feelings of rejection and depression
6.   T
7. a.   the age of onset of the obesity
 b.   presence of emotional disturbances or neuroses
 c.   a negative evaluation of the obesity by others
8. a.   the persistence of obesity into adulthood
 b.   narcolepsy
 c.   increased incidence of certain orthopedic problems
 d.   psychosocial problems from rejection and ridicule
.   F
.   diet; exercise
.   a
. a.   an adolescent who is older
 b.   having lean parents who are married
 c.   having a good academic record
 d.   an absence of any affective disorders
 e.   lack of a recent stressful life event
.   Anorexia nervosa
.   menarche
. a.   upper or middle class
 b.   academic high achievers
 c.   conforming and conscientious
 d.   high energy levels
 a.   a relentless pursuit of thinness
 b.   a fear of fatness
 a.   disturbed body image and body concept of delusional proportions
 b.   inaccurate and confused perception and interpretation of inner stimuli
 c.   paralyzing sense of ineffectiveness that pervades all aspects of daily life
 a.   parental conflict with possibility of divorce
 b.   a sibling who is rebellious and more outgoing
 a.   severe and profound weight loss
 b.   refusal to eat
 c.   preoccupation with food

	d.	strenuous exercise
	e.	self-induced vomiting and/or use of laxatives
	f.	self-imposed social isolation
	g.	physical signs of altered metabolic activity
20.	a.	reinstitution of normal nutrition or correction of the severe state of malnutrition
	b.	resolution of the disturbed patterns of family interaction
	c.	individual psychotherapy to correct deficits and distortions in psychologic functioning
21.		Bulimia
22.		self-induced vomiting, diuretics, laxatives
23.		d
24.	a.	those who consume vast quantities of food followed by purging but who, if unable to purge, still eat large amounts
	b.	those who restrict their caloric intake, especially when unable to purge
25.		T
26.	a.	monitoring of fluid and electrolyte alterations
	b.	observation for signs of cardiac complications
27.	a.	the turmoil associated with the pubertal changes of adolescence
	b.	limited problem-solving capacity
	c.	the struggle for independence
28.		T
29.	a.	act performed without any real attempt to cause either serious injury or death but rather to send out a signal that something is wrong
	b.	a deliberate act that is intended to cause injury or death
	c.	a rage response designed to punish or manipulate a loved person perceived as withdrawing that love
30.		b
31.	a.	developmental factors
	b.	family factors
	c.	psychoses
32.		Drug overdose
33.		T
34.	a.	relief of suffering
	b.	means of gaining comfort and sympathy
	c.	revenge against persons who have inflicted hurt
35.		F
36.	a.	occurrence as a predominant mood
	b.	persistence for an undue length of time
	c.	so disabling that normal tasks of life cannot be fulfilled
37.		d
38.	a.	social set
	b.	intent
	c.	method
	d.	history
	e.	stress
	f.	mental status
	g.	support
39.	a.	d
	b.	a
	c.	c
	d.	e
	e.	b
40.		legal, social, medical; individual
41.	a.	the type of drug used
	b.	the mode of administration
	c.	the duration of use
	d.	the frequency of use
	e.	whether use is of single or multiple drugs
42.		experimenters; compulsive users
43.	a.	social group
	b.	escapist group
	c.	punitive group
	d.	self-destructive group
44.	a.	the drug used and its purity

b.   the expectations of the user
c.   the context in which the drug is used
45.   Alcohol
46.   Hydrocarbons
47.   F
48.   psychologic; physical
49.   Cocaine
50.   environment
51.   function of the drug

Section IV A

1.   Because it is obvious to others, is difficult to treat, and has long-term effects on psychologic and physical health status.
2.   There is some evidence that general body growth is accelerated by overnutrition. Consequently, children who are obese from infancy may attain relatively greater height and body mass than those with later-onset obesity.
3.   a.   genetic
      b.   diseases
      c.   metabolic and endocrine
      d.   caloric disequilibrium
      e.   cellular structure
      f.   psychologic, social, and cultural
4.   a.   eat more at a given sitting than nonobese persons
      b.   eat more rapidly than nonobese persons
      c.   overeat when they are not hungry
      d.   tend to "gorge" at one meal, rather than eating intermittently over a period of time
      e.   tend to be night eaters
      f.   often skip meals, particularly breakfast
5.   a.   general appearance
      b.   comparison of height and weight with standard charts
      c.   height and weight history of child, parents, siblings
      d.   assessment of eating, appetite, and hunger patterns
      e.   description of physical activities
      f.   careful history regarding onset of obesity
      g.   physical examination to rule out organic etiology
      h.   psychologic assessment by interview and standard tests
6.   a.   alteration in nutrition: more than body requirements, related to obesity and overweight
      b.   knowledge deficit: nutritional, related to poor dietary practices
      c.   disturbance in self-concept: body image, related to obese appearance
      d.   social isolation, related to rejection by peers
7.   a.   teach to prepare and serve smaller portions, remove extra servings from the table
      b.   prepare low-caloric foods in an attractive way, remove junk foods from the house
      c.   encourage to eat slowly, provide activities that are not associated with food

Section IV B

.   A period of a year or two of mood disturbances and behavior changes. The weight loss may be triggered by an adolescent crisis such as the onset of menstruation or a traumatic interpersonal incident.
2.   The current emphasis on slimness as a standard for beauty and femininity.
3.   a.   alteration in self-concept: body image, related to denial of abnormality of emaciated appearance
      b.   alteration in nutrition: less than body requirements, related to denial of hunger and self-starvation
      c.   powerlessness, related to self-doubt and overconformity
.   a.   B
      b.   A, B
      c.   A
      d.   B
      e.   A
      f.   A
      g.   B
      h.   A, B
      i.   B
      j.   B
      k.   A, B

l.   A
5. a.   consistency
    b.   teamwork
    c.   continuity
    d.   communication
    e.   support of client, family, and staff
6. a.   assist adolescent to normalize eating behaviors
    b.   promote development of realistic perceptions and attitudes about food and the body
    c.   promote development of adaptive coping mechanisms to deal with perceptual distortions
    d.   promote a beginning identification and understanding of underlying issues and conflicts
    e.   provide for the development of adaptive interactions and relationships with family and other support systems
    f.   assist in identifying strengths in order to enhance self-worth and self-esteem
    g.   provide a comfortable, nonthreatening environment in which to practice new behaviors and explore sensitive or painful issues

Section IV C

1.   An impulsive act designed to punish or manipulate a loved person perceived as withdrawing that love.
2.   Girls make 4 to 8 times more unsuccessful suicide attempts than boys and are likely to ingest pills as the method
3.   A disturbed family situation, such as economic stresses, family disintegration, medical problems, psychiatric illness, abandonment, or alcoholism
4. a.   removal from the acute situation troubling her
    b.   provision of structure and security during crisis
    c.   provision of necessary surveillance
    d.   reinforcement of the perceived seriousness of the attempt
    e.   provision of warmth, support, and understanding
5. a.   determine what steps were taken to prevent rescue, and whether anyone was present during the attempt
    b.   determine how detailed the suicidal plan was
    c.   examine her understanding of the effects of the combination of barbiturates and alcohol
    d.   determine any previous attempts by Michelle and any family history of suicide
    e.   determine alternative methods available for coping with the loss of her boyfriend and previous coping methods Michelle has utilized
    f.   assess present status and compare it with preattempt status as described by others
    g.   evaluate support that could be expected from her family, friends, peers, teachers, etc.
6.   Marked mood changes, drinking rapidly to obtain a "high," emotional state, drinking alone, inability to predictably control their use of alcohol, protection of their alcohol supply, fear of being caught with alcohol, difficulty in remembering things done when intoxicated, and increasing alcohol tolerance.
7.   Careful assessment of the purpose alcohol serves for Michelle.

Chapter 22

QUESTION   **ANSWER**
Section III

1. a.   c
    b.   a
    c.   d
    d.   b
2.   T
3.   This refers to establishing a normal pattern of living.
4. a.   normalize the life of a child with special needs, including those with technologically complex care, in a family and community context and setting
    b.   minimize the disruptive impact of the child's condition on the family
    c.   foster the child's maximal growth and development
5.   Mainstreaming
6. a.   losing a perfect child
    b.   adjusting to and accepting the child and his condition
7. a.   shock and denial
    b.   adjustment
    c.   reintegration and acceptance
    d.   freezing-out phase

a.   guilt
b.   self-accusation
a.   parents fear letting the child achieve any new skill, avoid all discipline, and cater to every desire to prevent frustration
b.   the parents detach themselves emotionally from the child but usually provide adequate physical care or constantly nag and scold the child
c.   the parents act as if the disorder does not exist or attempt to have the child overcompensate for it
d.   the parents place necessary and realistic restrictions on the child, encourage self-care activities, and promote reasonable physical and social abilities
     T
a.   available support systems
b.   perception of the event
c.   coping mechanisms
     Coping mechanisms
a.   the child's developmental level
b.   available coping mechanisms
c.   the reactions of significant others to him
d.   the condition itself
     T
a.   males are more vulnerable than females
b.   children between ages 6 months and 4 years are considered at greatest risk
c.   temperament
d.   genetic factors
e.   intelligence
a.   denial
b.   guilt
c.   anger
a.   education of the parents regarding the disorder
b.   developmental needs of the child
c.   realistic goal setting

ction IV A

a.   assume responsibility for assuring immunization programs
b.   identify infants and mothers who may be at risk prenatally or postnatally
c.   identify disabilities early
d.   implement innovative health education programs
a.   care is now focused on the child's developmental age rather than chronologic age
b.   increased use of the principle of normalization
c.   earlier discharge of children from acute or chronic care facilities to the family and community
d.   trend toward mainstreaming, or integrating children with special needs into regular classrooms
a.   Using the developmental approach emphasizes the child's abilities and strengths rather than his disability. Under the developmental model, attention is directed to the child's functional development, changes, and adaptation to the environment.
b.   By applying the principles of normalization, the environment for the child is "normalized" and "humanized."
c.   Home care represents the return to a system and set of priorities in which family values are as important in the care of a child with a chronic health problem as they are in the care of the well child
d.   The school has now become an essential component of the child's overall physical, intellectual, and social development.

ction IV B

a.   to provide emotional support to the family
b.   to anticipate and prevent potential problems
c.   to foster growth despite the disorder
a.   this is a period of intense emotion and is characterized by shock, disbelief, and sometimes denial, especially if the disorder is not obvious.
b.   this follows shock and is usually characterized by an open admission that the condition exists. This stage is one of "chronic sorrow" and only partial acceptance and is manifested by several responses such as guilt and self-accusation, bitterness, or anger.
c.   this stage is characterized by realistic expectations for the child and reintegration of family life, with the child's condition in proper perspective. The family also broadens its activities to include relationships outside the home, with the child being an acceptable and participating member of the group.

d.   not all families reach the stage of acceptance and reintegration. If strategies of coping can't be employed to minimize the stress and disorganization of maintaining the child within the home, the child may be placed outside the home. Thi phase is not necessarily one of maladjustment

3. a.   physician shopping
    b.   attributing the symptoms of the actual illness to a minor condition
    c.   refusal to believe the diagnostic tests
    d.   delay in agreeing to treatment
    e.   acting very happy and optimistic despite the revealed diagnosis
    f.   refusing to tell or talk to anyone about the condition
    g.   insisting that no one is telling the truth regardless of others' attempts to do so
    h.   denying the reason for admission
    i.   asking no questions about the diagnosis, treatment, or prognosis

4. a.   It allows individuals to distance themselves from the onslaught of a tremendous emotional impact and to collect and mobilize their energies toward goal-directed, problem-solving behaviors.
    b.   It allows the individual to maintain hope in the face of overwhelming odds.

5. a.   in addition to grieving for the loss of a perfect child, they are less likely to receive positive feedback from transaction with their child. Parenting such children may be a series of unrewarding experiences, which continually support the parents' feelings of inadequacy and failure. Excessive demands on parents' time place additional strain on the couple. This may lead to feelings of resentment, anger, and bitterness toward the other for having their life style disrupted by the child's condition.
    b.   the child's reaction to his condition depends to a great extent on the reactions of significant others to him and to his disability, the child's developmental level, his available coping mechanisms, and to a lesser extent on the condition itself. Children with special needs frequently learn to use aspects of their illness or disability to control members of th family. They may also feel responsible for much of the stress created by their condition.
    c.   they often feel anger and resentment toward the child and the parents for the loss of routine and parental attention. Their perception is often of a sibling who has the undivided attention of their parents, who is showered with special privileges, and who is the focus of everyone's concern. Siblings are likely to show symptoms of irritability, social withdrawal, and fear for their own health.

6.   Assessing which families are at greater or lesser risk for succumbing to the effects of this crisis.

Section IV C

1. a.   status of the marital relationship
    b.   alternate support systems
    c.   ability to communicate

2.   This aids in evaluating the individual's ability to cope with various aspects of the crisis and identifies possible areas fc intervention.

3.   This will often indicate the family's possible reactions to the present stressful event.

4. a.   finds achievement in a variety of compensatory motor and intellectual pursuits
    b.   functions well at home, at school, and with peers
    c.   has an understanding of his disorder that allows him to accept his limitations, assume responsibility for care, and assist in treatment and rehabilitation regimens
    d.   expresses appropriate emotions
    e.   is able to identify with other similarly affected individuals

5.   To help the family to remain intact and functioning at maximum levels throughout the child's life.

6. a.   invites the parents' early input
    b.   encourages parents to be more accountable and responsible for the child's care
    c.   reinforces the fact that the family's ability to cope successfully with the child's problems affects the child's progress and developmental outcomes

7. a.   the family members' individual strengths
    b.   coping mechanisms
    c.   reactions to the disorder
    d.   parents' reaction to the child
    e.   parents' and child's understanding of the condition

8. a.   assess and respond to the variety of reactions displayed by family members
    b.   ensure that the parents understand the information provided

9. a.   be attentive to the family's responses to the child; encourage communication among all family members; encourage parents to discuss their feelings toward the child, the impact of this event on their marriage, and associated stresses; encourage parents to express their expectations for the child; provide with available resources
    b.   observe the child's responses to his disorder, ability to function, and adaptive behaviors; explore the child's own und standing of the nature of his illness or condition; support the child while he learns to cope with his feelings

   c.   provide anticipatory guidance to the parents regarding sibling reactions; encourage parents to discuss the condition with them; encourage parents to be sensitive to the reactions of siblings

0.   a.   provide accurate information in language that the parents can understand; provide guidance in how the condition may interfere with activities of daily living; stress the importance of communicating the child's condition in the event of a medical emergency.

   b.   assist the child to fully realize his potential in preparation for the next phase of development; evaluate the child's developmental progress at regular intervals; teach parents successful methods of controlling behaviors before they become problems

   c.   encourage the parents to determine realistic expectations for the child; encourage genetic counseling; encourage independence

Chapter 23

QUESTION		ANSWER

Section III

1. | | T
2. | | preadolescence
3. | | separation from parents
4. | | T
5. | | shock; disbelief

6.   a.   Truth dispels hope.
   b.   It unnecessarily increases anxiety.
   c.   It destroys the will to survive.

   a.   developmental age
   b.   previous knowledge
   c.   honesty

   a.   develops within hours to days and is characterized by somatic symptoms and intense subjective distress
   b.   refers to the lengthy process which begins with acute grief and extends into a period of reorganization of psychologic life, with attachment to new people and interests

   a.   denial
   b.   anger
   c.   bargaining
   d.   depression
   e.   acceptance

   a.   It is a definite syndrome with psychologic and somatic symptomatology.
   b.   The syndrome may appear immediately after a crisis, be delayed, be exaggerated, or apparently be absent.
   c.   In place of the normal syndrome, there may appear distorted reactions that represent one special aspect of the syndrome.
   d.   Through intervention, distorted reactions can be transformed into normal grief work with successful resolution.

   a.   shock and disbelief
   b.   expression of grief
   c.   disorganization and despair
   d.   reorganization
          Hospice

   a.   The family members are the primary caregivers and are supported by a team of professional and volunteer staff.
   b.   The priority of care is comfort that considers the child's physical, psychologic, social, and spiritual needs.
   c.   The needs of the family are considered as important as those of the patient.
   d.   Hospice is concerned with the family's postdeath adjustment and care may continue for a year or more.

   a.   revelation and dawning reality: diagnosis and treatment
   b.   reprieve: remission and maintenance therapy
   c.   recovery: cessation of therapy and possible cure
   d.   recurrence: relapse and death
   e.   the beginning: postdeath
          T
          burnout

Section IV A

   a.   They see death as a departure.
   b.   They may recognize the fact of physical death but do not separate it from living abilities.

	c.	They view death as temporary and gradual.
2.		as punishment for his thoughts or actions
3.		9; 10
4.		the reactions and attitudes of others, particularly their parents.
5.		because, developmentally, the adolescent's task is to establish an identity by finding out who he is, what his purpose is and where he belongs. Any suggestion of being different or nonbeing is a tremendous threat to the answers to such questions. The adolescent's concern is for the present much more than the past or the future.
6.	a.	structure the hospital admission to allow for maximum self-control and independence
	b.	allow the adolescent the opportunity to learn to know the nurse
	c.	answer the adolescent's questions honestly
	d.	treat the adolescent as a mature individual
	e.	respect the adolescent's need for privacy, solitude, and personal expressions of emotions
	f.	assist parents to communicate with their adolescent children by acting as a role model
	g.	avoid alliances with either parent or child
	h.	allow parents the opportunity to ventilate their feelings of frustration, incompetence, or failure in an atmosphere of acceptance and nonjudgment.
7.	a.	counsel parents regarding children's age-specific understanding of death and appropriate ways to handle behaviors
	b.	encourage parents to take advantage of "small deaths" to help children become familiar and more comfortable with loss
	c.	participate in organized programs on death education, especially in the schools
	d.	serve as resources to parents and others involved with children in answering questions about children and death

Section IV B

1.		Because children frequently speak in symbolic or nonverbal language. Even when asked direct questions and given the opportunity to discuss their thoughts, children may answer in a way that must be interpreted and understood by others in view of the child's age and cognitive abilities.
2.	a.	it avoids the entire issue of how to explain the illness
	b.	it solves the problem of the child asking parents or the hospital staff any difficult, probing questions
	c.	after induction therapy most children attain a remission and are physically well and ready to resume prehospital activities. For parents, it seems easier to return to normalcy if the diagnosis has been hidden.
3.	a.	following the course of remission therapy, there are future courses of treatment and evaluatory procedures which the child is likely to question
	b.	there is always the threat of relapse or recurrence of the illness and the child will then require an explanation
4.	a.	he realizes from the reactions of others that something is very wrong, yet knows that no one wants to talk about it; he is deprived of the truth and forced to supply his own answers or interpretations to events; he will often learn the truth by accidentally overhearing someone discuss his illness
	b.	they will regard the sick child as responsible for the family's disruption and inconvenience; they may feel resentful, angry and jealous of the child's special treatment
	c.	it robs parents of potential support from relatives or friends; it isolates and closes the family off from the world

Section IV C

1.	a.	In this first stage, the family responds with shock and disbelief. The duration of this stage depends on coping mechanisms utilized by the family in previous crises and on the support systems available. The most effective method to deal with denial is support and usually involves active listening by the nurse.
	b.	When denial fails and the reality of the situation penetrates the consciousness, the family's reaction is "Why did this happen to my child?" Families may react with anger, rage, hostility, envy, or resentment which is often directed at the medical and nursing staff. The nurse needs to encourage family members to express their feelings without making them feel guilty or judging them.
	c.	This is the third stage and the one that is most difficult to identify. It is the family's attempt to postpone the inevitable. Because bargaining may be associated with guilt, it is important for the nurse to explore the reasons behind the expressed wish.
	d.	Generally, there are two types of depression: the type experienced for past losses, and the type experienced for anticipated or impending losses. The nurse must help the family deal with the loss in a constructive and positive manner and investigate reasons for guilt, shame, or self-punishment.
	e.	This is the final stage of dying. The family is no longer angry or depressed, and if bargaining occurs, it is usually for a peaceful, painless death rather than for prolongation of life. It is often signaled by the family not planning for future events involving the child and not being preoccupied with past events. The nurse should respect parental wishes and concerns regarding the acceptance of death in their child.
2.	a.	The period of shock following the death is less; grief becomes chronic—parents mourn the loss of their child long before he dies; family members are unable to resolve their grief until the child is considered cured or dead; it provides families with the opportunity to complete all "unfinished business."

b. The family members are deprived of any of the advantages of anticipatory grief; they have no opportunity to prepare themselves for the death; they often feel guilt and remorse for not having done something additional or different with the child.

a. It is during this phase that parents learn of the life-threatening diagnosis. The usual response is one of disbelief and guilt, followed by grieving for the loss of a perfect, healthy child. Almost immediately after the diagnosis is confirmed, induction therapy begins and much of the parents' energy is directed toward waiting for the confirmation of a remission. Nursing considerations that are important at this time include: providing and explaining relevant information; encouraging parents to participate in the child's care; and providing reassurance.

b. This phase occurs once the child is in remission and there is hope for an eventual recovery. During this phase parents commonly react by overprotecting the child, encouraging dependency, and liberalizing discipline. Nursing considerations during this phase include: advising parents to continue appropriate discipline of the child by resuming pre-illness rules and limits; encouraging parents to allow the child to resume school and other daily activities as soon as possible; and preparing parents for the common responses of friends and relatives to the child's illness.

c. Often the maintenance period is followed by a cessation of therapy in the hope of a permanent recovery. Although this is usually a very happy time, it is mixed with feelings of grief, ambivalence, and concern for the future. Nursing considerations include: accepting the parents' need to regress to earlier forms of coping; encouraging the parents to call the nurse or clinic about any concerns; and encouraging family members to verbalize their feelings regarding cessation of therapy.

d. During this phase, there is intense anticipatory grieving, loss of hope, and depression. Nursing considerations include: helping the parents and child formulate realistic short-term goals and establish reasonable priorities of care; discussing the parents' wishes and expectations for the terminal phase; and preparing parents to deal with their fears.

e. Although families can prepare themselves for the expected loss, there is a period of acute grief when it actually occurs. This is usually followed by an extended phase of mourning. Nursing considerations include: providing follow-up care for the family and assisting parents in their grief.

Although some reactions may help the nurse provide care by protecting the dying child and his family from the emotional impact of the event, others may interfere with the establishment of a therapeutic relationship.

a. protects nurses from the overwhelming reality of death and is necessary to prevent feelings of failure

b. occurs because the exposure to potential failure in a fatal illness is extremely threatening; also may result from the nurse having to subject the child to painful procedures while being unable to relieve his physical and emotional suffering

c. occurs because a nurse may be unable to deal with a fatally ill child or may occur because the nurse became angry and depressed while providing care

d. occurs as a result of the nurse's personal needs

The nurse is continuously involved in a situation that is emotionally demanding.

a. The first step is to make a deliberate choice to become involved; the nurse must also investigate personal motivations for choosing to work in such an area and have an understanding of the stresses inherent in the role.

b. The nurse must be able to base nursing practice on sound theoretic formulations; ethical issues surrounding the definition of death, the use of extraordinary lifesaving measures, and patients' rights to know and to choose their own destiny must also be explored by the nurse.

c. These must be present to allow for regeneration of energies by sharing feelings and concerns with others.

d. The nurse should maintain good general health practices and should participate in diversionary activities that are of personal interest beyond the workplace.

Chapter 24

QUESTION   **ANSWER**

Section III

Mental retardation

Significantly subaverage general intellectual functioning existing concurrently with deficits in adaptive behavior and manifested during the developmental period.

It implies that intelligence alone is not the criterion for mental retardation.

after a period of suspicion by professionals and/or the family that the child's developmental progress is delayed.

standard intelligence tests

a. genetic
b. biochemical
c. viral
d. developmental
a. infection and intoxication
b. trauma or physical agents
c. metabolism or nutritional factors

    d.   gross postnatal brain disease
    e.   unknown prenatal influences
    f.   chromosomal abnormalities
    g.   conditions such as prematurity, low birth weight, and postmaturity that originate in the perinatal period
    h.   psychiatric disorders
    i.   environmental influences

8. a.   These are designed to eliminate the occurrence of the condition that causes the retardation.
    b.   These are designed to identify the condition early and institute treatment to avert cerebral damage.
    c.   These are concerned with treatment to minimize long-term consequences.

9.   This act requires local departments of education to provide education programs for handicapped children 3 years of age or older.

10.   because this is the normal sequence of development

11. a.   sit quietly for 3 to 5 minutes while working on a task
    b.   watch what he is doing while working on a task
    c.   follow physical gestures or cues
    d.   follow verbal commands
    e.   relate clothing to the appropriate body part

12.   Safety
13.   Down syndrome
14.   21
15.   through a chromosomal analysis
16.   F

17. a.   decreased muscle tone
    b.   an underdeveloped nasal bone that causes a chronic problem of inadequate drainage of mucus
    c.   constant stuffy nose which causes the child to mouth-breathe

18.   Because of their large, protruding tongues and decreased muscle tone.

Section IV A

1.   improved support
2. a.   rubella immunization; genetic counseling, especially in terms of Down or fragile X syndrome; education regarding the dangers of alcohol during pregnancy; adequate prenatal nutrition; and reduction of nonintentional and intentional cerebral injuries
    b.   prenatal diagnosis or carrier detection of disorders; newborn screening for treatable inborn errors of metabolism
    c.   early identification of conditions; provision of appropriate therapies and rehabilitation services
3.   promoting the child's optimum development as an individual within a family and community
4.   his learning abilities and deficits
5. a.   This model uses a didactic approach in which parents are taught behavioral strategies for teaching their children specific skills and competencies.
    b.   This model seeks to promote competent parenting through counseling and guidance techniques by focusing on resolving feelings related to the child's impairment.
    c.   This model focuses on the quality of the parent/child relationship and considers a mutually satisfying interaction as the prime requisite for the infant's optimum development.
6. a.   perform a task analysis prior to initiating the program to determine the child's capabilities; assess the child's physical capabilities and developmental readiness for self-feeding; assess for dietary deficiencies by encouraging parents to maintain a diet history; encourage parents to provide the child with supportive feedback
    b.   assess the child's physical and psychologic readiness; interview parents regarding their readiness for toilet training; evaluate any past attempts at toilet training
    c.   assess the child's readiness by doing a task analysis; maintain a detailed record of the child's abilities and accomplishments; teach parents to select clothing that the child will be able to manipulate
    d.   assess the child's level of readiness; assess parents' willingness to participate; encourage parents to provide the child with supportive feedback
7. a.   guide parents toward the selection of suitable toys and interactive activities; encourage parents to use every opportunity to expose the child to different sounds, sights, and sensations; stress the need for parents to supervise the child during play
    b.   teach shaping techniques to foster meaningful vocalization; instruct parents to record all meaningful vocalizations that the child learns; when speech acquisition is not possible, encourage parents to learn nonverbal methods of communication
    c.   teach parents to employ limit-setting measures that are simple, consistent, and appropriate for the child's mental age; teach parents to use behavior modification and time-out to control behavior
    d.   encourage parents to teach the child socially acceptable behavior; encourage parents to expose the child to various situations to practice these skills; stress the need for parents to allow the child to socialize with peers

Section IV A

1.   He is often unable to proceed past parallel play within a group because of his inability to follow directions during cooperative play. Also, his deficit may not allow him to interpret enough of the conversation to join in. As a result, he learns to stay on the periphery or to avoid social interactions altogether.

2.   a.   treat existing ear infections and prevent recurrences; encourage periodic auditory testing for children at risk; stress the need for routine immunizations; administer ototoxic agents cautiously; counsel pregnant women regarding the necessity of early prenatal care

     b.   screen all children for auditory function; observe for behaviors that indicate a hearing loss; isolate children who are at risk

     c.   assist the family in adjusting to the child's loss of hearing; help parents set realistic goals; explain the effects of the hearing loss on the child's development; encourage parents to provide appropriate stimulation; assist parents in maximizing the child's communication skills

3.   a.   the neonate's response to auditory stimuli as evidenced by reflexes; findings on the Brazelton Neonatal Behavior Assessment which evaluates the infant's orientation response to the sound of a voice; or any failure by the infant to orient to a sound or attempt to localize it by age 6 months

     b.   the presence of any difficulties in learning; any parental concerns regarding loss or change in hearing

4.   a monotone, flat type of speech

5.   a.   may speak fairly clearly but in a loud voice

     b.   usually there is difficulty in articulation; the child's speech is a reflection of the distortion of sound

     c.   by 18 months of age, the child behaves as if deaf; he can often give stereotyped responses to questions for which he has learned a patterned response; he often has difficulty in learning the correct usage of pronouns

6.   because speech is learned through a multisensory approach and the usual mechanisms are not available to the deaf child

7.   a.   facilitate the understanding of reasons for admission and procedures

     b.   promote the intactness of the family unit

     c.   facilitate continuity of care

     d.   promote socialization of the child

8.   a.   facilitate preparation with tactile and visual aids; constantly reassess the child's understanding of explanations

     b.   encourage parents to room with the child; encourage parents to participate in the child's care

     c.   alert other health care members and patients to the child's special needs; provide consistent caregivers

     d.   introduce the child to roommates; encourage the child to engage in play activities

Section IV B

  a.   screen pregnant women at risk; provide adequate prenatal and perinatal care to prevent prematurity; institute periodic screening of all children; ensure adequate immunization of all children; counsel parents and children regarding the common causes of ocular trauma

  b.   provide periodic visual screening for all children; observe for behaviors which indicate visual impairment; be attentive to parents' concerns

  c.   assist the parents and child to gain a realistic concept of the problem; encourage family members to investigate stimulation and educational programs; provide an environment that fosters security; encourage the child to participate in play activities; assist in the selection of appropriate play materials

  a.   discuss with the child the importance of the treatment in preserving eyesight

  b.   allow the child an opportunity to discuss his feelings regarding the treatment

  c.   assist the child to overcome difficulties associated with treatment such as unkind remarks by peers

  a.   avoid excessive eyestrain; when doing close work, periodically look into the distance to relax the muscles of accommodation

  b.   use proper lighting; light should not be glaring or cast shadows on reading material

  c.   get sufficient amounts of rest

  d.   have eyes check at least yearly by a licensed optometrist or ophthalmologist

  a.   help the family and child adjust to the impairment

  b.   promote parent-child attachment

  c.   foster optimum development and independence

  d.   provide for play/socialization

  e.   be aware of educational facilities

  a.   reassure the child and family throughout every phase of treatment

  b.   orient the child to his surroundings

  c.   provide a safe environment

  d.   encourage independence

  a.   talk to the child about everything the nurse is doing; identify oneself when entering the room; encourage parents to room-in and participate in care; encourage parents to bring to the hospital familiar objects from home

b. as soon as the child can be out of bed, familiarize him with the room; position things so that they are easily accessible
c. place furniture in the same position; place side rails up; remove objects from the floor
d. set up equipment and have child participate in care; explain where items are; praise child for his efforts

Section IV C

1. a. detection of communication disorders
   b. prevention of primary problems or development of further difficulties
   c. promotion of optimum educational opportunities
2. a. recognize infants and children at risk early so treatment may be initiated; provide families with education that fosters communication; provide parents with information regarding normal language development
   b. assess the child's speech and language development; initiate appropriate referrals
   c. encourage parents to talk to the child and praise him; teach the child the meaning of new words; provide the child with listening activities
3. Failure to detect communication disorders during early childhood affects the development of social relationships and emotional interactions, increases difficulty in developing academic skills, and lessens the chances for successful correction of deficit skills.
4. a. knowledge of normal language and speech development
   b. awareness of clues that indicate language and speech impairment
5. a. direct observations of the child's verbal skills
   b. questioning of the parents
   c. testing
6. This test employs the word-imitative procedure and is one of the most frequently used tests. The child repeats 22 word‐ but pronounces 30 different sound elements. The raw score, or the number of correctly pronounced sounds, is then compared with the percentile rank for children in that age group. The child is also scored on intelligibility.

Chapter 26

QUESTION   **ANSWER**

Section III

1. a. developmental age
   b. previous experience with illness, separation, or hospitalization
   c. available support system
   d. innate and acquired coping skills
   e. seriousness of diagnosis
2. Separation
3. protest; despair; detachment
4. peers
5. physical restriction; altered routine; rituals; dependency
6. a. a
   b. b
   c. b
   d. a
   e. c
   f. d
   g. a
   h. d
   i. c
   j. b
7. a. disbelief
   b. anger; guilt
   c. fear; anxiety; frustration
   d. depression
8. denial; intellectualization; regression; projection; displacement; introjection
9. a. d
   b. c
   c. a
   d. b
10. anger; jealousy; resentment
11. decrease

12.   a.   simple descriptive scale
        b.   numeric scale
        c.   faces scale
        d.   glasses scale
        e.   chips scale
        f.   color scale
13.   a.   c
        b.   c
        c.   c
        d.   x
14.   Fear of the unknown (fantasy) exceeds fear of the known.
15.   a.   T
        b.   F
        c.   T
        d.   F
        e.   T
        f.   T
        g.   F
16.   increases
17.   observation; questioning; measurement tools
18.   behavioral changes; physiologic responses.
19.   information
20.   work
21.   parent-child relationships; educational opportunities; self-mastery; socialization
22.   aloofness toward parents; attachment to parents; fears; nightmares; insomnia; withdrawal and shyness; hyperactivity; temper tantrums; attachment to toy; resistance to going to bed; and regression
23.   a.   Nursing Admission History
        b.   physical assessment
        c.   placing the child

Section IV A

1.   protest
2.   a.   allow the child to cry
        b.   provide support through physical presence in room even when child rejects strangers
        c.   acknowledge to the child that it is all right to miss her parents and it is all right to cry
        d.   encourage parents to stay with the child as much as possible

Section IV B

1.   a.   Encourage parents to room-in
        b.   Encourage parents to participate in the care of the child.
        c.   Assign a consistent primary nurse to care for Amy.
        d.   Accept Amy's separation behavior.
        e.   Help parents to understand Amy's separation behavior.
        f.   Ask parents to bring some of the child's favorite toys and articles to the hospital.
2.   a.   Utilize the minimum amount of restraint of physical activity.
        b.   Set schedules and routines as close to that of the child as possible.
        c.   Decrease dependency of the child by allowing the child to do things for herself and allowing the child to make decisions.

Section IV C

1.   a.   Be willing to stay and listen to parents' verbal and nonverbal messages.
        b.   Stay with the child to allow parents some time alone.
        c.   Accept cultural, socioeconomic, and ethnic values of parents.
        d.   Help parents to accept their own feelings toward the child
        e.   Provide information to the parents
        f.   Encourage parents to keep rest of family informed.
        g.   Prepare parents for posthospitalization behaviors of the ill child.
        h.   Warn parents of reaction of siblings to the ill child.
2.   a.   Encourage parents to give information to siblings.
        b.   Incorporate siblings into hospital admission programs.

    c.   Liberalizing visiting regulation.

    d.   Extending parent participation programs to include siblings.

    e.   Developing programs designed specifically for siblings.

    f.   Assist parents to cope with siblings reactions to the hospitalized child

3.   large puzzles, blocks, dress-up materials, puppets, scissors and paper, and crayons

Section IV D

1.   a.   Take a Nursing Admission History.

    b.   Perform a physical assessment.

    c.   Assess variables influencing placement of the child on the unit.

2.   a.   Assess the family's desire and capability in assuming responsibilities of care.

    b.   Develop teaching plan for those skills that parents or children are expected to continue at home.

    c.   Teach skills according to teaching plan

    d.   Provide an opportunity for a transition period from hospital to home.

    e.   Evaluate the discharge plan.

    f.   Provide for professional support after discharge.

Chapter 27

QUESTION	ANSWER

Section III

1.   The legal and ethical requirement that the patient clearly, fully, and completely understands the medical treatment performed and all risks, consequences, or results that may or may not occur from medical treatment.

2.   a.   The person must be capable of giving consent, must be over the age of majority, and must be considered competent.

    b.   The person must receive the information needed to make an intelligent decision.

    c.   The person must act voluntarily when exercising freedom of choice without force, fraud, deceit, duress, or other form of constraint or coercion.

3.   a.   one who is legally underage but is recognized as having the legal capacity of an adult under circumstances prescribed by law; for example, marriage

    b.   one who has attained the specific age (usually 15 or 16) at which a minor may consent to medical or surgical treatment without parental consent; for example, contraceptive services

    c.   considered in most states to be the age of 18

4.   preparation

5.   a.   Determine the details of the exact procedure to be performed.

    b.   Review the parents' and child's present level of understanding.

    c.   Plan the actual teaching based on the child's developmental age and existing level of knowledge.

    d.   Involve parents in the teaching if they so desire, especially if they plan to participate in the care.

    e.   While preparing the child, allow for ample discussion to prevent information overload and ensure adequate feedback.

6.   a.   Use concrete, not abstract, terms and visual aids to describe the procedure.

    b.   Emphasize that no other body part will be involved.

    c.   Use words appropriate to the child's level of understanding.

    d.   Avoid words or phrases with dual meanings.

    e.   Clarify all unfamiliar words, for example "anesthesia is a special sleep."

    f.   Allow the child to practice those procedures that will require his cooperation, such as turning, coughing, or using a blow bottle.

    g.   Emphasize the sensory aspects of the procedure, that is, what the child will feel, see, etc.

    h.   If the body part is associated with a specific function, stress the change or noninvolvement of that ability.

    i.   Introduce anxiety-causing information, such as the preoperative injection, last.

    j.   Be honest with the child about unpleasant aspects of a procedure, but avoid creating undue concern.

    k.   Emphasize the end of the procedure and any pleasurable events afterward.

7.   a.   teach

    b.   express feelings

    c.   achieve a therapeutic goal

8.   the extent to which the patient's behavior coincides with the prescribed regimen

9.   a.   clinical judgment

    b.   self-reporting

    c.   direct observation

    d.   monitoring appointments

    e.   monitoring therapeutic response
    f.   pill counts
    g.   chemical essay

10.   a.   organizational strategies
    b.   educational strategies
    c.   behavioral strategies

11.   widely spaced teeth; pomade

12.   a.   high-calorie fluids such as colas, carbonated drinks, fruit juice, fruit punch, sweetened water, and milkshakes
    b.   frozen or formed liquid such as popsicles, jello, sherbet, ice cream
    c.   small amounts of favorite fluids at frequent intervals

13.   fever

14.   a.   c
    b.   a
    c.   b

15.   antipyretics

16.   increase

17.   time-out

18.   a.   age
    b.   condition
    c.   destination

19.   The nurse must cleanse the genital area for the child instead of the child doing it himself. The nurse may hold the child over a sterile container, or she may apply a sterile plastic collecting bag. The start and stopping of urine stream (midstream) usually is impossible.

20.   Tincture of benzoin

21.   body surface area

22.   check his hospital identification band

23.   a.   vastus lateralis muscle
    b.   ventrogluteal muscle

24.   a.   inserted nasally or orally to the stomach: gastric gavage
    b.   inserted nasally or orally to the jejunum: enteral gavage
    c.   inserted directly into the stomach: gastrostomy
    d.   inserted directly into the jejunum: jejunostomy

25.   Slide the tube through a sterile disposable nipple whose tip is cut off and whose base is then taped to the abdomen.

26.   rapid fluid shift and fluid overload

27.   a.   Osmotic effect of the enema may produce diarrhea, which can lead to metabolic acidosis.
    b.   Extreme hyperphosphatemia, hypernatremia, hypocalcemia, which may lead to neuromuscular irritability and coma, may occur.

28.   1 gram = 1 milliliter.

29.   prevent skin breakdown and to facilitate adherence

30.   a.   admission
    b.   the blood test
    c.   the afternoon of the day before surgery
    d.   injection of preoperative medication
    e.   before and during transport to the operating room
    f.   return from the recovery room

31.   a.   a
    b.   c
    c.   b

32.   a.   hurt, discomfort
    b.   make better
    c.   special sleep
    d.   special opening
    e.   special place in body

Section IV A

1.   a.   The nurse who explains the procedure should be the one who supports the child throughout the procedure.
    b.   Assemble all equipment before beginning procedure.
    c.   Do not perform procedure in a ''safe'' room.
    d.   Avoid lengthy conversation during procedure.
    e.   Inform child when procedure is nearing completion.

Section IV B

1. a. repetition, written notes, pamphlets, ask patient to repeat the regimen
   b. provide emotional support, try to elicit patient's feelings, offer hope, avoid "sledgehammer" method of sharing diagnosis
   c. explain skills, demonstrate skills, then have patient perform skills

Section IV C

1. Measure the rectal temperature 30 minutes after the antipyretic is given to assess whether the temperature is lowered.
2. Use minimal clothing, expose skin to air, reduce room temperature, increase air circulation, administer cool applications to the skin or give a cooling bath.
3. crib sides

Section IV D

1. a. provides a snug fit with minimum danger of becoming too tight
   b. prevents muscle injury and psychologic stress

Section IV E

1. a. Use a small amount of liquid or food—the child may refuse to take the entire amount and thus receive only a partial dose of the medication.
   b. Avoid essential food items—child may become conditioned against them and refuse these foods.

Section IV F

1. a. because this entry causes less distress (since infants are obligatory nose breathers) and helps stimulate sucking.
   b. because the esophagus is situated behind the trachea, the tube is more easily inserted when the head is in this position and the chance of the tube entering the trachea is reduced
   c. so that the fluid and electrolyte balance won't be upset by removing the fluids and electrolytes
   d. because of possible damage to the nostril
   e. to prevent nausea and regurgitation
   f. to clear formula from tube and prevent souring
   g. to minimize the possibility of regurgitation and aspiration
2. a. attaching a syringe to the feeding tube and attempting to aspirate stomach contents.
   b. injecting with the syringe, 0.5 ml of air into the tube while listening with a stethoscope to the stomach area for sounds of gurgling or growling. Withdrawn air.
3. a. return residual aspirated fluid to the stomach
   b. provide a pacifier during feeding

Section IV G

1. a. potential for injury related to surgical procedure or anesthesia
   b. anxiety related to separation from support system and unfamiliar environment
   c. alteration in comfort related to pain
   d. alteration in family process related to surgical procedure.
2. to avoid glycogen depletion and dehydration
3. Lungs remain clear.

Chapter 28

QUESTION	ANSWER

Section III

1. F
2. c
3. 950–1100 ml
4. when the total output of fluid exceeds the total intake of fluid
5. T
6. c
7. d

8.   degree of hydration; type of dehydration; physical signs; serum sodium; other electrolytes; and presence of acid-base imbalances

9.   from accumulation of acid or loss of base

10.   27–41

11.   c

    a

    d

    b

12.   poor gas exchange

13.   T

14.   a.   gain of exogenous acid

    b.   incomplete oxygenation of fatty acids

    c.   incomplete oxygenation of carbohydrates

    d.   inability of the kidneys to excrete acids

    e.   losses from the GI tract

    f.   inappropriate excretion of bicarbonate in the kidney

15.   Pyloric stenosis

16.   observation

17.   T

18.   b

19.   T

20.   decreased

21.   F

22.   a microdrip and a calibated volume control chamber

23.   a.   chronic intestinal obstruction

    b.   bowel fistulas

    c.   chronic severe diarrhea

    d.   burns

    e.   abdominal tumors

24.   high concentrations of glucose protein and other nutrients

25.   superior vena cava and the subclavian veins

26.   infection

Section IV A

1.   a.   increased metabolic rate

    b.   inability of the kidney to concentrate urine

    c.   increased surface area

2.   It is made on the bases of a normal serum sodium, the presence of signs such as decreased blood pressure and poor skin turgor, and a 10% loss of weight as compared with present weight.

3.   The first priority is the restoration of circulation. This is usually accomplished by intravenous infusion of a saline solution.

4.   a.   a quiet environment while the infusion is inserted

    b.   introducing Michael to another child receiving intravenous therapy

    c.   using dolls to illustrate the procedure

    d.   informing the parents of the procedure and allowing them to be present if they wish

    e.   allowing Michael to help out during the procedure

5.   because children are prone to fluid disturbances, the use of a volume control chamber limits the amount of fluid that can be infused so that accidental overloads do not occur.

6.   The nurse observes that Michael's appearance is drawn, his expression is flaccid, his eyes lack luster, his appetite is diminished, and his activity level is decreased.

7.   Michael's vital signs are taken upon admission to determine whether shock is present. His weight is taken to provide a baseline to determine the adequacy of the fluid therapy.

8.   The nurse should assess the presence of tingling in the fingers or toes, abdominal cramps, muscle cramps, thirst, nausea, hypotonia, weakness, twitching, tremors, and seizures.

9.   a.   immobilizing of the site

    b.   restraining the child

    c.   monitoring the flow rate

    d.   monitoring the site for redness or swelling

    e.   checking dependent areas near the infusion site for presence of fluid

10.   The nurse can determine whether redness, inflammation and/or pain are present at the site. The absence of these indicates that interventions were successful.

Section IV B

1.   The laboratory test used to assess the presence of an acid/base disturbance is the arterial blood gas which includes the determination of the PCo_2, pH, and TCo_2

2.   It indicates the presence of respiratory acidosis.

3.   You should monitor the patient for signs of calcium and potassium imbalance, such as tingling in the fingers, abdominal and/or muscle cramps, twitching, and weakness or tremors. In addition, a urine pH should be obtained.

4.   The rationale for waiting until the patient voids is that serious imbalances of potassium are usually present with acid/base imbalances. You should wait until you are sure there is proper perfusion to the kidneys, so that excretion of excess potassium can occur.

5.   Interventions to prevent complications from immobilization might include:
- a.   frequent removal of the restraints
- b.   providing the child with the opportunity to move the extremity
- c.   holding or cuddling the child
- d.   encouraging the child to perform range of motion exercises
- e.   encouraging the child to move arms

Section IV C

1.   The rationale for infusion into a large vessel is that the solution should be diluted rapidly because the high glucose concentration is irritating.

2.   a.   hyperglycemia
     b.   acid/base imbalances
     c.   dehydration
     d.   overhydration
     e.   coma
     f.   liver disease—hepatomegaly, jaundice, increased alkaline phosphatase

3.   a.   vital signs
     b.   daily weights
     c.   monitoring acid/base imbalances
     d.   dextrostix, and monitoring urine for the presence of glucose
     e.   monitoring the infusion rate

4.   It is often difficult for the body to adapt to the high glucose concentration and hyperglycemia often occurs.

5.   While you change the solution and care for the line, you observe the line for kinks, catheter displacements, loose sutures, and signs of inflammation such as redness, edema, or sediment in the line. The absence of these would indicate that interventions were effective.

6.   TPN solutions are maintained at a uniform rate to insure proper utilization of glucose and amino acids. Speeding up the rate to compensate might overload the patient, and hyperglycemia and a metabolic acid/base imbalance might occur.

Chapter 29

QUESTION   **ANSWER**

Section III

1.   It is defined as a noticeable or sudden increase in the number of stools, as a reduction in their consistency, and as stools that are green in color.

2.   a.   osmotic factors
     b.   diminished absorption or increased secretion of water and electrolytes
     c.   reduction in anatomic or functional surface area
     d.   altered motility

3.   F

4.   a

5.   b

6.   a.   history
     b.   age of the child
     c.   presence of other family members with the illness
     d.   presence or absence of symptoms such as fever, vomiting, and abdominal cramps
     e.   laboratory tests such as CBC

	f.	examination of stool for color, red blood cells, and pH
7.		50 ml/kg body weight; 100 ml/kg body weight
8.		Opiates are not used because they have little or no effect on the course of the disease, and they can cause toxicity. Absorbents also have little effect on the disease because they do not reduce the amount of the fluid loss.
9.		rapid replacement of the fluid deficit, abnormal ongoing losses, and normal ongoing losses
10.		assessment; therapy; education
11.		F
12.		fecal-oral route; person-to-person contact
13.		F
14.	a.	higher cortical centers
	b.	a chemosensitive trigger zone in the fourth ventricle
	c.	vagal and sympathetic afferent nerves
15.		The circular muscle of the pylorus is grossly enlarged as a result of hypertrophy and hyperplasia and an obstruction occurs leading to projectile vomiting.
16.		d
17.		radiographic studies and a palpable olive mass in the right upper quadrant
18.		T
19.		restoring hydration and correcting electrolyte imbalance
20.		hypotension, tissue hypoxia, and metabolic acidosis
21.	a.	compensated
	b.	uncompensated
	c.	irreversible
22.		F
23.		Impaired perfusion to the peripheral tissue reduces the oxygen available. These tissues in turn revert to anaerobic metabolism producing large amounts of lactic acid leading to an acidosis.
24.		a
25.	a.	ventilation
	b.	fluid administration
	c.	improved pumping of the heart
26.		c
27.		to assure adequate tissue oxygenation
28.		interaction between an allergen and preexisting specific immunoglobin E
29.		Shock is seen because the allergic reaction releases histamine which causes vasodilation, bronchoconstriction, and increased capillary permeability. This leads to increased venous capacity and pooling, reduced arterial pressure, and a rapid loss of fluid into the interstitial space.
30.		T
31.	a.	percentage of body surface burned
	b.	depth of the burn
	c.	location of the burn
32.		Children have different body proportions especially in their heads and extremities, so the rule is not appropriate.
33.		c
34.		F
35.		b
36.		Anemia is a common occurrence because red blood cells are destroyed by heat, are lost in the zone of stasis, and are lost through direct bleeding and bone marrow depression.
37.		asphyxia
38.		to stop the burning process, cover the burn, transport the child to medical aid, and reassure the parents
39.	a.	shock
	b.	pulmonary complications
	c.	sepsis
	d.	Curling's ulcer
	e.	central nervous system problems such as seizures and delirium
40.	a.	establish and maintain an adequate airway
	b.	establish a lifeline for fluid resuscitation
	c.	care of the burn wound
	d.	provide adequate nutrition
	e.	prevent contractures
	f.	correct anemia and hypoproteinemia
	g.	promote rehabilitation
41.		c
		b

a

d

Section IV A

1.   Leah's diarrhea is of short duration (3 days), and the diarrhea appears to have been of acute onset.
2.   The age of the patient (under 2 years) and the season (winter) are factors that were considered.
3.   a.   prevent the spread of infection
      b.   prevent complications from restraining devices
      c.   observe for signs of complications
4.   a.   maintain accurate record of intake
      b.   weigh child daily or as ordered
      c.   apply urine restraining devices
      d.   measure urine volume and specific gravity
5.   nutrition, alteration in: less than body requirements, related to NPO status and diarrheal loss
6.   The skin exhibits no evidence of discoloration or irritation.
7.   The blood pressure is monitored to prevent or monitor a complication of dehydration, shock. It happens because losses of electrolytes and water occur as a result of diarrhea. These losses cause dehydration, and if the losses are severe, vascular volume is lost, leading to shock.
8.   a.   provide pacifier
      b.   bubble child
      c.   hold infant frequently
      d.   touch, talk, and otherwise provide comfort if the child is unable to be held
      e.   provide sensory stimulation
      f.   encourage family members to visit and allow them to comfort and care for child
9.   You will ask Leah's mother questions which would indicate her understanding of the instructions.

Section IV B

1.   a.   provide fluids
      b.   assess adequacy of intake
2.   a.   give small frequent feedings
      b.   bubble before and frequently during feedings
      c.   position in high Fowler's and slightly on right side after feedings
      d.   handle minimally and gently after feedings.
3.   This position facilitates the passage of formula through the pylorus and prevents vomiting from occurring.
4.   anxiety, related to separation from accustomed routine and environment
5.   You would have the parents demonstrate the infant's care in the hospital to see whether they provide optimum care.
6.   The rationale or reason behind these actions is to monitor the patient for signs of shock. Shock occurs in such patients as a result of electrolyte and water losses from vomiting, leading to dehydration. If vascular volume is compromised shock may occur.

Section IV C

1.   Tina's age, her use of tampons, and the presence of her menstrual period aid in the diagnosis. The presence of the high fever, hypotension, and red macular rash are also used.
2.   a.   monitor the intravenous infusion
      b.   monitor intake and output
      c.   monitor vital signs
      d.   monitor blood gases and hematocrit
      e.   support Tina and her parents
3.   It has been shown that the Trendelenberg position is not effective in shock patients, and that elevating the lower extremities decreases pooling in the extremities, thereby returning blood supply to the heart.
4.   a.   to modify her use of tampons (i.e., to use them intermittently)
      b.   not to use super absorbent tampons
      c.   not to leave any tampons in body for more than 12 hours
      d.   general hygiene measures
      e.   signs of toxic shock syndrome
5.   They occur because of a previous sensitization to an allergen. This sets up a generalized reaction leading to the signs Tina exhibited.
6.   The most important drug is epinephrine.
7.   The nurse could have asked Tina and her parents if she is allergic to any drugs or foods.

Section IV D

1. a. implement care
   b. obtain baseline information
   c. obtain history of burn injury
   d. prevent eye damage
   e. prevent respiratory failure
   f. prevent fluid overload
   g. prevent circulatory impairment
   h. assess cardiac function
   i. assess renal function
   j. prevent heat loss
2. Interventions to prevent fluid overload include:
   a. monitoring vital signs frequently
   b. observing for signs of overhydration
   c. being alert for altered behavior or sensorium
3. You determine the normal output for a child of your patient's age, then compare the normal output to your patient's output.
4. Infection is a leading cause of death in the patient with thermal injury and is a serious complication. Adhering to sterile technique lessens the chance of infection.
5. Nutrition, alteration in: less than body requirements related to loss of appetite.
6. a. perform range of motion exercises
   b. encourage mobility
   c. ambulate as soon as possible
   d. encourage and promote self-help activities
7. Constipation is a frequent complication of immobility. Because the patient is probably on bed rest, it is important to monitor bowel function to prevent the bowel from getting impacted.
8. Interventions that could be used are:
   a. convey a positive attitude to the child
   b. encourage parents to visit
   c. encourage as much independence as the condition allows
   d. arrange for continued schooling
   e. promote peer contact
9. The family demonstrates an understanding of the needs of the child (diet, rest, and activity), demonstrates the wound care, and sets realistic goals.
10. Shock is a common occurrence in the burn patient due to a loss of intracellular fluid leading to losses of vascular volume. These interventions are designed to prevent shock or to catch the occurrence of shock early.

Chapter 30

QUESTION	ANSWER

Section III

1. F
2. sodium
3. vomiting; poor feeding; failure to gain weight; frequent urination; pallor; fever; persistent diaper rash; dehydration; enlarged kidney or bladder
4. d
5. creatinine
6. urinary stasis
7. obstruction; constipation; pregnancy; catheters; antimicrobial administration; tight clothing and diapers; poor hygiene; local inflammation
8. F
9. a. eliminate infection
   b. detect and correct functional or anatomic abnormalities
   c. prevent recurrence
10. b.
11. c.
12. Corticosteroids

13.   a
14.   Cytoxan
15.   T
16.   b; b; a; b; a
17.   a.   hypertensive encephalopathy
       b.   cardiac decompensation
       c.   acute renal failure
18.   a.   history of a sore throat and/or skin infection
       b.   urine analysis
       c.   ASO titer
       d.   elevated AHase and ADNase-B titers
       e.   decreased serum complement levels
19.   F
20.   b
21.   proximal tubules; glomeruli
22.   b
            d
            c
            a
23.   the inability of the distal tubules and collecting duct to be sensitive to the actions of vasopressin.
24.   a.   vomiting
       b.   failure to thrive
       c.   dehydration
       d.   hypernatremia
       e.   copious output of dilute urine
25.   d
26.   T
27.   Hemolytic uremic syndrome
28.   the lining of the small glomerular arterioles
29.   a.   anorexia
       b.   pallor
       c.   bruising
       d.   rectal bleeding
       e.   anuria
       f.   anemia
       g.   hypertension
       h.   thrombocytopenia
30.   the damage to the red blood cells in the arterioles and the subsequent hemolysis
31.   c
32.   T
33.   oliguria
34.   F
35.   treating the underlying cause, management of the complications of renal failure, and provision of supportive therapy
36.   decrease serum potassium
37.   a.   renal hypoplasia
       b.   vesicoureteral reflux
       c.   chronic glomerulonephritis
       d.   Alport's syndrome
       e.   polycystic kidney disease
       f.   chronic pyelonephritis
38.   a.   retention of waste products
       b.   water and sodium retention
       c.   acidosis
       d.   calcium and phosphorus imbalance
       e.   hyperkalemia
       f.   anemia
       g.   growth disturbances
       h.   renal osteodystrophy
39.   F
40.   correcting calcium and phosphorus imbalance and the administration of supplemental calcium and vitamin D

Section IV A

1.
   a.   fever
   b.   frequent urination
   c.   poor feeding
   d.   failure to gain weight
   e.   dehydration
2.   The incidence of UTI in males is greater in infancy. This is usually the result of some sort of obstruction which results in urinary stasis. Also, the presence of a large or greater than normal output is suggestive of obstructive uropathy.
3.   prevention
4.
   a.   injury: potential for, related to presence of infected organism and anatomic abnormality
   b.   family process, alterations in, related to situational crisis
5.
   a.   collect of specimen
   b.   prepare Barry's parents for diagnostic procedures
   c.   administer antimicrobials as ordered
   d.   monitor vital signs
   e.   monitor urine output
   f.   teach Barry's parents how to prevent recurrences
   g.   teach Barry's parents how to perform his home care
6.   You would observe Barry's parents caring for him to see if they are putting the diaper on too tight and if they are cleaning his genitals well.

Section IV B

1.   fluid volume, alteration in: deficit related to protein loss and fluid excess
2.   Prevent and control acute infection.
3.
   a.   offer high protein, high carbohydrate diet
   b.   enlist the aid of the child and parents in formulation of diet
   c.   provide a cheerful, relaxed environment
   d.   provide special and preferred foods
   e.   serve foods in an attractive manner
4.   The presence of edema may predispose the child to skin breakdown and may make routine care more difficult. Also, because of low protein levels, the child is predisposed to infection and breakdown.
5.
   a.   maintaining bed rest
   b.   balance rest and activity
   c.   plan and provide quiet activities
   d.   instruct the child to rest when fatigued
.   Teach the family urine testing, administration of medications, signs of relapse, side effects of drugs, and prevention of infection.
.   The parents are able to test the urine and administer the medications correctly. They understand your instructions concerning prevention of infection, signs of relapse, and side effects of drugs.

Section IV C

.   The nurse should have instructed Tina's mother to continue the antibiotics for the total prescribed time, even if Tina should feel better.
   a.   visual disturbances
   b.   vomiting; motor disturbances
   c.   seizure activity
   d.   changes in behavior
         prevent fluid accumulation
   a.   encourage her parents to visit
   b.   spend time with the child
   c.   provide an opportunity to socialize with noninfected children
   d.   provide appropriate play activities
   a.   monitor fluid balance
   b.   weigh child daily
   c.   measure intake and output
   d.   measure specific gravity of urine
   e.   observe for signs of dehydration and overload
   f.   monitor vital signs
         Protein is restricted in children with acute renal failure to prevent the accumulation of nitrogenous wastes.

7.   The family members demonstrate an understanding of the information presented, and express their feelings and concerns.

Section IV D

1.   recognizing the possibility of RTA in Brad, referring him for medical supervision, and teaching his parents the importance of administration of citrate solution.
2.   a.   monitoring intake and output
      b.   monitoring vital signs
      c.   monitoring urine pH
      d.   administering of medication
      e.   monitoring Brad for signs of dehydration
3.   Brad will need to take the citrate solution on a long-term basis, because the tubular disease is usually permanent.

Section IV E

1.   She probably exhibited anemia, rectal bleeding, anorexia, bruising, hypertension, elevated serum creatinine levels, thrombocytopenia, and anuria.
2.   potential for infection related to diminished body defenses
3.   a.   promote self-care
      b.   determine the extent of disturbance
      c.   improve self-concept
4.   a.   assess home situation
      b.   teach the family home care
      c.   help family acquire needed drugs and equipment
      d.   assist family in problem solving
      e.   assist family in diet planning
      f.   prepare the child and family for home peritoneal dialysis
      g.   maintain periodic contact
5.   The kidney has a role in the activation of vitamin D. Vitamin D aids in the reabsorption of calcium. Failure to administer vitamin D may result in the development of renal osteodystrophy.
6.   a.   monitor fluid intake
      b.   provide low sodium diet
      c.   administer diuretics
      d.   administer antihypertensive medications
7.   Betsy would:
      a.   engage in activities appropriate for her age
      b.   discuss her feelings and concerns
      c.   comply with medication, diet and dialysis regimen

Chapter 31

QUESTION   **ANSWER**
Section III

1.   T
2.   a.   a smaller respiratory tract
      b.   a chest whose shape is different; round
      c.   abdominal respirations
      d.   little smooth muscle in the airways
      e.   a rib cage that is more compact
      f.   a diaphragm that is stretched, so it is unable to contract as far or as forcefully
      g.   less alveolar surface area for exchange
3.   increased
4.   of the presence of cartilaginous tissue limiting constriction
5.   b
6.   a.   rate
      b.   rhythm
      c.   symmetry
      d.   amplitude
      e.   effort
      f.   use of accessory muscles

	g.	alterations, such as pain, color, wheezing, retractions, rhonchi, rales, cough
7.		F
8.		c
9.	a.	type
	b.	progress
	c.	pattern
	d.	associated symptoms
	e.	presence of secretions
0.		T
1.		d
2.		to obtain lung aspirate for histologic study
3.		on the concentration needed and the ability of the child to cooperate
4.		T
5.		excessive fluid or mucus in the bronchi is not removed by normal ciliary activity and cough
6.		b
		c
		c
		a
7.	a.	develop more effective diaphragmatic breathing
	b.	relax all muscles
	c.	attain a good easy posture
8.		T
9.		a preset pressure in the delivery of gas
0.		suctioning, positioning, and providing support for the child
1.	a.	mechanical obstruction of the upper airways
	b.	disease of the CNS
	c.	neuromuscular disease
	d.	secretional obstruction
	e.	conditions such as smoke inhalation
	f.	prophylaxis for radical neck or head injury
2.		F
3.		F
4.		The cardinal signs are restlessness, tachypnea, tachycardia, and diaphoresis. The early signs are mood changes, headache, altered pattern of respiration, anorexia, increased cardiac and renal output, CNS symptoms, flaring nares, retractions, expiratory grunts, and wheezing. The severe signs are hypotension, dimness of vision, stupor, coma, dyspnea, depressed respirations, bradycardia, and cyanosis.

Section IV A

a.	rate
b.	regularity of respirations
c.	depth of respiration
d.	presence of retractions
e.	color
f.	type of sounds heard in the chest
g.	presence of pain in the older child
h.	clubbing
i.	cough
j.	nasal flaring
a.	recognize the signs which indicate the need to monitor blood gas, including changes in color, depth, and rate of respirations
b.	transport the specimen quickly
	Cold air may trigger the diving reflex, leading to bradycardia and shunting of blood from the peripheral to central circulation.
a.	allow Meghan to see that there is always someone nearby
b.	allow her to have a favorite toy inside the tent
c.	if she is well enough, remove Meghan from the tent for feeding and bathing
d.	reassure her that she will not be left alone
	Infants are abdominal breathers, and a tight diaper may hamper respiration.
a.	open the tent as little as possible
b.	check to see that the tent is tucked in securely
c.	check to see that the temperature is correct

    d.   monitor the oxygen concentration
    e.   check to see that Meghan is warm and dry
7.   This minimizes the chance of vomiting.
8.   You would auscultate the chest prior to treatment, then after treatment to hear whether the chest sounds clearer.

Section IV B

1.   Ramon probably had severe retractions, nasal flaring, cyanosis, dyspnea, tachypnea, tachycardia, and adventitious sounds such as a wheeze or rhonchi.
2.   The bronchoscopy was performed to see where the bronchi were obstructed.
3.   a.   change the dressing around the stoma three times daily
      b.   maintain aseptic technique
      c.   suction frequently
      d.   keep an extra tracheostomy set at the bedside
      e.   check patency of tube frequently by auscultating the chest
      f.   monitor the child for problems such as pallor, cyanosis, changes in pulse and/or blood pressure, and bleeding around the site.
4.   You would assess Ramon for the presence of noisy breathing, bubbling, or coughing.
5.   This is done to loosen secretions and crusts to facilitate aspiration.
6.   a.   assure adequate hydration
      b.   provide adequate nutrition
      c.   provide support to the child and parents
7.   Ramon should have been placed over the rescuer's arm with the head lower than his trunk, then placed supine while four chest thrusts were applied in rapid succession.

Chapter 32

QUESTION		ANSWER

Section III

1.   Respiratory failure
2.   a.   nature of the agent
      b.   age of the child
      c.   resistance of natural defenses
3.   viruses
4.   lack of specific antibodies against common viral pathogens for the first year of life
5.   a.   The diameter of the respiratory tract is smaller and therefore subject to narrowing from edematous mucous membranes and from increased production of secretions.
      b.   The distance between structures within the tract is anatomically shorter; therefore, organisms move more rapidly down the respiratory tract for more extensive involvement.
      c.   The short and open eustachian tube in infants and young children allows pathogens easy access to the middle ear.
6.   a.   T
      b.   T
      c.   F
      d.   T
      e.   F
      f.   T
      g.   F
      h.   T
      i.   F
      j.   F
7.   Saline nose drops
8.   The moisture soothes inflamed membranes and assists in liquefying secretions.
9.   using a hot shower for a few minutes
10.   symptomatic
11.   Depression of the cough reflex may increase the risk of aspiration.
12.   Antihistamines; stimulate
13.   Group A hemolytic streptococcus.
14.   a.   *Viral*
              gradual onset
              low-grade fever

        headache, rhinitis, cough, and hoarseness occur after 1 or 2 days of fever

        slight erythema of pharynx and enlargement of tonsils

        firm, tender cervical lymph nodes may be present

        moderately ill

b. *Bacterial*

        abrupt onset

        increased fever to 104°

        headache, severe sore throat and abdominal pain more common

        white exudate on tonsils, erythema and enlargement of tonsils

        localized firm, tender cervical lymph nodes are common

        acutely ill

5.   throat culture

6.   oral penicillin G for at least 10 days

7.   erythromycin

8.   few hours after initiation of penicillin therapy

9.   to filter and protect the respiratory and the alimentary tracts from invasion by pathogenic organisms

0.   palatine tonsils

1.   adenoids

2.   inflammation; swallowing; breathing

3. a. blockage of the eustachian tube which interferes with normal drainage and frequently results in otitis media and difficulty in hearing

4. a. a child has massive hypertrophy that results in difficulty eating or extreme discomfort when breathing

    b. a child has recurrent otitis media, especially when associated with hearing loss and in those children where hypertrophied adenoids obstruct nasal breathing

5. a. blood loss may be excessive

    b. possibility of regrowth or hypertrophy of lymphoid tissue

6.   hemorrhage

7. a. an inflammation of the middle ear without reference to etiology or pathogenesis

    b. a rapid and short onset of signs and symptoms lasting approximately 3 weeks

    c. an inflammation of the middle ear in which a collection of fluid is present in the middle ear space

    d. middle ear effusion lasting from 3 weeks to 3 months

    e. middle ear effusion that persists beyond 3 months

       Streptococcus pneumoniae; Hemophilus influenzae; Staphylococcus aureus

       blocked eustachian tubes

 a. The eustachian tubes are short, wide. and straight, and lie in a relatively horizontal plane.

    b. The cartilage lining is undeveloped, making the tubes more distensible and therefore more likely to open inappropriately.

    c. The normally abundant pharyngeal lymphoid tissue readily obstructs the eustachian tube openings in the nasopharynx.

    d. Immature humoral defense mechanisms increase the risk of infection.

    e. The usual lying-down position of infants favors the pooling of fluid, such as formula, in the pharyngeal cavity.

       hearing loss

       intact membrane that appears bright red and bulging, with no visible landmarks or light reflex

       amoxicillin; ampicillin

       hearing impairment

       Tympanostomy tubes

       the primary anatomic area affected

       laryngeal obstruction

       airway; adequate respiratory exchange

       to liquefy respiratory secretions and decrease edema of the respiratory tract

       an obstructive inflammatory process

       cherry-red edematous

       it could precipitate a complete obstruction

       Respiratory syncytial virus (RSV)

       a narrowing of the respiratory passages on expiration, which prevents the air from leaving the lungs

       there are repeated attacks; there is a family history of asthma; the child responds favorably to an administration of epinephrine

       viruses, bacteria, mycoplasmas; pneumonia associated with aspiration of foreign substances

       the clinical history, the child's age, the child's general health history, the physical examination, radiography, and the laboratory examination

       whooping cough; *Bordetella pertussis*

       Mycobacterium tuberculosis

50.   physical examination; history; reaction to tuberculin tests; radiographic examinations

51.   chemotherapy

52. a.   Isoniazid (INH)

      b.   Rifampin (RMP)

      c.   Ethambutol (EMB)

53.   avoid contact; Bacillus Calmette-Guerin

54.   they are naturally curious and tend to put everything into their mouths

55.   choking, gagging, wheezing, or cough

56.   laryngoscopy; bronchoscopy

57.   back blows; Heimlich maneuver

58.   cannot speak; becomes cyanotic; collapses

59.   secondary bacterial infection

60.   pneumonitis

61.   because of the renewed danger of aspiration

62.   prevention of aspiration

63. a.   heat

      b.   local chemical

      c.   systemic

64.   Carbon dioxide

65.   100% oxygen

66.   Passive smoking

67.   allergens

68.   skin testing

69. a.   desensitization injections

      b.   antihistamines

      c.   alpha-adrenergic decongestants

70.   a reversible process that is characterized by variations in central and/or peripheral airway obstruction over short period of time, with a decrease in the degree of airway obstruction demonstrated clinically and physiologically as a direct response to bronchodilator drugs

71.   allergic hypersensitivity to foreign substances.

72. a.   edema of mucous membranes

      b.   accumulation of tenacious secretions from mucous glands

      c.   spasm of the smooth muscle of the bronchi and bronchioles, which decreases the caliber of the bronchioles

73.   Gas trapping; higher and higher lung volume

74.   infection resulting from diminished efficiency of defenses and mucous growth media; atelectasis; emphysema; pneumothorax; collapsed lung; status asthmaticus; cor pulmonale; misuse of medications; emotional and behavior problems

75.   large numbers of eosinophils; Charcot-Leyden crystals.

76.   prevent disability; minimize physical and psychologic morbidity

77.   Allergen

78.   control the acute attack; maximum

79.   Rapid-acting bronchodilators

80. a.   beta-adrenergics

      b.   methylxanthines

81.   methylxanthine

82.   It has been found that moderate exercise or even strenuous exercise is advantageous for children with asthma.

83. a.   chest physical therapy

      b.   breathing exercises

      c.   physical training

      d.   inhalation therapy

84.   theophylline; Serum levels

85.   children who continue to display respiratory distress despite vigorous therapeutic measures

86.   The side effects are tachycardia, elevated blood pressure, pallor, weakness, tremors, and nausea.

87.   fever, restlessness, nausea, vomiting, hypotension, abdominal discomfort that may progress to convulsions and coma

88.   rejection; overprotection

89.   generalized dysfunction of the exocrine glands

90.   autosomal-recessive trait

91.   mechanical obstruction caused by the increased viscosity of mucous gland secretions

92.   Pulmonary complications

93.   Because essential pancreatic enzymes are unable to reach the duodenum, digestion and absorption of nutrients, particularly fats, proteins, and to a lesser degree, carbohydrates, are markedly impaired

94.   steatorrhea; azotorrhea

95.   meconium ileus

96.   large, frothy, and extremely foul smelling
97. a.   history of the disease in the family
     b.   absence of pancreatic enzymes
     c.   increase in electrolyte concentration of sweat
     d.   chronic pulmonary involvement
98.   sweat test
99.   higher in calories and protein
00.   pancrease
01.   prevention and treatment of pulmonary infection by improving aeration, removing mucopurulent secretions, and administering antimicrobial agents
02. a.   chest physiotherapy
     b.   breathing exercises
     c.   humidification of air
03.   pulmonary involvement

Section IV

  a.   potential for secondary infection related to hospital environment
  b.   potential for airway obstruction related to the inflammatory process
  c.   alteration in body temperature related to the inflammatory process
  d.   potential fluid volume deficit related to increased metabolic rate, insensible fluid loss, and anorexia
  e.   alteration in nutrition related to difficulty swallowing and loss of appetite
  f.   ineffective breathing pattern due to infective process
  g.   potential for activity intolerance related to imbalance between oxygen supply and demand
  h.   fear of separation related to hospitalization
  i.   alteration in family process related to hospitalization of child

Section IV B

  a.   take pulse and respiration frequently; assess skin color; be alert for signs of covert bleeding; inspect throat for signs of oozing, inspect any vomitus for evidence of fresh bleeding
  b.   discourage child from coughing frequently or clearing her throat; avoid use of gargles or hard objects in the mouth.
      no evidence of bleeding
      cool water, popsicles, dilute fruit juices, jello (Avoid fluids with red or brown color.)

Section IV C

    child would be irritable and pull on her ears or roll her head from side to side; she may have a fever of as much as 104°F; lymph glands may be enlarged; rhinorrhea, vomiting and diarrhea, signs of respiratory or pharyngeal infection, and anorexia may be present
    maintain regularity of administration of antibiotic and continue therapy for at least 10 days

Section IV D

    monitor respirations; auscultate lungs; observe color of skin and mucous membranes; observe for presence of hoarseness, stridor, and cough; monitor heart rate and regularity; observe behavior
  a.   assess respiratory status and detect any impending airway obstruction
  b.   ease respiratory efforts
  c.   prevent dehydration
  d.   be prepared to assist with tracheostomy
  e.   provide nutrition
  f.   reduce parental anxiety
    to liquefy respiratory secretions and decrease the edema of the respiratory tract

Section IV E

    Respiratory syncytial virus (RS) accounts for largest percentage
    Mycoplasma pneumoniae
    Pneumococcus, Streptococcus, Staphylococcus
    Mild fever, slight cough, and prostration. Whitish sputum.
    Fever, chills, headache, malaise, anorexia, myalgia, rhinitis, sore throat, dry hacking cough; mucopurulent or blood-streaked sputum
    Pneum.—Follows URI, poor feeding, fever, pleurisy pain; Strep.—Tachypnea, chills, similar to pneumococcus.
    Staph.—Fever, lethargy, anorexia, retractions, cyanosis
    Symptomatic

8.   Symptomatic
9.   Antimicrobial therapy directed at causative organism

Section IV F

1.   a.   Never leave various forms of hydrocarbons accessible to children.
     b.   Refrain from use of talcum powder with infants.
     c.   Refrain from using oily nose drops and oil-based vitamin preparations.
     d.   Position infants and debilitated children on the right side or the abdomen after feedings.

Section IV G

1.   the history of eczema as a baby; maternal history of hay fever; paternal history of asthma during childhood
2.   hacking, nonproductive cough, shortness of breath
3.   productive cough; audible wheezing upon expiration; restlessness and apprehension; sweating; use of accessory muscles; rapid respirations; upright position with hunched shoulders
4.   a.   relief of bronchospasm
     b.   tachycardia, increased blood pressure, pallor, weakness, tremors, and nausea
5.   skin color for cyanosis; character of respirations; presence of retractions; nasal flaring; breath sounds; and mental status.

Section IV H

1.   a.   to remove the stigma of self-fault for the condition
     b.   to integrate the reality of asthma into the life style of the individual's choice
     c.   to learn management skills to avoid or minimize conditions which cause asthma attacks

Section IV I

1.   a.   potential for infection related to impaired body defenses
     b.   alteration in nutrition related to inability to digest nutrients
     c.   activity intolerance related to decreased oxygen
     d.   ineffective airway clearance related to secretion of thick tenacious mucus
     e.   ineffective breathing pattern related to tracheobronchial obstruction
     f.   sleep pattern disturbance related to frequent coughing and ineffective breathing
     g.   disturbance in self-concept related to body image
     h.   alteration in family process related to situational crisis
     i.   anticipatory grieving related to perceived potential loss of child
     j.   impaired social interaction related to hospitalization
2.   Dennis manages secretions with minimum distress.
3.   a.   obstruction of bronchioles and bronchi with abnormally thick mucus
     b.   lack of trypsin, amylase, and lipase causes large amounts of undigested food which are excreted
     c.   because so little food is absorbed from intestine, the child tries to compensate
     d.   appetite can't compensate for fecal wastage
     e.   inability to absorb fat-soluble vitamins
4.   a.   postural drainage technique
     b.   breathing exercises

Chapter 33

QUESTION   **ANSWER**

Section III

1.   a.   processes and absorbs nutrients necessary to maintain metabolic processes and to support growth and development
     b.   performs an excretory function for both digestive residue and other waste products
     c.   provides detoxification while other routes of elimination (kidneys, liver, skin) are still immature
     d.   participates in maintaining fluid and electrolyte balance in infancy
2.   rapidity
3.   Peristalsis
4.   the catabolism of foodstuffs from their original complex form to simple, assimilable nutrients
5.   small intestine
6.   a.   lower GI series
     b.   upper GI series
7.   the habitual, purposeful, and compulsive ingestion of nonfood substances in the environment

. esophagus
. Malabsorption syndrome
. intestinal mucosal transport system
. gluten
. fat absorption (soaps and fatty acids)
. protein, carbohydrates, calcium, iron, folic acid, and vitamins
. failure to gain weight, anorexia, steatorrhea, diarrhea, constipation, vomiting, abdominal pain, and behavioral changes such as irritability, uncooperativeness, or apathy
. celiac crisis
. colicky abdominal pain, nausea, vomiting, abdominal distention, and constipation
. vomiting; constipation
. an abdomen that is rigid and boardlike, with moderate to severe tenderness; bowel sounds that gradually diminish and cease; respiratory distress that occurs as the diaphragm is pushed up into the pleural cavity
. an invagination or telescoping of one portion of the intestine into another
. red, currant-jelly-like
. barium enema

a. obstipation
b. encopresis
c. constipation

Environmental change
autonomic parasympathetic ganglion cells
absence of propulsive movement (peristalsis)
rectal biopsy
surgical correction
vomiting, weight loss, respiratory problems, and bleeding
barium esophagram
outpouching of the ileum
omphalomesenteric; vitelline duct fails to completely obliterate
the diverticulum contains gastric mucosa, which produces hydrochloric acid, which irritates the bowel and erodes the intestinal surface
Rectal bleeding
history
surgery
delay in treatment

a. colicky abdominal pain
b. abdominal tenderness
c. fever
d. decreased peristalsis

McBurney's point; anterior superior iliac crest and the umbilicus
sudden pain at the point of tenderness elicited by pressing firmly over a part of the abdomen distal to the area of tenderness

a. chronic abdominal pain especially when stomach is empty
b. recurrent vomiting after meals
c. chronic anemia with occult blood in the stools
d. vague G.I. complaints with a positive family history of peptic ulcer

a. potential for injury related to susceptibility to gastric hypersecretion
b. alteration in comfort related to pain
c. potential knowledge deficit related to unfamiliarity with resources
d. alteration in family process related to illness and/or hospitalization of child

a. Hepatitis A virus (HAV)
b. Hepatitis B virus (HBV)
c. Hepatitis D virus (HDV)
d. Non-A, non-B virus (NANBV)

a. 15 to 40 days
b. 6 weeks to 6 months
c. unknown
d. variable
e. oral, fecal
f. parenteral
g. parenteral
h. oral-, venereal-, saliva-fetal transfer

    i.   usually rapid
    j.   more insidious
    k.   present after one attack, no cross-over to Type B
    l.   present after one attack, no cross-over to Type A
    m.   none
    n.   yes

44.   a.   hepatitis B surface antigen
      b.   antibody to hepatitis B surface antigen
      c.   hepatitis B core antigen
      d.   antibody to core antigen
      e.   E antigen which is closely associated with the HBV infection
      f.   antibody to the E antigen

45.   T, F, F, T, T

Section IV A

1.   prevention of foreign body ingestion through preventive family teaching
2.   esophagus

Section IV B

1.   a.   explaining why she must be NPO for 4 to 8 hours prior to the procedure
      b.   explaining why a tube is passed through the mouth
      c.   supporting Patricia during the test
2.   foods containing wheat, rye, barley and oats; cereal; baked goods; processed foods containing hydrolyzed vegetable protein

Section IV C

1.   a.   (1) Explain diagnosis; (2) encourage parents to room-in; (3) explain procedures and equipment; and (4) support parents through this sudden emergency.
      b.   (1) Explain and demonstrate why this is being performed; (2) assure the parents that you will accompany Jason to x-ray and support the child through the procedure.
      c.   (1) Prepare infant and parents as for all surgeries; (2) ask parents to assist you in monitoring all stools prior to surgery to report a normal brown stool, (3) instruct parents in postoperative care; (4) explain to parents that Jason might be kept in hospital for 2 to 3 days for observation.
2.   a small stomach capacity with rapid transit time

Section IV D

1.   a.   accurate history of bowel habits
      b.   diet and events that may be associated with the onset of constipation
      c.   consistency, color, frequency, and other characteristics of the stool
2.   milk and milk products, apples, apple juice, carrots, bananas, juice, and jello

Section IV E

1.   a.   listen carefully to the history given by the parents
      b.   inquire particularly about history of stools
2.   a.   creation of temporary colostomy
      b.   surgical correction—''pulling through''
      c.   closure of colostomy
3.   a.   to empty the bowel
      b.   to prevent abdominal distention
      c.   to decrease bacterial flora in intestine
      d.   to detect discrepancies
      e.   to allow for escape of accumulated fluid and gas
      f.   to prevent damage to mucosa
4.   a.   keep NPO until bowel sounds return and colostomy and/or anastomosed bowel are ready for feedings
      b.   monitor IV therapy
      c.   change abdominal dressing prn
      d.   monitor nasogastric suctioning
      e.   change perineal dressing prn

Section IV F

. Position infant in prone position with 30 degree angle for 24 hours/day. Maintain position with a body harness.
. Reassuring them of benign nature of gastroesophageal reflux and its relationship to physiologic maturity.

Section IV G

. perforation of the appendix
. assist in establishing a medical diagnosis
. degree of change in his behavior
. a. listen for return of bowel sounds
  b. observe for passage of stool

Section IV H

. chronic inflammatory reaction involving mucosa and submucosa of large intestine; mucosa becomes hyperemic and edematous with formation of patchy granulations over intestinal surface that bleed easily and lead to development of superficial ulcerations
. affects the terminal ileum and involves all layers of bowel wall; acute edema and inflammation progress to deep ulcerations often associated with fissure formations leading to obstruction

  a. common
  b. often severe
  c. less frequent
  d. mild to moderate
  e. moderate
  f. usually mild
  a. uncommon
  b. moderate to absent
  c. common
  d. can be severe
  e. severe
  f. often marked

Section IV I

  a. severity of hepatitis
  b. rigidity of medical regime.
  c. factors influencing control and transmission of the disease
  a. providing small frequent snacks rather than large meals
  b. developing a realistic activity schedule with parents
  c. encouraging child to take frequent tepid baths
  d. observing for behavioral changes
  e. instructing parents not to administer any medications to Samuel without physician's knowledge

Chapter 34

QUESTION	ANSWER

Section III

. the sinoatrial node, the atrioventricular node, the atrioventricular bundle, and the Purkinje fibers
  a. oxygen saturation of the blood within the chambers and great vessels
  b. pressure changes within these structures
  c. changes in cardiac output and stroke volume
  d. anatomic abnormalities such as septal defects or obstruction to flow
      a
      foramen ovale; ductus arteriosus
      F
      acyanotic; cyanotic
      left; right
      right; left
  a. a
  b. b

c. a, g
d. c
e. e
f. d.
g. b
h. g
i. f
j. d

10.   ventricular septal defect; atrial septal defect; patent ductus arteriosus; coarctation of aorta; pulmonic stenosis; aortic stenosis

11.   the inability of the heart to pump an adequate amount of blood to the systemic circulation to meet the body's metabolic demands

12.   increased blood volume and pressure

13. a. right-sided failure
     b. left-sided failure

14.   sympathetic nervous system; renal system

15.   tachycardia

16.   dyspnea; retractions; tachypnea; orthopnea; cyanosis

17.   hepatomegaly; edema; weight gain

18. a. improve cardiac function
     b. remove accumulated fluid and sodium
     c. decrease cardiac demands
     d. improve tissue oxygenation

19. a. allow a period of grief
     b. assess the level of understanding
     c. help the family cope with the effects of the defect
     d. foster growth-promoting family relationships

20. a. ventricular septal defect
     b. pulmonary stenosis
     c. overriding aorta
     d. right ventricular hypertrophy

21.   mitral valve

22.   group A streptococcal

23.   Jones; streptococcal; ASO

24.   blood pressure

25.   Surgery; hypertensive drug

26.   Kawasaki disease; cardiovascular

27.   temperature

28.   aspirin

Section IV A

1. a. The groin is cleansed with an antiseptic solution.
    b. A local anesthetic is injected into the site of entry.
    c. A catheter is inserted into a blood vessel, usually one in the groin.
    d. Dye is injected into the cardiac catheter.
    e. The room is dimmed for viewing the angiograph screens.

2. a. This detects rate and rhythm irregularities caused by introduction and placement of the catheter into the heart.
    b. In infants, it is done to monitor the potential loss of heat through conduction and convection; in all patients, it is done to monitor the effects of the injected dye.

Section IV B

1. a. level of understanding, especially cognitive skills
    b. past experiences
    c. understanding and perception of the situation

2. a. provide physical preparation
    b. provide psychologic preparation (explanation)

3. a. detects abnormalities in rate and rhythm
    b. detects cardiac hemorrhage from perforation or bleeding at the site of the initial catheterization
    c. detects vessel obstruction
    d. detects possible vessel obstruction

e.   detects evidence of bleeding or hematoma formation

4.   a.   whether she is fully reactive

       b.   whether she is experiencing nausea

5.   The child is usually kept in bed for 8 hours after the procedure.

Section IV C

1.   a.   C

       b.   X

       c.   C

       d.   C

       e.   C

       f.   X

       g.   C

       h.   C

       i.   X

       j.   C

2.   a.   maternal rubella; poor nutrition; diabetes; maternal age over 40 years

       b.   increased risk of congenital heart disease in a child who (1) has a sibling with a heart defect, (2) has a parent with congenital heart disease, (3) has a chromosomal aberration, (4) is born with other noncardiac congenital anomalies

3.   a.   a loud, harsh, pansystolic murmur

       b.   signs and symptoms of congestive heart failure (poor feeding, diaphoresis, tachypnea, tachycardia)

4.   a.   congestive heart failure

       b.   endocarditis

       c.   aortic insufficiency

       d.   pulmonary stenosis

       e.   progressive pulmonary vascular disease

Section IV D

.   a.   improves cardiac functioning by such beneficial effects as increased cardiac output, decreased heart size, decreased venous pressure, and relief of edema

       b.   remove accumulated fluid and sodium

.   a.   count the apical pulse for one full minute before administering digitalis, and withhold dose if pulse is lower than either 90–100 in infants or 70 in older children

       b.   calculate dosage accurately

       c.   use correct preparation of digitalis (use digoxin)

       d.   monitor serum potassium levels

.   a.   If the child vomits within 15 minutes of receiving the digoxin, repeat the dose once.

       b.   If more than 15 minutes have elapsed since the child has vomited, do not give a second dose.

       c.   If more than two consecutive doses have been missed, notify the physician.

       d.   Do not increase or double the dose to compensate for missed doses.

           Low potassium increases the cardiac effects of digitalis.

.   a.   recording of fluid intake and output

       b.   monitoring of body weight

       a.   administer digitalis; observe for signs of digitalis toxicity; institute teaching regarding drug administration at home

       b.   provide for optimal rest periods; conserve child's energy for feeding; minimize child's crying and stress; maintain child's body temperature

       c.   position in semi- to high-Fowler's position; carefully assess child's respiratory status

       d.   provide small, frequent feedings; feed with a nipple that has a hole large enough to permit entry of milk without danger of aspiration

       e.   administer diuretics as ordered; carefully monitor intake and output; monitor body weight

       f.   lessen parents' anxiety through anticipatory guidance; communicate frequently with parents regarding the child's progress; encourage parents to participate in the child's care.

Section IV E

    a.   a, c, i

    b.   a, d

    c.   a, f

    d.   b, e, g

    e.   f, h

Section IV F

1. a. fluid volume deficit, actual, related to increased body temperature
   b. sensory perceptual alterations, visual, related to inflammation of the eyes
   c. alteration in nutrition, less than body requirements, related to inadequate intake
   d. impairment of skin integrity, potential, related to irritation of edematous tissues and denuded skin
   e. alteration in comfort, pain and itching, related to rash
   f. alteration in comfort, related to swelling in cervical region
2. a. perivasculitis of the small blood vessels
   b. coronary artery stenosis
   c. inflammation of the heart and its surrounding tissues
   d. phlebitis of the large veins
   e. coronary artery thrombosis
   f. aneurysm formation
3. a. administer aspirin, teach the family signs of aspirin toxicity, monitor the temperature frequently, promote rest, give tepid sponge baths
   b. encourage fluids, keep accurate intake and output records, take and record daily weight, monitor temperature status, assess skin turgor, monitor urine specific gravity
   c. administer aspirin as ordered, observe for signs of myocarditis and congestive heart failure, monitor vital signs frequently, observe for behavioral changes, teach parents the need for close follow-up care

Chapter 35

QUESTION   **ANSWER**

Section III

1. a. produces cells without specific functions
   b. provides for oxygenation and distribution of nutrients and other chemicals to the cells
   c. collects wastes from the cells
   d. regulates heat
2. plasma; formed elements
3. red bone marrow; lymphatic system; reticuloendothelial system
4. hemocytoblast; red bone marrow
5. a. basophils
   b. normoblast
   c. reticulocyte
   d. mature erythrocyte
6. reticulocyte count
7. tissue oxygenation; hemopoietin
8. transport hemoglobin
9. Granulocytes; agranulocytes
10. neutrophils; basophils; eosinophils
11. Polys
12. Bands
13. monocytes; lymphocytes
14. a. monocytes, lymphocytes
    b. neutrophils, monocytes
    c. eosinophils
    d. neutrophils
    e. basophils, eosinophils
    f. basophils
    g. eosinophils
15. thrombocytes; clot formation
16. serotonin; vasoconstriction
17. a. red blood cell (RBC)
    b. white blood cell (WBC)
    c. hematocrit (Hct)
    d. hemoglobin (Hgb)
    e. differential white blood count
    f. mean corpuscular hemoglobin (MCH)
    g. mean corpuscular hemoglobin concentration (MCHC)

	h.	peripheral smear
	i.	reticulocyte count
	j.	platelet count
8.		history; physical examination
9.		reduction of red cell
0.	a.	Etiology and physiology—the causes of erythrocyte and hemoglobin depletion
	b.	Morphology—the characteristic changes in red cell size, shape, and color
1	a.	blood loss
	b.	increased destruction of RBCs
	c.	impaired or decreased rate of production
2.	a.	macrocytic
	b.	extracorpuscular factor
	c.	intracorpuscular
	d.	normocytic
	e.	microchromic
	f.	hemolysis
	g.	normochromic
	h.	hypochromic
	i.	microcytic
3.	a.	replacement of bone marrow by fibrosis or by neoplastic cells
	b.	depression of marrow activity
	c.	interference with bone marrow activity from other systemic diseases
4.	a.	deficient iron supply
	b.	supplement iron with oral iron and foods high in iron
	c.	gastric mucosa fails to secrete sufficient amounts of intrinsic factor which is essential for absorption of vitamin B.
	d.	administration of vitamin B_{12}
5.	a.	average or mean volume of a single RBC
	b.	mean quantity of hemoglobin in a single RBC
	c.	mean concentration of hemoglobin in a single RBC
	d.	number of RBC/mm³ of blood
	e.	amount of Hgb/100 ml of whole blood
	f.	percentage or volume of packed RBC to whole blood
	g.	percentage of reticulocytes to RBCs
	h.	number of WBC/mm³ of blood
	i.	inspection and quantification of WBC types present in peripheral blood
	j.	cellular fragments which are necessary for clotting to occur
5.		decrease in the oxygen-carrying capacity of the blood
7.	a.	muscle weakness and easy fatigability; pale skin; growth retardation; anorexia
	b.	headache; dizziness and lightheadedness; irritability; slowed thought processes; decreased attention span; apathy and depression
	c.	increased heart rate and cardiac output; possible cardiac failure
3.	a.	determining the cause of the anemia
	b.	fostering appropriate supportive and therapeutic treatments
	c.	decreasing tissue oxygen requirements
.		Iron
.		Children become anemic because they drink milk, a poor source of iron, almost to the exclusion of solid foods.
	a.	serum-iron concentration (SIC)
	b.	total iron-binding capacity (TIBC)
.		nausea, gastric irritation, diarrhea or constipation; anorexia
.		prevention of nutritional anemia through education of parents
.		tarry green color
	a.	sickle cell trait—the heterozygous form of the disease (HbA + HbS, or HbSA)
	b.	sickle cell anemia—the homozygous form of the disease (HbSS)
	c.	sickle cell hemoglobin C disease—a variant of sickle cell anemia including HbS and HbC
	d.	Sickle cell and HbE disease—a variant of sickle cell anemia in which glutamic acid has been substituted for lysine in the number 26 position of the beta chain
.		sickle-shaped
.		oxygenation; hydration
.	a.	increased blood viscosity
	b.	increased red blood cell destruction
.		infection

40.   a.   vaso-occlusive crisis
      b.   splenic sequestration crisis
      c.   aplastic crisis
      d.   hyperhemolytic crisis
41.   Sickeldex
42.   oxygenation; maintenance of hemodilution
43.   no
44.   can depress bone marrow activity and further aggravate anemia
45.   sepsis; sequestration
46.   hemoglobin chain; Cooley anemia; not compatible
47.   red blood cells; anemia; life span; hemosiderin; hemochromatosis
48.   microcytosis; hypochromia; anisocytosis; poikilocytosis; target cells; basophilic stippling of immature erythrocytes
49.   Deferoxamine
50.   a.   Prothrombin activator is formed in response to extrinsic or intrinsic mechanism.
      b.   Prothrombin activator catalyzes the conversion of prothrombin into thrombin.
      c.   Thrombin acts as an enzyme to convert fibrinogen into the fibrin threads that enmesh the red blood cell and plasma to form a clot.
51.   a group of bleeding disorders in which there is a deficiency of one of the factors necessary for coagulation of blood
52.   Classic hemophilia
      a.   factor VIII
      b.   factor IX
53.   X-linked recessive disorder
54.   joint cavities; hemarthrosis
55.   warmth; redness; swelling; severe pain with considerable loss of movement
56.   intracranial hemorrhage
57.   replacement of the missing factor
58.   Cryoprecipitate
59.   Humoral immunity; cell-mediated immunity
60.   complement; B-lymphocyte
61.   G; M; A; D; E
62.   T-lymphocyte
63.   direct contact; intimate sexual contact
64.   perinatal
65.   failure to thrive; interstitial pneumonitis; hepatosplenomegaly; diffuse lymphadenopathy
66.   preventing transmission of the virus
67.   a.   ?HTLV-III virus
      b.   no cure; primarily supportive; prevention and management of the opportunistic infections
      c.   fatal

Section IV A

1.   a.   explaining the significance of each test
      b.   physically being with the child during the procedure
      c.   allowing the child to play with the equipment on a doll and/or participate in the actual procedure.
2a.   1.   the child's level of tolerance for activities of daily living and play
      2.   take vital signs during rest to establish baseline of nonexertion energy expediture
      3.   take vital signs during periods of activity to establish baseline of exertion energy expenditure
2b.   1.   Utilize the baseline observations to decide with which activities the child needs assistance, and how much assistance she needs.
      2.   Allow the child as much control of her environment as possible.
      3.   Schedule activities to occur throughout the day, with planned rest periods.
      4.   Institute diversional activities that avoid boredom but promote rest.
      5.   Choose a roommate who is of an appropriate age, and who also has energy restrictions.
3.   a.   potential for infection related to lowered body defenses
      b.   activity intolerance related to general weakness
      c.   alteration in family process related to hospitalization

Section IV B

1.   a.   avoid strenuous physical activity; avoid emotional stress; avoid environments of low oxygen concentration; avoid known sources of infection

   b.   calculate the child's daily fluid requirements; assess the child's actual fluid consumption; encourage fluids; assess signs of dehydration; teach parents how to assess fluid status; monitor output.
2. a.   ensure an adequate intake
   b.   increase tissue oxygenation
   c.   relieve pain
3. a.   observing for signs of transfusion reaction
   b.   observing for signs of cardiac failure

Section IV C

1.   signs of anemia and chronic hypoxia; unexplained fever; poor feeding; a markedly enlarged spleen, particularly in a child of Mediterranean extraction
2.   to maintain sufficient hemoglobin levels to prevent tissue hypoxia
3.   chills; shaking; fever; pain at needle site and along venous tract; nausea/vomiting; sensation of tightness in chest; red or black urine; headache; flank pain; shock

Section IV D

1.   headache; slurred speech; loss of conciousness; black tarry stools; hematemesis
2. a.   Apply pressure to area of bleeding for 10 to 15 minutes—to allow clot formation.
   b.   Immobilize and elevate area above the level of the heart—to decrease blood flow.
   c.   Apply cold—to promote vasoconstriction.
3. a.   control bleeding
   b.   decrease risk of injury
   c.   prevent crippling effects of joint degeneration

Section IV E

1. a.   Always wash hands after changing diapers.
   b.   Wrap diapers in plastic bag before discarding.
   c.   Wash child's eating utensils in a dishwasher by using hot water and detergent.
   d.   Wash or discard any article soiled with feces or blood.
   e.   Care for bleeding wounds must utilize aseptic technique.
2. a.   potential for infection related to immune deficiency
   b.   potential for deficit in sensory stimulation related to restricted environment
   c.   alteration in family process related to life threatening illness
   d.   anticipatory grieving related to potential loss of child

Chapter 36

QUESTION	ANSWER

Section III

1.   unknown
2. a.   environmental agents
   b.   viruses
   c.   familial/genetic factors
   d.   host factors—chromosome abnormalities, immune deficiencies
3. a.   C
   b.   A
   c.   B
4. a.   the lymphatic system
   b.   the blood-forming organs
   c.   from connective and supportive tissue
   d.   from epithelial tissue
   e.   from glandular tissue
5. a.   biologic characteristics of the tumor
   b.   the involvement of regional lymph nodes
   c.   the presence of metastasis
6.   surgery; chemotherapy; radiotherapy; immunotherapy; bone marrow transplantation
7.   cytotoxic

8.   alkylating agents, antimetabolites, plant alkaloids, antitumor antibiotics, hormones, enzymes, miscellaneous agents

9.   allogenic; autologous; syngeneic

10.   allopurinol

11.   the initial white blood count; the patient's age at diagnosis; the histologic type of the disease; sex

12. a. a low leukocyte count, but a greatly increased count of immature cells or "blasts"

     b. cellular destruction in the bone marrow by infiltration and subsequent competition for metabolic elements

13.   anemia: infection; bleeding tendencies

14.   fever; pallor; fatigue; anorexia; hemorrhage; bone and joint pain

15.   increased intracranial pressure

16.   bone marrow aspiration; biopsy

17.   induction; sanctuary: maintenance

18.   the central nervous system: the testes

19. a. corticosteroids; vincristine; and L-asparaginase, with or without doxorubicin

     b. methotrexate and cranial irradiation, and bilateral testicular irradiation

     c. 6-Mercaptopurine, methotrexate, prednisone, and vincristine

20.   Hodgkin disease originates in the lymphoid system and primarily involves the lymph nodes. It predictably metastasizes to non-nodal or extralymphatic sites, especially the spleen, liver, bone marrow, and lungs. Non-Hodgkin lymphoma in children is strikingly different from Hodgkin disease. This disease is usually diffuse, rather than nodular; the cell type is either undifferentiated or poorly differentiated; dissemination occurs early, more often than in Hodgkin disease, and rapidly.

21. a. lesions limited to one lymph node area or only one additional extralymphatic site

     b. two or more lymph node regions on the same side of the diaphragm or one additional extralymphatic site or organ on the same side of the diaphragm is involved

     c. involved areas include lymph node regions on both sides of the diaphragm, one extralymphatic site, the spleen, or both of the latter two areas

     d. cancer has metastasized diffusely throughout the body to one or more extralymphatic sites with or without involvement of associated lymph nodes

22.   enlargement of lymph nodes; nonproductive cough, abdominal pain, low grade fever, anorexia, nausea, weight loss, night sweats and pruritus

23.   biopsy; Sternberg-Reed

24.   radiation; chemotherapy

25.   brain tumor and neuroblastoma

26.   because their sutures are still open and an increase in the size of the head is not readily detected

27.   CAT scan

28.   extirpation

29.   respiratory infection

30.   infectious process

31.   Mannitol

32.   cerebral edema

33.   gag reflex; suctioning

34.   abdomen

35.   invasiveness

36.   primary site; areas of metastasis

37.   by analyzing the breakdown products that are normally excreted in the urine, namely vanillylmandelic acid (VMA)

38. a. surgery

     b. radiotherapy

     c. chemotherapy

39. a. This tumor develops from embryonic neural crest tissue and may arise anywhere along the craniospinal axis. The majority of tumors arise from the adrenal gland or from the retroperitoneal sympathetic chain.

     b. This is the most frequent intraabdominal tumor of childhood and the most common type of renal cancer.

     c. This is the most common soft tissue sarcoma in children.
        Because striated muscle is found almost anywhere in the body, tumors occur in many sites. The most common sites are the head, neck, and especially the orbit of the eye.

40.   Osteogenic sarcoma; Ewing sarcoma

41. a. arises from bone-forming mesenchyme giving rise to malignant osteoid tissue

     b. arises in the marrow spaces of the bone rather than in osseous tissue

     c. radical surgical amputation followed by intensive chemotherapy

     d. intensive radiation of the involved bone combined with chemotherapy

42.   prosthesis

43.   Wilms tumor

44.   mass

45.		the site of the tumor and the compression of adjacent organs
46.		orbit
47.		congenital; retina
48.		secondary tumors
49.		a whitish glow in the pupil known as the cat's eye reflex or leukokoria
50.		indirect ophthalmoscopy employing scleral indentation
51.		irradiation; enucleation

Section IV

1. The nurse should play a supportive role in helping the family to understand the various therapies, preventing or managing expected side effects or toxicities, and observing for late effects of treatment.
2. fever, pallor, fatigue, anorexia, hemorrhage (usually petechiae), and bone and joint pain
3.
   a. institute protective isolation if ordered
   b. evaluate the child for any potential sites of infection
   c. monitor temperature elevation
   d. administer meticulous skin care, especially in the mouth and perianal regions
   e. prevent skin breakdown by frequent position changes
   f. encourage adequate calorie-protein intake
   g. avoid exertion or fatigue
   h. teach preventive measures at discharge (handwashing)
   i. stress importance of isolating child from any known cases of chickenpox or other childhood communicable diseases
4.
   a. administer antiemetics prior to the onset of nausea and vomiting
   b. administer drugs on an empty stomach when possible
   c. inform the child that this side effect is only temporary
   d. assess for dehydration
5. It prevents the metabolic breakdown of xanthine to uric acid to help prevent renal damage.
6.
   a. use scalp tourniquet to decrease effect
   b. introduce idea of a wig before hair loss
   c. administer good scalp hygiene
   d. provide adequate covering during sunlight, wind, or cold
   e. stress that hair begins to regrow in 3-6 months and may be a slightly different color or texture

Section IV B

1. Hodgkin disease
2. malaise or lack of energy

Section IV C

1. note time and amount of vomiting, relationship of vomiting to feeding, presence of nausea, and activity just before vomiting
2.
   a. prevent hyperthermia
   b. monitor vital functions
   c. prevent pneumonia
   d. maintain desired position
   e. prevent fluid overload or dehydration
   f. prevent eye damage
   g. provide special postoperative care
3. Amanda exhibits no signs of fluid overload or dehydration.
4.
   a. recording behavior at regular intervals
   b. noting sleep patterns
   c. noting response to stimuli
   d. assessing level of consciousness
5.
   a. to prevent pressure against the operative site
   b. to reduce intracranial pressure
   c. to avoid the danger of aspiration
6. gag and swallowing reflexes
7.
   a. provide a quiet, dimly lit environment
   b. restrict visitors to a minimum
   c. avoid any sudden jarring movement
   d. position properly
   e. prevent straining such as coughing, vomiting, or defecating

    f.   monitor stools to prevent constipation

    g.   apply ice bag to forehead to relieve headache

Section IV D

1.   a.   Keep explanations simple, and repeat them often.

    b.   The·nurse should be present during physician-parent conferences in order to answer questions that arise after the conference.

2.   a.   monitor bowel movements

    b.   auscultate for bowel sounds

    c.   monitor for abdominal distention or vomiting

Section IV E

1.   a.   identify the signs of retinoblastoma

    b.   prepare the family for diagnostic/therapeutic procedures and home care

    c.   provide emotional support to the child and his family

2.   a.   observe for signs of retinoblastoma

    b.   explain to parents about the procedures performed and the expected reactions of their child

    c.   prepare parents for enucleation

    d.   prepare parents for the child's appearance postoperatively

    e.   describe and explain the use of a prosthesis

    f.   encourage parents to seek genetic counseling for themselves and for the child after he reaches puberty

Chapter 37

QUESTION   **ANSWER**

Section III

1.   a.   central nervous system

    b.   peripheral nervous system

    c.   autonomic nervous system

2.   a.   irritability; high-pitched cry; cries when held or rocked; bulging fontanels; separated cranial sutures; increased occipital-frontal circumference; change in feeding patterns

    b.   headache; nausea; vomiting; diplopia; drowsiness; diminished physical activity and motor performance; fatigue; memory loss; seizures

3.   pupils become fixed and dilated, papilledema, decreased motor response to painful stimuli, decreased motor response to command, and the level of consciousness progressively deteriorates from drowsiness to eventual coma

4.   a.   observation of spontaneous and elicited reflex responses

    b.   observation of the development of increasingly complex locomotor and fine motor skills

    c.   eliciting of progressively more sophisticated communicative and adaptive behaviors

    d.   observing for the presence of a primitive reflex beyond the time it would normally disappear

5.   history; physical examination

6.   an estimation of the level of development

7.   ataxia, spastic paraplegic gait, spastic hemiplegic gait, cerebellar gait, and extrapyramidal gait

8.   a.   alertness—an aroused or waking state that includes the ability to respond to stimuli

    b.   cognitive power—the ability to process stimuli and produce verbal and motor responses

9.   the patient's responses to his environment

10.   sleep, confusion, delirium, pseudowakeful states, and comatose states

11.   a.   eye opening

    b.   verbal response

    c.   motor response

12.   Harvard criteria

13.   a.   unreceptivity and unresponsivity

    b.   no movement or breathing

    c.   no reflexes

    d.   flat electroencephalogram

    e.   all tests if repeated at least 24 hrs later show no change

    f.   the cause of coma is not hypothermia or central nervous system depressants

14.   establish an accurate, objective baseline of neurologic function

15.   vital signs, skin, eyes, motor function and posturing, and reflexes

16.   neurosurgical emergency

17.   a.   electroencephalogram
      b.   auditory and visual testing
      c.   tomography
      d.   brain scan
      e.   roentgenography
      f.   miscellaneous sophisticated tests

18.   patent airway

19.   a.   concussion—a transient and reversible neuronal dysfunction with instantaneous loss of awareness and responsiveness for minutes or hours.
      b.   contusion and laceration—visible bruising and tearing of cerebral tissue
      c.   fracture—a break in the skull that is linear, depressed, compound, basilar, and diastotic

20.   a.   hemorrhage
      b.   infection
      c.   edema
      d.   herniation through the tentorium

21.   Accumulation of blood between the skull and cerebral surfaces is dangerous because it can compress the underlying brain and produce effects that can be rapidly fatal or insidiously progressive.

22.   the middle meningeal artery

23.   hematoma

24.   between the dura and the cerebrum; cortical veins

25.   a.   irritability, headache, vomiting; lasts longer than 48 hours; increased intracranial pressure
      b.   seizure, vomiting, irritability, drowsiness, or other personality changes, headache, increased intracranial pressure

26.   cerebral edema

27.   Intracranial pressure exceeds arterial pressure and fatal anoxia ensues and/or the pressure causes herniation of a portion of the brain over the edge of the tentorium, compressing the brain stem and occluding the posterior cerebral arteries.

28.   the length of submersion, the physiologic response of the victim, and the development and degree of immersion hypothermia

29.   a.   *Hemophilus influenzae* (type B)
      b.   *Streptococcus pneumoniae*
      c.   *Neisseria meningitidis* (Meningococcus)

30.   Meningococcal meningitis is readily transmitted by droplet infection from nasopharyngeal secretions.

31.   antidiuretic hormone; retention of fluid

32.   examination of the cerebrospinal fluid by lumbar puncture

33.   a.   F
      b.   T
      c.   T
      d.   F

34.   symptomatic

35.   a.   may arise from central areas in the brain that affect consciousness immediately
      b.   may be restricted to one area of the cerebral cortex, producing manifestations characteristic of that particular anatomic focus
      c.   may begin in a localized area of the cortex and spread to other portions of the brain

36.   aura

37.   a.   clonic
      b.   tonic
      c.   jacksonian

38.   generalized seizures and partial seizures

39.   a period of altered behavior for which the individual is amnesic and during which he is unable to respond to his environment

40.   electroencephalogram (EEG)

41.   a.   control the seizures or reduce their frequency
      b.   discover and correct the cause of seizures
      c.   help the child to live as normal a life as possible

42.   The action of anticonvulsive drugs is to reduce the responsiveness of normal neurons to sudden high-frequency nerve impulses.

43.   The drug should be reduced gradually over 1 or 2 weeks.

44.   Dilantin causes gingival hyperplasia.

45.   The drugs are monitored by taking frequent blood levels.

46.   a series of seizures at intervals too brief to allow the child to regain consciousness between the time one attack ends and the next begins.

47.   a.   less than 30 sec
      b.   greater than 60 sec

    c.   may be sole manifestation of seizure
    d.   frequently
    e.   never
    f.   always
    g.   frequently
    h.   occasionally
    i.   occàsionally
    j.   frequently
    k.   frequently
    l.   common

48.   grand mal
49.   absence seizure; petit mal

Section IV A

1.   a.   muscular activity and coordination, including ocular movements and gait
    b.   pupillary response, facial movements, and mouth functions
    c.   testing reflexes, strength, presence and location of tremors, twitching, tics, or other unusual movements
2.   alteration in neurologic status related to increased intracranial pressure
3.   delirium

Section IV B

1.   a.   maintain patent airway
    b.   minimize intracranial pressure
    c.   prevent cerebral hypoxia
    d.   detect signs of cerebral hypoxia
    e.   assess neurologic status
    f.   assess level of consciousness
    g.   prevent cerebral edema
    h.   prevent or control hyperthermia
    i.   prevent respiratory complications
    j.   maintain skin integrity
    k.   protect child from injury
    l.   maintain limb flexibility and function
    m.   provide nutrition and hydration
    n.   assure adequate elimination
    o.   provide stimulation
    p.   support parents
2.   vital signs, central venous pressure, pupillary reactions, voluntary movements, muscle tone, tremors, twitching, seizures, nuchal rigidity, and posture
3.   elevate head of bed 10 to 15 degrees; avoid pressure on neck veins
4.   perform passive range of motion exercises; position to reduce contractures; splint if necessary
5.   to prevent pressure on prominent areas of the body

Section IV C

1.   vital signs, neurologic signs, and level of consciousness
2.   assure parents that everything possible is being done to treat the child; repeat message often

Section IV D

1.   Clinical manifestations include fever, vomiting, marked irritability, seizures, a high-pitched cry and a bulging fontanel. Nuchal rigidity may or may not be present. Brudzinski and Kernig signs are not usually used in making the diagnosis since they are difficult to evaluate in children in this age-group.
2.   a.   prevent the spread of infection
    b.   eradicate causative organisms
    c.   maintain optimal hydration
    d.   assess neurologic status
    e.   detect complications
    f.   maintain nutritional status
    g.   provide emotional support to parents
3.   monitor vitals signs, neurologic signs, level of consciousness, and behavior; observe for opisthotonos, seizures, high-pitched cry, and nuchal rigidity; measure head circumference daily and assess status of fontanels

Section IV E

1. a. description of child's behavior before and during a seizure
   b. the age of onset of first seizure
   c. the usual time at which the seizure occurs
   d. any factors that may have precipitated the seizure
   e. any sensory phenomena that the child can describe
   f. duration and progression of the seizure
   g. postictal feelings and behavior
2. a. observe the seizure carefully
   b. protect from view of others
   c. do not move or forcefully restrain her
   d. do not force object between clenched teeth
   e. protect her from injury on siderails
3. a. Help the family to establish time of administration of medication to coincide with the family routine.
   b. The tablet form of the drug is the preferred form; crush and administer in syrup or jelly.
   c. Emphasize that the medication must be continued for 2 to 3 years after the last seizure.
   d. Explain what will happen if doses are omitted.
   e. Teach what side effects may occur.
   f. Explain why periodic blood studies are necessary.

Chapter 38

QUESTION	ANSWER

Section III

1. a. the cell—sends a chemical message by means of a hormone
   b. target cell/end organs—receive the chemical message
   c. environment—medium through which the chemical is transported (blood, lymph, extracellular fluid)
2. energy production, growth, fluid and electrolyte balance, response to stress, and sexual reproduction
3. complex chemical substance; physiologic controlling
4. negative feedback; pituitary
5. a. endocrine system
   b. autonomic nervous system
6. a. gonadotropin deficiency with absence or regression of secondary sex characteristics
   b. retarded somatic growth
   c. hypothyroidism
   d. adrenal hypofunction
7. tumors
8. short stature
9. growth hormone
10. a. surgical removal or irradiation of tumor
    b. replacement of growth hormone
11. overgrowth of long bones; overgrowth in transverse direction; acromegaly
12. increasing intracranial pressure
13. early identification of children with inappropriate growth rates
14. diabetes insipidus; diuresis
15. polyuria; polydipsia
16. vasopression
17. Inappropriate secretion of antidiuretic hormone; fluid retention; hypotonicity
18. thyroid
19. to regulate the basal metabolic rate
20. an enlargement or hypertrophy of the thyroid gland; iodine; tyrosine
21. thyroid gland; exophthalmos
22. acute onset of severe irritability and restlessness; vomiting; diarrhea; hyperthermia; hypertension; severe tachycardia; prostration
23. hypoparathyroidism; parathyroid
24. calcium; phosphate
25. hyperparathyroidism
26. a. A

	b.	B
	c.	B
	d.	A
	e.	A
27.	a.	A
	b.	B
28.		iatrogenic Cushing syndrome
29.		dexamethasone (cortisone) suppression
30.		aldosterone; cortisol
31.		sexual
32.		genotype
33.		adrenogenital syndrome
34.	a.	strong
	b.	weak
	c.	weak
	d.	strong
	e.	---
	f.	increases
	g.	increases
	h.	---
	i.	increases more than Norepinephrine.
	j.	---
35.		familial; dominant
36.		increased production of catecholamines
37.	a.	glucagon—stimulates liver to release stored glucose
	b.	insulin—facilitates metabolism of carbohydrates, fats, and proteins, and their entry into the cells; facilitates entry of glucose into muscle and fat cells; mobilizes fat from fat cells; facilitates storage of glucose as glycogen in cells of liver and muscle
	c.	somatostatin—regulates release of insulin and glucagon
38.		IDDM; NIDDM; MODY
39.	a.	less than 20 years
	b.	over 40 years
	c.	5–8%
	d.	85–90%
	e.	sometimes
	f.	frequently
	g.	three Ps* common
	h.	may be none
	i.	underweight
	j.	overweight
	k.	usually 0; low to absent; minimum
	l.	over 50% normal; high or low; marked
	m.	always; ineffective; ineffective
	n.	20–30% of patients; often effective; often effective
	o.	common
	p.	infrequent
40.	a.	glucose is unable to enter cells, causing hyperglycemia
	b.	glucose accumulates in bloodstream causing an osmotic gradient to occur, which results in fluid moving from the intracellular to the extracellular space
	c.	fluid is filtered through the glomerulus into the renal tubule; the renal tubule reabsorbs the glucose and most of the water in the filtrate; when glucose concentrate exceeds the threshold, the glucose is excreted in the urine
	d.	water is also excreted as part of the osmotic diversion
	e.	urinary fluid losses cause the individual to experience thirst
	f.	because glucose is unable to enter the cells, the body burns fats for energy but also utilizes protein
	g.	the liver metabolizes protein and converts it to glucose for energy use
	h.	when fats are metabolized, they are broken down into fatty acids and ketone bodies; the ketone bodies are excreted in the urine and in the lungs
	i.	the production of ketone bodies, which are organic acids, and the dehydration that results from the osmotic diuresis, lead to a metabolic acidosis
	j.	because the body cannot utilize glucose, and fat and protein stores are depleted, the patient experiences hunger and increased food intake

41.   polyphagia; polydipsia; polyuria
42.   a.   ½–1 hr
      b.   2–4 hrs
      c.   6–8 hrs
      d.   ½–1 hr
      e.   2–4 hrs
      f.   8–10 hrs
      g.   1–2 hrs
      h.   6–8+ hrs
      i.   12–14 hrs
      j.   1–2+ hrs
      k.   8–12 hrs
      l.   14–16 hrs
      m.   4–6 hrs
      n.   8–12 hrs
      o.   24–36 hrs
      p.   4–6 hrs
      q.   18+ hrs
      r.   36–72 hrs
43.   lowers
44.   a.   rapid
      b.   gradual
      c.   too much insulin; increased exercise with no increase in food intake; diminished food intake; gastroenteritis
      d.   too little insulin; improper diet; reduced exercise with no reduction in food; emotional stress; physical stress; drugs; illness
      e.   lability of mood; irritability; shaky feeling; headache; impaired vision; hunger; convulsions
      f.   weakness; increased thirst; polyuria; signs of dehydration; nausea; abdominal pain; acetone breath; rapid and deep respirations
      g.   shock; coma; death
      h.   acidosis; coma; death
      i.   glucose negative; acetone negative
      j.   glucose positive; acetone positive
      k.   decreased: 60 mg per 100 ml, or less
      l.   increased: 250 mg per 100 ml, or more
45.   a physiologic reflex response to a decreased blood glucose level which results in release of counterregulatory hormones (epinephrine, growth hormone, and corticosteroids) and a rebound hyperglycemia
46.   a.   rapid assessment
      b.   adequate insulin to reduce the elevated blood glucose
      c.   fluids to overcome dehydration
      d.   electrolyte replacement, especially potassium and bicarbonate
47.   potassium
48.   regular short-acting insulin
49.   a.   microvascular changes
            1) nephropathy
            2) retinopathy
            3) neuropathy
      b.   macrovascular changes
      c.   alteration in thyroid function
      d.   limited mobility of small joints of hand

Section IV A

1.   a.   short stature but proportional height and weight
      b.   delayed epiphyseal closure
      c.   retarded bone age proportional to height age
      d.   premature aging
      e.   increased insulin sensitivity
2.   a.   overgrowth of long bones; reaches height of 8 feet
      b.   rapid and increased development of muscles and viscera
      c.   proportional enlargement of head circumference
3.   a.   polyuria

    b.   polydipsia

    c.   irritability

    d.   dehydration signs

4.   cessation or retardation of growth in an infant whose growth has previously been normal

5.   early identification of children with hypothyroidism

6.   a.   institute seizure precautions

    b.   institute safety precautions

    c.   reduce environmental stimuli

    d.   observe for signs of laryngospasm

7.   Because of problems with calcium utilization, the child is prone to fractures and muscular injury.

Section IV B

1.   to monitor the hyperpyrexia and shocklike state

2.   Overdosage can produce hypotension and a sudden fall in temperature.

3.   cardiac irregularities; poor muscle control; and inappropriate serum electrolyte levels

Section IV C

1.   immediate recognition of ambiguous genitalia in the newborn

2.   to suppress the abnormally high secretion of adrenocorticotropic hormone

3.   increased

Section IV D

1.   a.   1) recognize diabetic ketoacidosis

        2) treat associated problems

        3) detect alteration in status

        4) ensure adequate hydration

    b.   child exhibits adequate hydration

2.   home blood glucose monitoring

3.   ensure day-to-day consistency in total calorie, protein, fat, and carbohydrate

4.   a.   irritability; shaky feeling; headache, impaired vision, hunger, pallor, and sweating

    b.   Give child simple sugar

Section IV E

1.   a.   Child and family will understand nature of diabetes.

    b.   Child and family will understand principles of meal planning.

    c.   Child and family will understand the insulin medication.

    d.   Child and family will be able to demonstrate an appropriate injection procedure.

    e.   Child and family will be able to demonstrate appropriate testing of urine.

    f.   Child and family will be able to monitor blood glucose level.

    g.   Child and family will be able to identify signs of hyperglycemia.

    h.   Appropriate exercise program will be planned.

    i.   Child and family will demonstrate accurate method of record keeping.

Chapter 39

QUESTION	ANSWER

Section III

1.   a nonspecific term applied to impaired muscular control resulting from a nonprogressive abnormality in the pyramidal motor system

2.   no

3.   a.   delayed motor development

    b.   abnormal motor performance

    c.   alterations in muscle tone

    d.   abnormal postures

    e.   reflex abnormalities

4.   One third of the children with cerebral palsy have normal intelligence; one third are mildly retarded; and one third are moderately retarded or below.

5. a.   Spastic cerebral palsy—an upper motor neuron type of muscular weakness, characterized by hypotonia
   b.   Dyskinetic cerebral palsy—abnormal involuntary movements that originate in the basal ganglia and the nuclei of cranial nerve VIII and of other cranial nerves
   c.   Ataxic cerebral palsy—caused by a defect in the cerebellum or its pathways, and characterized by nonprogressive failure of muscle coordination and irregular muscle action
   d.   Mixed-type cerebral palsy—a combination of spasticity and athetosis
   e.   Rigid, tremor, and atonic types of cerebral palsy—both rigid and atonic types have a poor prognosis
6. a.   to establish locomotion, communication, and self-help
   b.   to gain optimum appearance and integration of motor functions
   c.   to correct associated defects as effectively as possible
   d.   to provide educational opportunities adapted to the needs and capabilities of the individual child
7.   physical therapy
8.   acute polyneuropathy in which motor dysfunction predominates over sensory disturbance
9.   In most patients, paralysis ascends from the lower extremities, frequently involving the muscles of the trunk, upper extremities, and those supplied by cranial nerves. The seventh (facial) cranial nerve is almost universally affected.
10.   assisted ventilation
11.   an acute, preventable, and often fatal disease caused by an exotoxin produced by the anaerobic, spore-forming, gram-positive bacillus, *Clostridium tetani.*
12.   trismus (difficulty in opening the mouth)
13.   administration of either tetanus toxoid or tetanus antitoxin; human tetanus immune globulin
14.   the chance of infection
15. a.   provide a quiet environment that reduces external stimulation from sound, light, and touch
    b.   administer the prescribed sedatives or muscle relaxants
16.   muscle fibers; progressive weakness and wasting of skeletal muscles with increasing disability and deformity
17.   muscle groups affected, age of onset, rate or progression, and inheritance patterns
18.   Pseudohypertrophic muscular dystrophy or Duchenne muscular dystrophy
19.   respiratory tract infection or cardiac failure
20.   Contractures
21.   to maintain function in unaffected muscles for as long as possible
22.   structural and functional
23.   external or internal fixation techniques
24.   Bracing
25.   Traction
26.   Stryker frame; bed
27.   The advantage to this procedure is that the patient is able to ambulate within a few days, and no postoperative immobilization is required. The disadvantage is the possibility of spinal nerve damage.
28.   infectious process of bone; exogenous; hematogenous
29.   intravenous therapy; antibiotic; 3 to 4 weeks
30.   bed rest; immobilized
31.   negative
32.   stiffness, swelling, and loss of motion develop in the affected joints. They are swollen and warm to the touch, but seldom red.
33. a.   Growth is retarded during active disease.
    b.   Corticosteroid therapy is a contributing factor.
34.   At least 75% of affected children enter long remissions without significant residual deformity or impaired function.
35. a.   to preserve joint function
    b.   to prevent physical deformities
    c.   to relieve symptoms without iatrogenic harm
36.   inflammation of the iris and ciliary body
37.   the nonsteroidal antiinflammatory drugs; the desired effects are analgesic, antipyretic, and antiinflammatory
38.   there is a narrow margin between the effective and the toxic dose
39.   the slower-acting antirheumatic drugs
40.   Corticosteroids are not the drug of choice because of their chronic and serious side effects.
41.   a chronic inflammatory disease of the collagen or supporting tissues
42.   An erythematous blush, or an outbreak of scaly erythematous patches, that appears over the bridge of the nose and symmetrically extends to each cheek, and that may extend to the scalp, neck, chest and extremities. It is called a "butterfly" rash.
43.   the presence of renal involvement and consequent kidney failure
44. a.   to reverse the autoimmune and inflammatory processes
    b.   to prevent exacerbations and complications

45.   The principal drugs utilized are corticosteroids.
46.   to help the child and family adjust to the limitations and treatments of the disease and to prevent exacerbations and complications
47.   The exact relationship between SLE and rest is unclear, but fatigue, stress, or sudden exertion brings about a relapse of symptoms.

Section IV A
1.   a.   teach and reinforce the methods utilized for physical therapy, proper handling, and home care
      b.   teach them how to provide optimal nutrition and rest
      c.   teach safety measures to prevent accidents
      d.   teach methods to prevent respiratory infections
      e.   assist them to provide meticulous dental care
      f.   help parents to reduce their frustration
      g.   support their psychological and emotional needs
2.   a.   potential for traumatic injury related to neuromuscular impairment
      b.   alteration in nutrition related to greater than normal energy expenditure
      c.   activity intolerance related to decreased energy, fatigue, and perceptual/cognitive impairment
      d.   impaired physical mobility related to neuromuscular impairment
      e.   self-care deficit related to neuromuscular impairment
      f.   impaired verbal communication related to neuromuscular impairment
      g.   disturbance in self-concept: body image, related to appearance of physical disability
      h.   alteration in family process related to birth of handicapped child

Section IV B
1.   to prevent complications of the disease
2.   a.   observe for difficulty in swallowing and for respiratory involvement
      b.   take frequent vital signs
      c.   monitor level of consciousness
      d.   maintain good postural alignment
      e.   change position frequently
      f.   perform passive range of motion every 4 hours

Section IV C
1.   help parents to develop a balance between limiting the child's activity because of muscular weakness, and allowing him to accomplish things by himself.
2.   encourage parents to seek genetic counseling

Section IV D
1.   a.   disturbance in body image related to the defect in body structure
      b.   alteration in self-concept related to immobility
2.   a.   accentuate positive aspects of appearance
      b.   motivate Jane to have good habits of personal hygiene
      c.   encourage Jane to wear attractive clothes and hairstyle
      d.   emphasize positive long-term outcome
      e.   help devise positive ways to deal with reactions of others

Section IV E
1.   He would appear very ill, would be irritable, and would have an elevated temperature, rapid pulse and signs of dehydration. He would complain of localized tenderness, increased warmth, and diffuse swelling over the involved bone. The extremity would be painful, especially upon movement, and the child would hold it in semiflexion.
2.   a.   monitor rate, amount, and type of IV solution
      b.   assess the integrity of the infusion site
      c.   protect IV from dislodgement
      d.   change IV set-up every 24 hours
      e.   explain to child the importance of the IV in order to elicit his cooperation
      f.   record infused amounts accurately

Section IV F
1.   a.   joint flexibility improves in relation to baseline findings
      b.   child develops no contractures

2.   potential for more than body requirements related to decreased mobility
3.   a.   hyperventilation—a sign of acidosis
      b.   bleeding—from decreased clotting capacity
      c.   tinnitus—sign of cranial nerve VIII involvement
      d.   undue drowsiness—may indicate CNS depression

Chapter 40

QUESTION   **ANSWER**

Section III

1.   a.   significant loss of muscle strength, endurance, and muscle mass
      b.   bone demineralization leading to osteoporosis
      c.   loss of joint mobility and contractures
2.   atelectasis, hypostatic pneumonia, and respiratory acidosis
3.   participate in his or her own care
4.   Trauma
5.   a.   accidental injury
      b.   child abuse injury
      c.   birth injuries
6.   hazardous environmental factors
7.   identify and treat the precise injury and prevent any additional injury to the child
8.   a loss of sensation or motor function
9.   a.   airway—assure open airway
      b.   breathing—promote breathing; if not breathing, begin pulmonary resuscitation
      c.   circulation—check pulse; if no pulse, begin cardiac compression
10.   a.   The growth plate serves to absorb shock and protect joint surfaces from injury.
      b.   The periosteum of a child's bone is thicker, stronger, and has more osteogenic potential.
      c.   The bones of growing children are more porous, which causes them to bend, buckle, and break in a "greenstick" manner.
      d.   Healing is more rapid in children.
      e.   Stiffness is unusual.
      f.   Children only complain when something is wrong.
11.   a.   bends—a child's flexible bone can be bent 45° or more before breaking
      b.   buckle fracture—compression of the porous bone produces a buckle, or torus, fracture
      c.   greenstick fracture—occurs when a bone is angulated beyond the limits of bending
      d.   complete fracture—those types that divide the bone fragments
12.   a.   reduction—to regain alignment and length
      b.   immobilization—to retain alignment and length
      c.   to restore function to the injured parts
13.   traction; closed manipulation; casting
14.   pain, swelling, discoloration of exposed portions, lack of pulsation and warmth, or inability to move the exposed parts
15.   presence of any foul odors; increased temperature; lethargy; discomfort
16.   a.   to fatigue the involved muscle and reduce muscle spasm so that bones can be realigned
      b.   to position the distal and proximal bone ends in desired realignment to promote satisfactory bone healing
      c.   to immobilize the fracture site until realignment has been achieved and sufficient healing has taken place to permit casting or splinting
17.   a.   manual traction
      b.   skin traction
      c.   skeletal traction
18.   a.   e
      b.   c
      c.   d
      d.   b
      e.   a
19.   fat emboli
20.   a.   paralysis of two extremities, usually the lower limbs
      b.   functional disuse in all four extremities
21.   neurologic; clinical
22.   a.   Initial response to acute injury is flaccid paralysis below the level of the damage caused by the sudden disruption of

central and autonomic pathways. Signs of spinal shock include: absence of reflexes at or below the cord lesion resulting in flaccidity in the involved muscles, loss of sensation and motor function, and autonomic dysfunction manifested by hypotension, low or high body temperature, loss of bladder and bowel control, and autonomic dysreflexia. Spinal shock lasts for 1 to 6 weeks.

    b.   Flaccid paralysis is replaced by spinal reflex activity and increasing spasticity. Spasticity leads to contractures of the hip adductor, hip and knee flexor muscles, and heel cords. The atonic bladder now becomes hypertonic. Paralysis of autonomic function is replaced by autonomic dysreflexia. Sensory stimuli may produce a sudden generalized increase in sympathetic activity.

    c.   Neurologic signs are stabilized and the major emphasis is on rehabilitation. A problem unique to children is progressive spinal deformity beginning at this point.

23. a.   maximizing function and minimizing the disabling effects of the pathology

    b.   assisting the child and family in setting realistic goals for him, learning to be good problem solvers, and using the assets he has

    c.   helping the child to cope with the stigma of being different and to build a positive self-concept

Section IV A

1. a.   change position frequently
    b.   elevate extremity without knee flexion
    c.   ensure adequate fluid intake
    d.   perform passive range of motion
    e.   ask doctor to prescribe antiembolic stockings for older child or wraps for younger child
    f.   measure circumference of extremity periodically
    g.   administer anticoagulant drugs if ordered
    h.   promptly intervene to maintain adequate oxygen if signs and symptoms of pulmonary emboli appear
2.   to monitor any change in the function of the cardiac or respiratory systems, and to identify possible development of an infection.
3. a.   apply pressure to skin; if hyperemia does not disappear after thirty minutes, you would suspect a developing pressure sore
    b.   increase in temperature in affected area
    c.   blistering or swelling
    d.   color, especially dark purple or black
    e.   drainage

Section IV B

1. a.   Make certain the child is not in immediate danger of additional trauma.
    b.   Do not move the child unless absolutely necessary.
    c.   If you must move the child, then move as a log with the head and neck held firmly in a neutral position.
2.   Apply direct pressure to the wound or to the appropriate pressure point.
3. a.   pain and point of tenderness
    b.   pulse—distal to the fracture site
    c.   pallor
    d.   paresthesia sensation distal to the fracture site
    e.   paralysis—movement distal to fracture site
4.   Immobilize the limb, including the knee and ankle.

Section IV C

1. a.   Keep the extremity elevated on pillows for the first day.
    b.   Avoid indenting the cast until it is thoroughly dry.
    c.   Encourage frequent rest for a few days, keeping the injured extremity elevated while resting.
    d.   Avoid allowing the affected limb to hang down for any length of time.
2. a.   Do not allow the child to put anything in the cast.
    b.   Keep clear path for ambulation.
    c.   Use crutches appropriately.

Section IV D

1. a.   Understand function of traction.
    b.   Check desired line of pull frequently to maintain alignment.
    c.   Check function of component parts.

    d.   Make sure ropes move freely through pulleys.
    e.   Make sure weights hang free.
    f.   Maintain total body alignment
    g.   Do not remove traction.
2.   potential for injury related to immobility due to traction
3.   bleeding; inflammation

Section IV E

1.   a.   prevention of complications
    b.   maintenance of functions
2.   a.   turn every two hours as a log
    b.   place on alternating pressure mattress
    c.   inspect skin once a day for signs of pressure, such as warmth, firmness, redness
    d.   keep skin clean and dry
3.   To keep the urine acidic in order to decrease the likelihood of stone formation and to inhibit bacterial growth.